INTERNAL MEDICINE
FOR ADVANCED
PHARMACIST PRACTITIONERS

VOLUME I

INTERNAL MEDICINE FOR ADVANCED PHARMACIST PRACTITIONERS - VOLUME I

Copyright © 2024 by Huynh Wynn Tran

Cover: Artist Dinh Khai - Book designer: Tien Minh Nguyen

United Buddhist Publisher (UBF)

First printed in California, USA, September 2024

ISBN-13: 979-8-8693-0545-9

© All rights reserved. No part of this book may be reproduced by any means without prior written permission.

HUYNH WYNN TRAN, MD, FACP, FACR

INTERNAL MEDICINE

FOR ADVANCED PHARMACIST PRACTITIONERS

VOLUME I

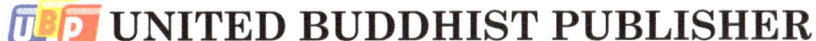 UNITED BUDDHIST PUBLISHER

This book is dedicated to all my patients, who have been my greatest teachers and sources of inspiration.

**Additionally, I wish to dedicate this book to my parents,
Ms. Nhung Huynh and Mr. Dang Tran,
whose unconditional love has been a constant source of strength throughout my journey as a physician.**

Preface

The role of the clinical pharmacist has evolved significantly in recent years, with California leading the way by establishing the first Advanced Practice Pharmacist (APh) separate license in 2017 through Bill SB493. This initiative has paved the path for pharmacists to assume expanded responsibilities and become integral members of primary care teams.

In 2020, Wynn Medical Center embarked on a groundbreaking collaboration with the University of Southern California and 986 Pharmacy to establish a pioneering APh residency program aimed at training PharmD residents to become fully-fledged healthcare providers within a physician clinic setting.

This comprehensive guide is designed to equip Advanced Practice Pharmacists and APh residents with a foundation of 350 common conditions encountered in primary care. Spanning across 24 chapters, this book addresses the APh profession, major disorders in internal medicine, common disorders in pregnancy and pediatrics, post-surgical and wound care, laboratory, imaging, biostatistics, and preventive measures.

I extend my heartfelt gratitude to a dedicated team of international expert reviewers, editors, and students who have contributed their time, expertise, and insights to the creation of this textbook.

Huynh Wynn Tran, MD, FACP, FACR
Associate Professor of Medicine and Pharmacy
Founder/CEO of Wynn Medical Center Clinics, Los Angeles, USA

Reviewers:

Alvin Wong, MBBS, MD, MRCP
Consultant Dermatologist
NHS Stafford, United Kingdom

Dean Nguyen, MD, RN
Ottawa, Canada

Helen Tran, DO
Assistant Professor, Core Faculty, Department of Family Medicine
Charles R. Drew University of Medicine and Science
Los Angeles, California

Hoang Henry Nguyen, RPH, APh, MD, PhD, FACHE
Assistant Dean of Preclinical Education
Nova Southeastern University Dr. Patel College of Osteopathic Medicine, Tampa, Florida

Huynh Wynn Tran, MD, FACP, FACR
Associate Professor of Medicine and Pharmacy
Founder/CEO of Wynn Medical Center Clinics, Los Angeles, USA

Ken Thai, PharmD, APh
Vice-President of National Community Pharmacist Association
CEO 986 Pharmacy Corporation
Los Angeles, California

Loan Vo, MD, RRT, ACCS
Clinical Instructor, Foothill College Respiratory Therapist Program
San Jose, California

Long To, PharmD, APh, BCPS
Clinical Pharmacy Specialist
Residency Program Director, Pharmacotherapy, Henry Ford Hospital
Detroit, Michigan

Micah Hata, PharmD, APh
Program Director, Pharmacy residency and fellowship
Western University College of Pharmacy
Pomona, California

Minh Do, MD
Attending Physician at Parkland Health
Dallas, Texas

Philip Phuc Tran, DO, FACC, FACOI
Associate Professor of Medicine and Cardiology, Midwestern University Phoenix, Arizona

Quan-Vinh Nguyen, MD
Internist and Attending Nephrologist
Fribourg and Lausanne, Switzerland

Quy Pham Nguyen, MD, PhD
Attending Oncologist, Chief Physician
Kyoto Miniren Central Hospital
Clinical researcher, Department of Clinical Oncology
Kyoto University, Japan

Richard Dang, PharmD, APh
Program Director, PGY-1 Community Pharmacy Residency
University of Southern California Mann School of Pharmacy
Los Angeles, California

Sunil Prabhu, BPharm, PhD
Dean and Professor
Western University College of Pharmacy
Pomona, California

Tanya Thuy Nguyen, MD, FAAP
Attending Pediatrician at Wynn Medical Center
Los Angeles, California

Thanh Hoang, DO, FACP, FACE, CAP (US Navy)
Professor of Medicine and Endocrinology
Program Director, Endocrinology Fellowship, Uniformed Services
University Bethesda, Maryland

Tuan Nguyen, DO
Attending Nephrologist at Wynn Medical Center
Los Angeles, California

Student Editors:

Molynna Duong Nguyen, BS (Team Lead)
University of Toledo College of Medicine, Toledo, Ohio

Nancy Dinh, BS
Thomas Jefferson University Sidney Kimmel Medical College
Philadelphia, Pennsylvania

Nidhi Lakshmanan, BS
Wynn Medical Center, Los Angeles, California

Tam Do (Tammy), BS
Wynn Medical Center, Los Angeles, California

Tri Huynh, BS
Western University College of Pharmacy, Pomona, California

CONTENTS

VOLUME I

Part I:
The Advanced Pharmacist Practitioners (APPs) Profession

Chapter 1: Definition and Roles of Advanced Pharmacist Practitioners 23
- 1.1. APh Definition by California Board of Pharmacy 23
- 1.2. APh Scope of Practice 23
- 1.3. APh Roles in Clinical Practice 23
- 1.4. Billing and Coding for the APh 24

Chapter 2. Current APh Licensure and Training 29
- 2.1. APh Licensure in California 29
- 2.2. APh Licensure in Other States 29
- 2.3. Collaborative Practice Agreement (CPA) with a Physician: 30
- 2.4. Current Challenges of APh Training Model 31

Chapter 3. Future of APh 33
- 3.1. APh and Primary Care Provider Shortage: 33
- 3.2. Proposed a National Title for APh: APP 33
- 3.3. Primary Care Residency Curriculum for the APh 34
- 3.4. APh Credentials and National Board Certification 35
- 3.5. Evidence based practice for the APh 35

Part II:
Common Disorders in General Practice for the APh

Chapter 4. Cardiovascular Disorders 41
- 4.1. Hypertension 42
- 4.2. Chest Pain 47
- 4.3. Coronary Artery Disease 50
- 4.4. Heart Failure 52
- 4.5. Arrhythmias 54
- 4.6. Atrial Fibrillation 56
- 4.7. Bradycardia 59

4.8. Tachycardia 61
4.9. Valvular Heart Disease 62
4.10. Mitral Valve Prolapse 64
4.11. Mitral Valve Regurgitation 67
4.12. Aortic Stenosis 69
4.13. Peripheral Artery Disease (PAD) 71
4.14. Stroke and Transient Ischemic Attack 73
4.15. Deep Vein Thrombosis and Pulmonary Embolism 76
4.16. Aortic Aneurysm 78
4.17. Myocardial Infarction 80
4.18. Cardiomyopathy 83
4.19. Rheumatic Heart Disease 85
4.20. Congenital Heart Defects 89
4.21. Endocarditis 92
4.22. Pericarditis 96
4.23. Atrial Septal Defect 98
4.24. Cardiac Arrest 100
4.25. Thrombophlebitis 102
4.26. Varicose Vein 104
4.27. EKG Findings in Common Cardiac Conditions 106

Chapter 5. Respiratory Disorders 113
5.1. Common Cold 114
5.2. Influenza 115
5.3. Sinusitis 117
5.4. Pharyngitis 120
5.5. Tonsillitis 122
5.6. Community Acquired Pneumonia 124
5.7. Healthcare-Associated Pneumonia 126
5.8. Bronchitis 129
5.9. Bronchiolitis 131
5.10. Tuberculosis 133
5.11. Chronic Obstructive Pulmonary Disease 135
5.12. Bronchiectasis 137

5.13. Asthma 140
5.14. Interstitial Lung Diseases 142
5.15. Sarcoidosis 145
5.16. Hypersensitivity Pneumonitis 147
5.17. Obstructive Sleep Apnea 150
5.18. Cystic Fibrosis 153
5.19. Pleural Effusion 156
5.20. Pulmonary Hypertension 159

Chapter 6. Gastrointestinal Disorders 165
6.1. Abdominal Pain 166
6.2. Gastroesophageal Reflux Disease 169
6.3. Peptic Ulcer Disease 171
6.4. Cirrhosis 173
6.5. Inflammatory Bowel Disease - Crohn's disease 175
6.6. Inflammatory Bowel Disease - Ulcerative colitis 177
6.7. Gastroenteritis 179
6.8. Appendicitis 181
6.9. Diverticulitis 183
6.10. Cholelithiasis 185
6.11. Constipation 187
6.12. Hemorrhoids 189
6.13. Celiac Disease 191
6.14. Non-Alcoholic Fatty Liver Disease 193
6.15. Acute Pancreatitis 195
6.16. Chronic Pancreatitis 197
6.17. Gallstones 199
6.18. Functional Dyspepsia 202
6.19. Anal Fissure 204
6.20. Anal Abscess 206
6.21. Eosinophilic Esophagitis 207
6.22. Gastrointestinal Bleeding 209
6.23. Barrett's Esophagus 211
6.24. Intestinal Obstruction 213

6.25. Small Intestinal Bacterial Overgrowth 215
6.26. Malabsorption Syndromes 217
6.27. Gastrointestinal Motility Disorders 219
6.28. Inguinal Hernia and Ventral Hernia 221

Chapter 7. Endocrine and Metabolism Disorders 227
7.1. Diabetes Mellitus Type 2 228
7.2. Diabetes Mellitus Type 1 230
7.3. Hypothyroidism 232
7.4. Hyperthyroidism 234
7.5. Thyroid Nodules 236
7.6. Hashimoto's Thyroiditis 239
7.7. Addison's Disease 241
7.8. Cushing's Syndrome 243
7.9. Hyperparathyroidism 246
7.10. Hypoparathyroidism 249
7.11. Pituitary Adenoma 252
7.12. Hypopituitarism 256
7.13. Growth Hormone Deficiency 260
7.14. Hyperaldosteronism 264
7.15. Congenital Adrenal Hyperplasia 266
7.16. Pheochromocytoma 269
7.17. Multiple Endocrine Neoplasia Syndrome 272
7.18. Hypercalcemia 274
7.19. Hypocalcemia 277
7.20. Mixed Hyperlipidemia 280
7.21. Metabolic syndrome 282

Chapter 8. Infectious Disorders 287
8.1. Urinary Tract Infections 288
8.2. Pyelonephritis 290
8.3. Chlamydia 292
8.4. Gonorrhea 294
8.5. Syphilis 296
8.6. Genital Herpes 299

8.7. Lyme Disease 301
8.8. Hepatitis A 303
8.9. Hepatitis B 305
8.10. Hepatitis C 307
8.11. Hepatitis D 310
8.12. Hepatitis E 312
8.13. Chickenpox 315
8.14. Measles 317
8.15. Mumps 319
8.16. Shingles 321
8.17. Dengue Fever 323
8.18. Malaria 326
8.19. HIV/AIDS 328
8.20. Norovirus Infection 331
8.21. Rabies 334
8.22. Leprosy 336
8.23. Respiratory Syncytial Virus 339

Chapter 9. Neurologic and Psychiatric Disorders 343
9.1. General Headache 344
9.2. Migraine 346
9.3. Tension Headache 349
9.4. Cluster Headache 351
9.5. Transient Ischemic Attack 353
9.6. Epilepsy 355
9.7. Peripheral Neuropathy 357
9.8. Multiple Sclerosis 359
9.9. Parkinson's Disease 361
9.10. Alzheimer's Disease 363
9.11. General Vertigo 366
9.12. Peripheral Vertigo 368
9.13. Benign Paroxysmal Positional Vertigo 370
9.14. Ménière's Disease 371
9.15. Hearing Loss 373

9.16. Amyotrophic Lateral Sclerosis 375
9.17. Guillain-Barré Syndrome 377
9.18. Myasthenia Gravis 379
9.19. Other Neuromuscular Disorders 381
9.20. Neuralgia 383
9.21. Carpal Tunnel Syndrome 384
9.22. Restless Legs Syndrome 386
9.23. Essential Tremor 388
9.24. Depression 390
9.25. General Anxiety Disorder 392
9.26. Panic Disorder 394
9.27. Substance Use Disorder 396
9.28. Attention Deficit Hyperactivity Disorder 398
9.29. Bipolar Disorder 401
9.30. Post-Traumatic Stress Disorder 404
9.31. Obsessive-Compulsive Disorder 406
9.32. Eating Disorders 407
9.33. Insomnia 409
9.34. Personality Disorders 410

Chapter 10: Rheumatologic and Musculoskeletal Disorders 415
10.1. Osteoarthritis 416
    10.1.1. Knee Osteoarthritis 419
    10.1.2. Shoulder OA 420
    10.1.3. Hand and Wrist OA 422
10.2. Rheumatoid Arthritis 423
10.3. Reactive Arthritis 426
10.4. Gout Arthritis 428
10.5. Fibromyalgia 429
10.6. Systemic Lupus Erythematosus 431
10.7. Ankylosing Spondylitis 433
10.8. Enteropathic Arthritis 435
10.9. Psoriatic arthritis 437
10.10. Osteoporosis 438

10.11. Juvenile idiopathic arthritis 440
10.12. Sjögren's syndrome 442
10.13. Polymyalgia Rheumatica 444
10.14. Systemic Sclerosis 445
10.15. Temporal Arteritis 447
10.16. Polymyositis and Dermatomyositi 449
10.17. Paget's Disease of Bone 451
10.18. Behçet's Disease 453
10.19. Raynaud's Phenomenon 455
10.20. Ehlers-Danlos Syndrome 456
10.21 Lumbar Radiculopathy 458
10.22. Cervical Radiculopathy 460
10.23. Baker's Cyst 462
10.24. Ganglion Cyst 464
10.25. Frozen Shoulder 465
10.26. Hip Avascular Necrosis 467
10.27. Tennis Elbow 469
10.28. Falls in the Elderly 471
10.29. Low Back Pain 473
10.30. Vasculitis 476

Part I:

The Advanced Pharmacist Practitioners (APPs) Profession

Chapter 1: Definition and Roles of Advanced Pharmacist Practitioner

1.1. APh Definition by California Board of Pharmacy

An Advanced Practice Pharmacist (APh) or Advanced Pharmacist Practitioner (APP):

1. A licensed pharmacist who has been recognized as an advanced practice pharmacist by the Board of Pharmacy.
2. Has undergone advanced training and education that surpasses the conventional scope of pharmacy practice.
3. Holds a higher degree such as a Doctor of Pharmacy (PharmD)
4. Entitled to engage in the practice of advanced pharmacy, exercising autonomous decision-making within their defined scope of practice.

1.2. APh Scope of Practice

A board-recognized an advanced practice pharmacist provider may:

1. Perform patient assessments.
2. Order and interpret drug therapy-related tests.
3. Refer patients to other health care providers.
4. Participate in the evaluation and management of diseases and health conditions in collaboration with other healthcare providers.
5. Initiate, adjust, or discontinue drug therapy

1.3. APh Roles in Clinical Practice

A. Clinical Care

1. Identify and manage medication-related problems.
2. Collaborating with other healthcare professionals to optimize patient care.
3. Providing medication therapy management (MTM) services to improve patient outcomes.

B. Patient Education

1. Educating patients on proper medication use, potential side effects, and adherence strategies.

2. Conducting medication reviews and counseling sessions to enhance patient understanding.

C. **Preventive Care**
1. Participating in immunization programs and health screenings.
2. Promoting healthy lifestyle choices and disease prevention measures.

D. **Research and Scholarship**
1. Contributing to clinical research projects and publications.
2. Staying abreast of current literature and evidence-based practice guidelines.

E. **Leadership and Advocacy**
1. Serving as advocates for patients and the profession of pharmacy.
2. Providing leadership in pharmacy organizations and healthcare committees.

F. **Continuous Professional Development**
1. Ensuring completion of 10 hours of continuing education (CE) each renewal cycle. The subject matter shall be in one or more areas of practice relevant to the pharmacist's clinical practice.
2. Pursuing advanced certifications and credentials to expand clinical expertise.

1.4. Billing and Coding for the APh

Medical coding and billing for Advanced Pharmacist Practitioners (PharmD/APhs) in California require a thorough understanding of the services that are billable, the appropriate codes, and the regulatory requirements governing their practice. By maintaining detailed documentation, adhering to the collaborative practice agreement, and using the correct codes, the APh can ensure proper reimbursement while delivering high-quality care to patients.

A. Scope of Billable Services for Advanced Pharmacist Practitioners (APh)

APPs in California can provide a variety of services that are eligible for reimbursement under medical billing codes. These services include:

- **Medication Therapy Management (MTM)**
    - Comprehensive medication reviews.

- Development and implementation of personalized medication treatment plans.
- Monitoring and adjusting medication therapy.
- Educating patients on proper use of medications.
- **Chronic Disease Management**
  APPs can assist in managing chronic conditions like hypertension, diabetes, and cardiovascular disease by adjusting medications under physician protocols, performing patient education, and ordering related laboratory tests.
- **Preventive Health Services**
  - Immunization administration (vaccines, biologics).
  - Preventive medication counseling (e.g., smoking cessation, preventive cardiovascular care).
- **Laboratory Testing** APPs may order and interpret laboratory tests related to drug therapy monitoring, such as blood glucose levels, liver function tests, and kidney function tests.

B. Billable Codes for APh Services

Several Current Procedural Terminology (CPT) and Healthcare Common Procedure Coding System (HCPCS) codes are relevant for APPs performing billable services in California. Some examples include:

- **Medication Therapy Management (MTM) Codes:**
  - **99605**: Medication therapy management services provided by a pharmacist, initial 15 minutes, for a new patient.
  - **99606**: Medication therapy management services provided by a pharmacist, initial 15 minutes, for an established patient.
  - **99607**: Medication therapy management services provided by a pharmacist, each additional 15 minutes (used in conjunction with 99605 or 99606).
- **Evaluation and Management (E/M) Codes:** Depending on the level of service provided, APPs can use E/M codes in collaborative settings, which include:
  - **99211**: Office or outpatient visit for an established patient, typically 5 minutes.
  - **99212-99215**: Office or outpatient visits, varying complexity, and time (ranging from 10 to 40 minutes).

- **Preventive Services and Immunizations:**
  - **90471**: Immunization administration (single vaccine).
  - **90472**: Immunization administration (each additional vaccine).
  - **G0438**: Annual wellness visit, includes a personalized prevention plan.

- **Chronic Care Management (CCM):**
  - **99490**: Chronic care management services, 20 minutes of clinical staff time per calendar month, directed by a physician or other qualified healthcare professional.
  - **99487**: Complex chronic care management services, 60 minutes of clinical staff time per calendar month.
  - **99489**: Complex chronic care management, additional 30 minutes.

- **Telehealth Services:** APPs can also bill for services provided via telehealth, including:
  - **G2025**: Telehealth services, 5 minutes or longer of remote check-in.
  - **G2061-G2063**: Qualified non-physician healthcare professional assessment via telehealth.

C. Requirements for Billing

To bill for services, APh must meet the following requirements:

- **Collaborative Practice Agreement:**
  APh must have a formal collaborative practice agreement (CPA) with an attending physician, which clearly outlines the scope of services they are authorized to perform. The CPA must meet the regulatory requirements of the California Business and Professions Code Section 4052.6.
- **Licensing and Credentialing:**
  The APP must be licensed as a Pharmacist in California, hold the Advanced Practice Pharmacist (APh) credential, and have DEA registration for controlled substances, if applicable. They must also be credentialed with insurance payers (Medicare, Medi-Cal, or private insurers).

- **Documentation Standards:**
  APPs must document all services provided in the electronic health record (EHR) system in accordance with California law and payer guidelines. Documentation must include:
    - The date and time of the encounter.
    - The patient's history, examination, and assessments (where applicable).
    - Services rendered (e.g., medication review, adjustments, lab orders).
    - Follow-up recommendations or consultations with a supervising physician.
    - Signatures (electronic or physical) of the APP, as required.
- **Time-based Codes:**
  Many CPT codes used by APPs (e.g., MTM, CCM) are time-based. The APP must document the total time spent with the patient or managing their care to bill accurately for services. Each code specifies the amount of time required (e.g., 15 minutes for MTM).

D. How to Bill for APh Services

1. **Verify Insurance Coverage:**
   Before providing services, verify whether the patient's insurance plan covers services provided by an APP. APPs may bill Medicare, Medi-Cal, and private payers, depending on their scope and credentialing status.
2. **Determine the Appropriate CPT/HCPCS Code:**
   Based on the services provided, select the correct CPT or HCPCS code. For instance, if the APP is providing a 20-minute MTM session, the appropriate code would be **99605** for a new patient or **99606** for an established patient.
3. **Document the Encounter:**
   Properly document the patient encounter, including the service provided, the time spent, and the outcome. This documentation is essential for justifying the billed code.
4. **Submit the Claim:**
   Using an electronic billing system, submit the claim to the patient's insurance payer (Medicare, Medi-Cal, or a private insurance company) with the appropriate CPT/HCPCS codes and any necessary modifiers (e.g., for telehealth services).

5. **Follow-Up on Denials or Rejections:**
   In the event of claim denial or rejection, work with the billing department to address any issues (e.g., missing documentation, incorrect coding) and resubmit the claim if needed.

E. Billing Protocols and Compliance

1. **Collaborative Agreement Protocol:**
   - The attending physician and APP must define the protocols under which the APP operates, including which services they are authorized to bill.
   - The collaborative practice agreement must be reviewed regularly and updated as necessary to ensure compliance with current laws and billing regulations.
2. **Review of Billing Practices:**
   The billing practices of APPs must be reviewed by the attending physician to ensure compliance with the collaborative agreement, payer requirements, and California law. This includes:
   - Regular audits of APP billing claims.
   - Review of documentation to ensure that it supports the billed services.
   - Adjustments to protocols if issues arise with compliance or reimbursement.

Fraud and Abuse Compliance:
The APh must be cautious to avoid upcoding (billing for services at a higher level than provided) or billing for services not rendered. All billing must follow state and federal regulations to prevent fraud and abuse.

Chapter 2. Current APh Licensure and Training

2.1. APh Licensure in California

A pharmacist who seeks recognition as an advanced practice pharmacist (APh) in California shall meet all of the following requirements:

- A. Hold an active license to practice pharmacy issued pursuant to this chapter that is in good standing.
- B. Satisfy any two of the following criteria:
  1. Earn certification in a relevant area of practice, including, but not limited to, ambulatory care, critical care, geriatric pharmacy, nuclear pharmacy, nutrition support pharmacy, oncology pharmacy, pediatric pharmacy, pharmacotherapy, or psychiatric pharmacy, from an organization recognized by the Accreditation Council for Pharmacy Education or another entity recognized by the board.
  2. Complete a postgraduate residency through an accredited postgraduate institution where at least 50 percent of the experience includes the provision of direct patient care services with interdisciplinary teams.
  3. Have provided clinical services to patients for at least one year under a collaborative practice agreement or protocol with a physician, advanced practice pharmacist, pharmacist practicing collaborative drug therapy management, or health system.

The APh license is distinct from the standard pharmacist license. California is the only state by far that has a distinct APh license application process.

To attain an Advanced Practice Pharmacist (APh) license, licensed pharmacists must submit an application to the Board of Pharmacy along with a $300 fee.

2.2. APh Licensure in Other States

In other states, the pathway to becoming an Advanced Practice Pharmacist also varies, reflecting the unique needs and legislative environments of each state.

In **New Mexico**, the title of "Pharmacist Clinician" has been established to address the shortage of primary care providers. This role allows pharmacists to provide primary and specialty care services, prescribe medications including controlled substances, perform physical exams, and order lab tests.

To become a Pharmacist Clinician in New Mexico, a pharmacist must complete a 60-hour physical assessment course approved by the New Mexico Board of Pharmacy and a 150-hour, 300-patient-contact preceptorship supervised by a physician or other practitioner with prescriptive authority.

In **North Carolina**, a Clinical Pharmacist Practitioner (CPP) is a licensed pharmacist approved to provide drug therapy management, including controlled substances, under the supervision of a licensed physician.

To become a CPP, a pharmacist must be approved by the Pharmacy Board. The application process involves registering through the Board's Gateway and following specific instructions for collaborative practice agreement (CPA) protocol and site changes.

Other states have enacted legislation to enhance the scope of practice for advanced practice pharmacists. **Wyoming, Virginia, Maryland, Missouri, and North Dakota** have passed laws that increase pharmacists' ability to provide comprehensive medication management (CMM) services and ensure reimbursement for services provided within their scope of practice.

Alaska, Arizona, Connecticut, Florida, Montana, Oregon, Washington have broadened the scope of pharmacists' practices to include independent prescription and administration of vaccines, administration of emergency medication, engagement in clinical care, and collaborative drug therapy management.

As of August 2023, **Delaware** became the 50th state to pass legislation allowing pharmacists and physicians to enter into CPAs.

2.3. Collaborative Practice Agreement (CPA) with a Physician:

APhs may enter into collaborative practice agreements with physicians or other healthcare providers.

1. Clinical Services: APhs may provide a range of clinical services, which may include:

- Medication Therapy Management (MTM)
- Managing chronic diseases such as diabetes, hypertension, and asthma
- Providing immunizations
- Performing medication reconciliation and review
- Ordering and interpreting laboratory tests related to medication management
- Providing patient education and counseling on medication use and disease management

2. Prescriptive Authority: APhs may have limited prescriptive authority under certain conditions, such as:
   - Prescribing medications pursuant to a CPA or protocol established with a licensed physician
   - Prescribing and dispensing certain medications independently under specific circumstances, such as emergency contraception or travel medications

3. Record-Keeping and Documentation: APhs are required to maintain accurate patient records and documentation of their clinical interventions, assessments, and recommendations.

4. Continuing Education: APhs must comply with continuing education requirements set forth by the state Board of Pharmacy to maintain licensure and stay updated on best practices and emerging trends in pharmacy practice.

5. Collaboration and Referral: APhs must collaborate with other healthcare providers as appropriate and refer patients to physicians or specialists for further evaluation or management when necessary.

2.4. Current Challenges of APh Training Model

The challenges of the Advanced Practice Pharmacist (APh) training model in California:

- *Lack of residency training program:* Not enough postgraduate training programs for pharmacists could result in inconsistency in equipping the pharmacists as healthcare providers, leading to varied skill levels and competencies. In 2023, California had 397 general PGY-1 pharmacy residency positions available for 1,200 graduates, a significant shortage. Notably, only a limited number of these residency positions facilitated direct collaboration between pharmacists and physicians, with examples including programs at Wynn Medical Center/USC/986 Pharmacy.

- *Lack of national board certification:* Unlike nurse practitioners (NPs) who have a standardized national board examination, there is no equivalent for advanced pharmacist practitioners, making it challenging to establish a recognized standard of competence across the profession.
- *Limited dedicated clinical training sites:* The availability of dedicated clinical training sites specific for APh is a significant barrier to expanding APh programs, as evidenced by the scarcity of opportunities for APh residents in California, despite growing interest from pharmacists and medical clinics.
- *Title recognition:* the APh is a new title to the California healthcare system. In other states, APh uses different titles such as CPP (Clinical Pharmacist Practitioner Montana and North Carolina) or Pharmacist Clinician (New Mexico).

Addressing these challenges requires collaboration among stakeholders, including academic institutions, healthcare organizations, professional associations, and regulatory bodies, to develop standardized curricula, establish national board certification, and expand clinical training opportunities for APhs.

Chapter 3. Future of APh

3.1. APh and Primary Care Provider Shortage:

The recent increased interest among California pharmacists in clinical practice is evident in the increasing numbers of Advanced Practice Pharmacists (APh). By 2022, the state had 1,065 APh licensees, representing about 2% of its pharmacists. This shift signals a significant evolution toward more direct clinical roles within the profession.

In New Mexico, the adoption of the Pharmacist Clinician model by approximately 250 of 1,800 pharmacists underscores its success and the expanding role of pharmacists in direct patient care, reflecting a broader trend towards enhancing the clinical capabilities of pharmacists.

California is facing a significant shortage of primary care providers. Projections indicate that by 2025, California will require an additional 4,100 primary care providers, with this need rising to 4,700 by 2030. It's estimated that California will have between 78,000 and 103,000 primary care practitioners by then, with mild levels (NP/PA) making up about half of this workforce.

The US is anticipated to have a shortfall of 40,000 primary care providers within the next decade, as forecasted by the American Association of Medical Colleges.

The involvement of Advanced Practice Pharmacists, with their unique blend of pharmacy knowledge and clinical training, presents a viable solution to alleviate the primary care provider shortage in both California and the United States.

3.2. Proposed a National Title for APh: APP

Across different states, the title for advanced practice pharmacists varies, with terms like Clinical Pharmacist Practitioner and Pharmacist Clinician used.

To align with the recognition similar to Nurse Practitioners (NPs) and Physician Assistants (PAs), we suggest the unified title of **Advanced Pharmacist Practitioner (APP)** nationwide.

This title highlights their practitioner role, bridging the terminology with that of other health care providers. In this context, APh and APP refer to the same role, emphasizing the practitioner aspect in line with nurse practitioners.

3.3. Primary Care Residency Curriculum for the APh

In 2020, the Wynn Medical Center, in partnership with USC and 986 Pharmacy, initiated a residency program aimed at preparing Advanced Practice Pharmacists (APh) for primary care roles. In 2024, this collaboration extended to include Western University.

The comprehensive APh residency program spans 60 weeks, incorporating an initial 8-week pre-residency training at the pharmacy school followed by a 52-week residency at the medical and pharmacy clinic, structured in 4-week intervals.

Pre-APh Residency Training at Pharmacy School:
- PharmD students who wish to pursue APh residency should select electives in basic medical science such as anatomy, physiology or pathophysiology.
- Pre-Clinical Skills: Patient Interviewing, Documentation, Physical Exams, and Oral Presentations, BCLS, Technical Skills (Bandaging & Splinting, Drug Orders, Suturing, X-ray Interpretation), Informed care and telemedicine.

APh Residency at Medical and Pharmacy Clinic:
- Core Rotation in Primary Care 24 weeks (WMC) : Family Medicine/Internal Medicine (12 weeks), Pediatrics (4 weeks), OB/GYN (4 weeks), and General Surgery (4 weeks).
- Core Rotation in Clinical Pharmacy 12 weeks (at 986 Pharmacy)
- APh Profession 4 weeks (at Western or WMC/986)
- Elective Clinical Assignments 8 weeks (WMC affiliated clinics): Select 2 from Dermatology, Rheumatology, Nephrology, Cardiology, or Psychiatry.
- Advanced Topics Seminars 4 week: Research (Evidence-Based Medicine; Application of Medical Literature to Clinical Guidelines/Patient Education); Education (Community Health Promotion – Disease Prevention, Patient Education, Board Review Seminar); Medical Care Organizations (Health Care Structure; Financing; Billing and Coding).
- Vacation: 4 weeks

Reading Materials:
- Internal Medicine for Advanced Practice Pharmacist (this medical textbook)

- American College of Physicians (ACP) Internal Medicine Board Core Knowledge (MKSAP 19)
- ACP Internal Medicine Intern Curriculum
- WMC/WesternU/USC APh training protocols

3.4. APh Credentials and National Board Certification

While APhs have the option to obtain board certification in their area of specialization. There are currently 15 pharmacy board specialties. Examples of board certifications include Board Certified Pharmacotherapy Specialist (BCPS), Board Certified Ambulatory Care Pharmacist (BCACP), and Board Certified Critical Care Pharmacist (BCCCP).

There's currently no national board exam specific to the APh designation that assesses clinical practice competencies nationally, unlike the exams for Nurse Practitioners (NPs) and Physician Assistants (PAs).

Instituting a national board examination for APhs could enhance the profession's standardization and public trust in their clinical abilities, paralleling the certification processes of other mid-level healthcare providers.

3.5. Evidence based practice for the APh

Evidence-based practice (EBP) in medicine involves integrating the best available research evidence with clinical expertise and patient values to guide clinical decision-making.

Research Evidence:

> This involves systematically reviewing and critically appraising research literature to identify high-quality studies relevant to a specific clinical question or problem. Randomized controlled trials (RCTs), systematic reviews, and meta-analyses are often considered the highest level of evidence.

Clinical Expertise:

> The APhs bring their clinical experience, skills, and knowledge to the decision-making process. This expertise involves understanding the strengths and limitations of available evidence and applying it appropriately to individual patient situations.

Patient Values and Preferences:

> Patient-centered care involves considering patients' values, preferences, beliefs, and unique circumstances when making healthcare

decisions. Engaging patients in shared decision-making ensures that their preferences align with treatment recommendations.

Integration and Implementation:

EBP requires integrating research evidence, clinical expertise, and patient values into clinical practice. This may involve adapting guidelines or protocols to suit patient needs, preferences, and circumstances.

Continuous Learning and Improvement:

EBP involves an ongoing process of critically appraising new evidence, updating clinical knowledge and skills, and incorporating feedback to improve patient care outcomes over time.

References

- American College of Clinical Pharmacy (ACCP). (2016). Definition of clinical pharmacy. Pharmacotherapy, 36(10), e200-e203.
- American Society of Health-System Pharmacists (ASHP). (2019). ASHP statement on the pharmacist's role in clinical pharmacogenomics. American Journal of Health-System Pharmacy, 76(13), 977-981.
- Board of Pharmacy Specialties (BPS). (2019). Pharmacotherapy specialist content outline. McGivney, M. S., & Meyer, S. M. (Eds.). (2015). The pharmacist's role in health care. ASHP.
- Accreditation Council for Pharmacy Education (ACPE). (2016). Accreditation standards and key elements for the professional program in pharmacy leading to the Doctor of Pharmacy degree.
- American Society of Health-System Pharmacists (ASHP). (2018). ASHP residency accreditation standard for postgraduate year one (PGY1) pharmacy residency programs.
- Accreditation Council for Pharmacy Education (ACPE). (2019). Accreditation standards and key elements for the professional program in pharmacy leading to the Doctor of Pharmacy degree (Appendix D).
- California State Board of Pharmacy. (2021). Pharmacist licensure requirements.
- National Association of Boards of Pharmacy (NABP). (2021). NABP's Verified Pharmacy Program (VPP) - standards.
- California State Board of Pharmacy. (2021). Pharmacist collaborative practice agreement.
- American Pharmacists Association (APhA). (2020). Credentialing and privileging of pharmacists: A resource paper from the American Pharmacists Association. Journal of the American Pharmacists Association, 60(6), e185-e198.

- Adams, A. J., & Frost, T. P. (2023). Implementation of the California advanced practice pharmacist and the continued disappointment of tiered licensure. *Exploratory Research in Clinical and Social Pharmacy, 12*, Article 100353. https://doi.org/10.1016/j.rcsop.2023.100353

Part II:

Common Disorders in General Practice for the APh

Chapter 4. Cardiovascular Disorders

Reviewed by
Philip Tran, DO, FACC, FACOI

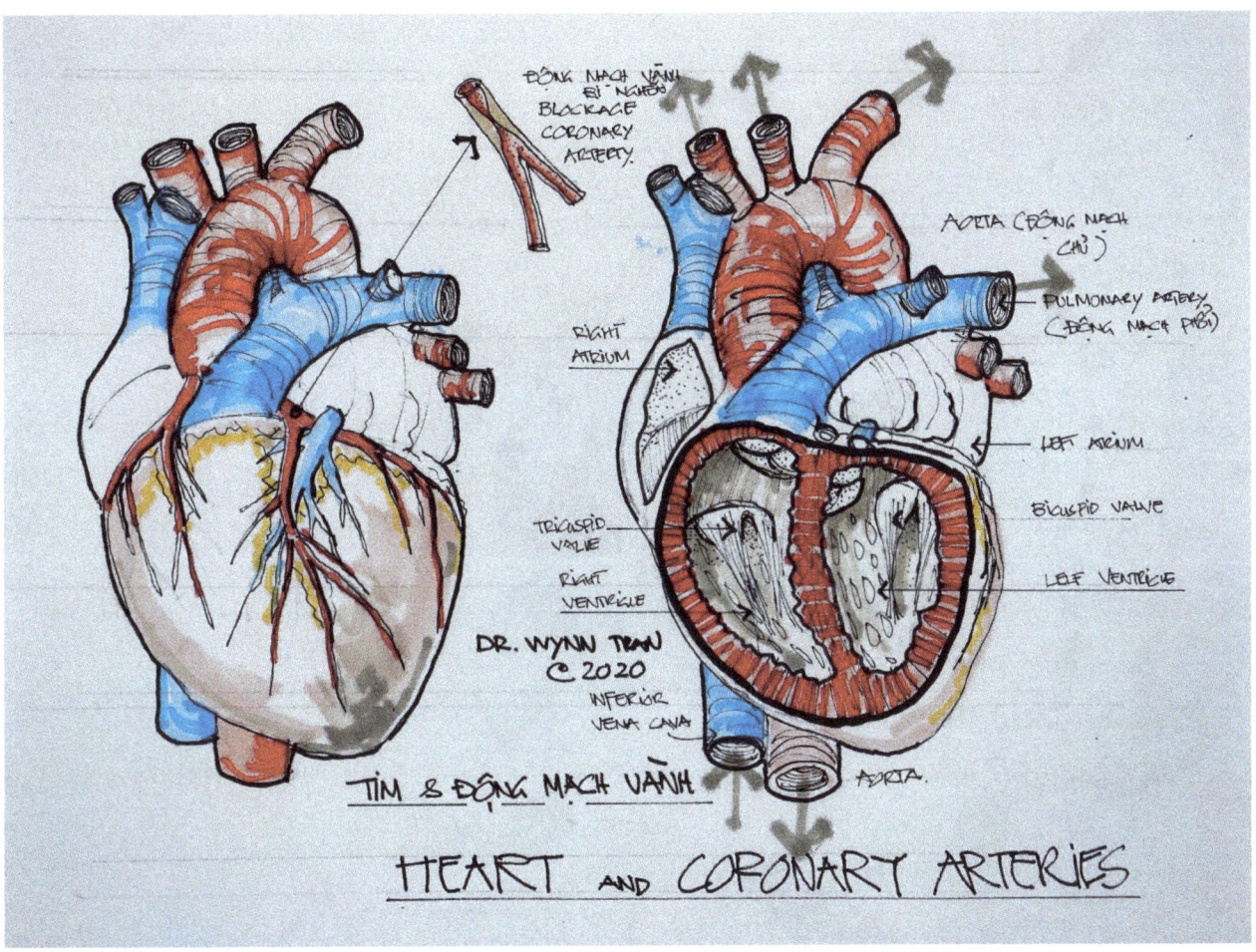

The APh should be familiar with the presentation, diagnosis, and management of these common cardiovascular disorders to provide appropriate care and referral to the cardiologist when necessary.

4.1. Hypertension

> ➢ *High blood pressure can lead to many complications such as stroke, heart attack, heart failure, and kidney failure.*
>
> ➢ *Risk factors include older age, overweight/obesity, family history, lack of physical activity, and unhealthy diet.*
>
> ➢ *Management involves lifestyle changes and medications to lower blood pressure and reduce the risk of associated complications.*

Hypertension (HTN), also known as high blood pressure, is a common condition characterized by elevated blood pressure levels in the arteries. It's often named as a "silent killer" because it typically does not cause noticeable symptoms until it reaches a severe or life-threatening stage.

Symptoms

- Headaches: Sometimes when blood pressure is very high, especially at the posterior head and in the morning.
- Shortness of breath: During physical exertion and strenuous activity.
- Chest pain: Usually related to complications like heart attack or aortic dissection.
- Blurred vision.
- Dizziness or fainting: Especially due to sudden changes in position.
- Nausea and vomiting.

Causes and Risk Factors

These conditions may increase the risk of developing hypertension:

- Age: older adults.
- A family history of hypertension.
- Obesity or being overweight.
- Lack of exercise.
- Smoking or chewing tobacco can damage arterial walls.
- Diet: High salt intake, excessive alcohol consumption, and a diet high in saturated fats and low in fruits and vegetables.
- Long-term stress.
- Other chronic conditions: Kidney disease, diabetes, and sleep apnea.

Workup and Diagnosis

- <u>Blood Pressure Measurement (primary diagnostic tool):</u>

Normal blood pressure is typically considered below 120/80 mm Hg. The APh needs to know the proper technique to measure blood pressure and compare with a patient's home blood pressure.

- Physical Examination: check for signs of organ damage, such as enlarged heart, abnormal heartbeats (S4), or hypertensive retinopathy.
- Lab Tests:

  Assess other risk factors of cardiovascular diseases like diabetes (fasting blood sugar or A1c), lipid panel, or complications of hypertension like kidney function test and microalbuminuria, left ventricular hypertrophy (LVH), reduced ejection fraction (EF) on the transthoracic echocardiogram (TTE).
- Electrocardiogram (EKG): evaluate signs of LVH.

Treatment
- Lifestyle Modifications:
  - Dietary Modifications: low sodium, DASH (Dietary Approaches to Stop Hypertension) diet
  - Weight Management: achieving and maintaining a healthy weight.
  - Regular Exercise: at least 30 minutes of moderate-intensity exercise on at least 5 days a week (at least 150 minutes a week)
  - Limit Alcohol: Moderation is key.
  - Quit Smoking: if applicable
- Medications :
  - **Diuretics:**
    - Thiazide Diuretics: often the first choice in hypertension treatment.
      - Hydrochlorothiazide (HCTZ)
      - Chlorthalidone
    - Loop Diuretics: usually used in patients with heart failure along with high blood pressure because they are more potent than thiazides.
      - Furosemide (Lasix)
      - Bumetanide

- Potassium-Sparing Diuretics: retain potassium while still promoting water elimination.
  - Spironolactone
  - Amiloride
  - Triamterene

Side effects of Diuretics include electrolyte imbalances, dehydration, dizziness, muscle cramps, increased urination, and changes in blood sugar levels.

- **ACE Inhibitors and ARBs:**
  - Lisinopril (Prinivil, Zestril): For HTN and heart failure.
  - Enalapril (Vasotec): For HTN, diabetic kidney disease, and heart failure.
  - Ramipril (Altace): For HTN and to improve survival after heart attacks.
  - Captopril (Capoten): For HTN and heart failure.
  - Benazepril (Lotensin)
  - Losartan (Cozaar): For HTN and CKD patients with diabetes.
  - Valsartan (Diovan): For HTN and heart failure, and to reduce cardiovascular mortality after MI.
  - Irbesartan (Avapro): For HTN and diabetic nephropathy.
  - Telmisartan (Micardis): For HTN and potential cardiovascular protection.
  - Olmesartan (Benicar): Often noted for its potency and efficacy.

Common side effects may include dry cough, dizziness, and fatigue. Rarely, they can cause more severe side effects such as kidney problems, high potassium levels, and angioedema.

- **Calcium Channel Blockers (CCB):**
  - Dihydropyridines: primarily affect the blood vessels
    - Amlodipine (Norvasc)
    - Nifedipine (Procardia, Adalat)
    - Felodipine
    - Nicardipine

- Non-dihydropyridines: affect both the heart rate and blood vessels. They are useful in both hypertension and angina.
    - Verapamil (Calan, Verelan)
    - Diltiazem (Cardizem, Tiazac)
  - **CCB side effects** may include dizziness, flushing, headache, and swelling in the lower legs in some cases.
  - **Beta-Blockers:**
    - Atenolol (Tenormin), also beneficial for heart rhythm disorders and chest pain.
    - Metoprolol (Lopressor, Toprol XL) Available in both immediate and extended-release forms, metoprolol is used for HTN, chest pain, and heart failure.
    - Propranolol (Inderal, Inderal LA), a non-selective beta blocker for HTN and preventing migraines and treating essential tremor.
    - Bisoprolol (Zebeta), for HTN and heart failure.
    - Nadolol (Corgard) for HTN and chest pain, it is less selective in the targeting of beta receptors.

    Common side effects include fatigue, cold extremities, sleep disturbances, bradycardia, mood changes, orr depressive symptoms. Additionally, beta blockers can affect respiratory function in patients with asthma or COPD and may lead to sexual dysfunction in some individuals
  - Other medications: depend on patient factors.
- Regular Monitoring: Blood pressure should be monitored regularly, even when under control.
- Stress Management: Techniques like mindfulness, yoga, or meditation can help manage stress, which can reduce blood pressure.

Treatment for Specific Patient Groups
- Patients with diabetes mellitus:
  - Antihypertensive therapy can help prevent microvascular and macrovascular complications associated with type 2 diabetes.
  - In patients with hypertension and diabetes, an ACE or ARB is recommended.

- The combination of an ACE inhibitor and ARB or the combination of an ACE inhibitor/ARB with a direct renin inhibitor is not recommended.
- Patients with chronic kidney disease (CKD):
  - In patients with hypertension and proteinuric CKD, an ACE inhibitor or ARB is recommended to slow the progression of kidney disease and preserve remaining kidney function.
  - A dual combination of an ACE inhibitor with an ARB is not recommended.
- Patients with coronary artery disease:
  - In patients with hypertension and coronary artery disease, an ACE inhibitor, ARB, or β-blocker is recommended for compelling indications (such as recent myocardial infarction or angina), in addition to other antihypertensive medications (such as dihydropyridine CCBs, long-acting thiazide diuretics, and/or mineralocorticoid receptor antagonists) as needed to optimize blood pressure control.
  - The combination of a β-blocker and nondihydropyridine CCBs (such as diltiazem or verapamil) should be avoided.
- Patients with heart failure:
  - In patients with hypertension and heart failure, an ARNI/ACEI/ARB, β-blocker, MRA, SGLT2i and diuretic (with symptoms of fluid overload) are recommended.
  - Nondihydropyridine CCBs should be avoided in patients with HFrEF because of their pronounced negative inotropic effect.

Treatment of Persistent Hypertension

The most effective combination therapy for persistent hypertension depends on various factors, including individual patient characteristics, comorbidities, tolerability, and response to treatment.

- ACE Inhibitor or Angiotensin II Receptor Blocker (ARB) + dihydropyridine for all CCB for HTN. Ex: dihydropyridine CCB + Calcium Channel Blocker (CCB)

    This combination is often recommended for patients with persistent hypertension, particularly those with diabetes or chronic kidney disease.

- ACE Inhibitor or ARB + Thiazide Diuretic:

    Combining an ACE inhibitor or ARB with a thiazide diuretic can effectively lower blood pressure by reducing fluid load and vasodilation. This combination is particularly useful for patients with heart failure or those at risk of developing it.

- CCB + Thiazide Diuretic:

    This combination is commonly used as first-line therapy for patients with persistent hypertension. CCBs and thiazide diuretics work synergistically to lower blood pressure by relaxing blood vessels and reducing fluid volume.

- Triple Therapy (ACE Inhibitor or ARB + CCB + Thiazide Diuretic):

    For patients with severe or resistant hypertension, triple therapy combining an ACE inhibitor or ARB with a CCB and thiazide diuretic may be necessary to achieve blood pressure control.

4.2. Chest Pain

> ➢ *Chest pain is a symptom that can be caused by a variety of conditions ranging from non-serious to life-threatening, including heart, lung, gastrointestinal, musculoskeletal, and psychological issues.*
>
> ➢ *It requires careful evaluation to determine the underlying cause, utilizing history, physical examination, and diagnostic tests.*
>
> ➢ *Treatment depends on the diagnosis, addressing the specific cause of the chest pain.*

Symptoms:

Chest pain can manifest in many forms, varying from sharp to dull aches, and may be accompanied by symptoms such as:

- Pressure or tightness in the chest
- Shortness of breath
- Nausea
- Fatigue
- Dizziness
- Palpitations
- Pain spreading to the jaw, back, or arms

Causes and Risk Factors:

Risk factors for chest pain can be related to cardiac, gastrointestinal, musculoskeletal, respiratory, or psychological causes:

- Cardiac-related: history of heart disease, hypertension, high cholesterol, diabetes, smoking, excessive alcohol use, sedentary lifestyle, and obesity

- Other causes: stress, panic attacks, acid reflux (GERD), pulmonary embolism, pneumonia, rib cage injuries, or muscle strain

Epidemiology:

The prevalence of chest pain varies widely depending on the underlying cause. It is a common symptom that leads people to seek emergency medical attention. The epidemiology of chest pain encompasses its occurrence across different populations, with cardiovascular diseases being a leading cause of severe chest pain worldwide.

Workup and Diagnosis:
- Medical history and physical examination: identify any risk factors or physical signs that could suggest a specific cause.
- Electrocardiogram (ECG): detect heart problems.
- Blood tests: look for markers of heart damage, infection, or inflammation.
- Chest X-ray: visualize the lungs, heart, and chest wall.
- Echocardiography: examine the heart's structure and function.
- CT scans or MRI: visualize detailed imaging of the chest structures.

Chest Pain Score (0-10)

The HEART score is a risk stratification tool used to assess the likelihood of major adverse cardiac events (MACE) in patients presenting with chest pain to the emergency department. It has five components.

HEART Score		
History	<ul><li>Highly Suspicious</li><li>Moderately Suspicious</li><li>Slightly or Non Suspicious</li></ul>	2 1 0
ECG	<ul><li>Significant ST-Depression</li><li>Nonspecific Repolarization</li><li>Normal</li></ul>	2 1 0
Age	<ul><li>$\geq$ 65 years</li><li>45 - 65 years</li><li>$\leq$ 45 years</li></ul>	2 1 0
Risk Factors	<ul><li>$\geq$ 3 Risk Factors or History of CAD</li><li>1 or 2 Risk Factors</li><li>No Risk Factors</li></ul>	2 1 0

Troponin	<ul><li>≥ 3x Normal Limit</li><li>1-3x Normal Limit</li><li>≤ Normal Limit</li></ul>	2 1 0

- **0 to 3 points**: low risk (0.6% to 1.7% risk of major adverse cardiac events)
- **4 to 6 points**: intermediate risk (16.6% risk)
- **7 to 10 points**: high risk (50.1% risk)

Differential Diagnosis for Chest Pain:

1. Cardiovascular Causes
    - Acute Coronary Syndrome (ACS): includes conditions like unstable angina or myocardial infarction.
    - Aortic Dissection: a serious condition involving a tear or rupture in the aorta's inner layer, causing severe, sudden chest pain.
    - Pericarditis: inflammation of the pericardium
    - Myocarditis: inflammation of the heart muscle, often due to viral infection
2. Pulmonary Causes
    - Pulmonary Embolism (PE): a blockage of the major pulmonary arteries in the lungs.
    - Pneumothorax: collapse of the lung due to air leaking into the space between the lung and chest wall.
    - Pneumonia: infection that inflames the air sacs in one or both lungs.
3. Gastrointestinal Causes
    - Gastroesophageal Reflux Disease (GERD): a condition where stomach acid frequently flows back into the esophagus, causing chest pain.
    - Esophageal Spasm: irregular, painful contractions of the esophagus
    - Peptic Ulcers: sores on the lining of the stomach or small intestine that cause pain
4. Musculoskeletal Causes
    - Costochondritis: inflammation of the cartilage that connects a rib to the breastbone
    - Muscle Strain: injury to the chest muscle from overuse or heavy lifting

5. Psychological Causes
   - Panic Attack: sudden episodes of intense fear that trigger severe physical reactions when there is no real danger or apparent cause
   - Anxiety: can cause chest pain through muscle tension or by mimicking symptoms of heart conditions.
6. Other Causes
   - Herpes Zoster (Shingles): A viral infection causes a painful rash, sometimes leading to chest pain before the rash appears.
   - Rib Fracture or Bruising: Direct trauma to the chest can cause pain that is sharp and worsens with deep breathing or movement.

Treatment:
- Cardiac causes may require immediate medications (like nitroglycerin, aspirin, or clot-busting drugs), surgical procedures (such as angioplasty or bypass surgery), and lifestyle changes.
- Gastrointestinal causes like GERD are treated with dietary modifications, antacids, or proton pump inhibitors.
- Musculoskeletal pain often improves with rest, physical therapy, or pain relievers.
- Psychological factors might be addressed with stress management techniques, counseling, or medication for anxiety or depression.

4.3. Coronary Artery Disease

> ➤ *Narrowing or blockage of the coronary arteries, reducing blood flow to the heart muscle which can lead to angina (chest pain) and myocardial infarction (heart attack).*
> ➤ *Risk factors include smoking, high cholesterol, high blood pressure, diabetes, and sedentary lifestyle.*
> ➤ *Prevention and management strategies include lifestyle modifications, medications, and in some cases, procedures such as angioplasty or bypass surgery.*

Coronary Artery Disease (CAD) is a condition characterized by the narrowing or blockage of the coronary arteries, which supply oxygen-rich blood to the heart muscle. It is the leading cause of heart attacks and other cardiovascular complications.

Symptoms:
- Angina: pressure, tightness or heavy, squeezing, or burning sensation in the chest
- Shortness of Breath: especially associated with physical exertion or during stress
- Fatigue: unexplained tiredness or weakness
- Nausea: sometimes accompanied by sweating and dizziness
- Pain or discomfort in other areas: arms, neck, jaw, or back

Causes and Risk Factors:
- Hypertension
- High Cholesterol Levels
- Smoking
- Diabetes
- Obesity
- Sedentary Lifestyle
- Family History of Heart Disease
- Age

Workup and Diagnosis:
- <u>Medical History and Physical Examination:</u> assessment of risk factors and symptoms.
- <u>ECG/EKG:</u> detects abnormal heart rhythms and signs of ischemia.
- <u>Blood Tests:</u> cholesterol levels, blood sugar, and cardiac enzymes
- <u>Stress Tests:</u> exercise stress test or pharmacological stress test to evaluate heart function and reversible or irreversible ischemic areas under stress
- <u>Echocardiogram:</u> assess heart structure, wall motions, and cardiac function.
- <u>Coronary Angiography:</u> invasive procedure using contrast and X-rays to visualize coronary arteries for blockages

Treatment:
- <u>Lifestyle Modifications:</u>
  - Healthy Diet: low in saturated fat, cholesterol, and sodium
  - Regular Exercise: at least 30 minutes of moderate-intensity exercise most days of the week
  - Smoking Cessation: reduces the risk of heart disease.

- o Weight Management: maintain a healthy weight.
- Medications:
  - o Aspirin and Antiplatelet Medications: reduce the risk of blood clots.
  - o Statins: lower cholesterol levels.
  - o Beta-blockers, ACE Inhibitors, Calcium Channel Blockers: manage blood pressure and reduce strain on the heart.
  - o Nitroglycerin: relieves chest pain.
- Medical Procedures:
  - o Angioplasty and Stenting: open blocked arteries to restore blood flow.
  - o Coronary Artery Bypass Grafting: a surgery to bypass blocked coronary arteries
- Cardiac Rehabilitation: structured program including exercise, education, and counseling to improve heart health and recovery

4.4. Heart Failure

> ➢ *Heart failure (HF) is a chronic condition where the heart is unable to pump blood effectively, leading to fluid buildup in the lungs and other tissues. Symptoms include shortness of breath, fatigue, and swelling in the legs.*
>
> ➢ *Risk factors include CAD, hypertension, diabetes, obesity, and certain medications.*
>
> ➢ *Treatment involves medications, lifestyle changes, and in some cases, interventions like device implantation or heart transplantation.*

Symptoms:
- Dyspnea: especially during physical activity or when lying down flat
- Fatigue and Weakness: even with minimal exertion
- Edema: fluid retention in the legs, ankles, or abdomen
- Rapid or Irregular Palpitations
- Persistent Coughing or Wheezing: especially when lying down
- Reduced Exercise Tolerance: inability to perform activities previously tolerated

Causes and Risk Factors:
- Coronary Artery Disease

- Hypertension
- Diabetes
- Obesity
- Smoking
- Family History of Heart Disease
- Age
- Heart Valve Disorders
- History of Heart Attack
- Cardiomyopathy

Workup and Diagnosis:
- Medical History and Physical Examination: assessment of symptoms and risk factors
- Blood Tests: assess kidney function, electrolyte levels, and biomarkers such as B-type natriuretic peptide (BNP) or N-terminal pro-B-type natriuretic peptide (NT-proBNP).
- ECG/EKG: evaluates heart rhythm and electrical activity.
- Echocardiogram: assesses heart structure and function, including ejection fraction.
- Chest X-ray: detects signs of fluid buildup in the lungs or enlarged heart.
- Cardiac MRI or CT Scan: further evaluates heart structure and function, and identify underlying causes.

Treatment:
- Medications:
    - Diuretics: reduce fluid retention.
    - ACE Inhibitors, ARBs, or ARNIs: improve heart function and reduce strain.
    - Beta-Blockers: help control heart rate and blood pressure.
    - Aldosterone Antagonists: reduce fluid retention and improve heart function.
    - Digoxin: helps strengthen heart contractions.
- Lifestyle Modifications:
    - Low-Sodium Diet: reduces fluid retention.
    - Fluid Restriction: as advised by PCP or APh
    - Regular Exercise: tailored to patient capabilities.

- Smoking Cessation: if applicable
- Medical Devices:
  - Implantable Cardioverter-Defibrillator (ICD): monitors heart rhythm and delivers shocks if needed.
  - Cardiac Resynchronization Therapy (CRT): improves heart function in certain cases.
- Surgery:
  - Heart Valve Repair or Replacement
  - Coronary Artery Bypass Grafting (CABG)
  - Heart Transplantation

4.5. Arrhythmias

> *Arrhythmias are abnormal heart rhythms that can cause the heart to beat too fast, too slow, or irregularly. Types include atrial fibrillation, ventricular tachycardia, and bradycardia.*
>
> *Risk factors include heart disease, electrolyte imbalances, and substance abuse.*
>
> *Treatment options include medication, lifestyle changes, cardiac procedures, or implantable devices to manage or correct the abnormal heart rhythms.*

Symptoms:

- Palpitations: sensation of rapid, fluttering, or irregular heartbeat.
- Dizziness or Lightheadedness: especially with exertion or sudden changes in position
- Syncope: often without warning
- Shortness of Breath: especially with exertion or during episodes of arrhythmia
- Chest Pain or Discomfort: sometimes mistaken for symptoms of a heart attack
- Unexplained tiredness or weakness

Causes and Risk Factors:

- Coronary Artery Disease
- Hypertension
- Heart Attack

- Heart Valve Disorders
- Heart Failure
- Congenital Heart Defects
- Electrolyte Imbalance
- Thyroid Disorders
- Obstructive Sleep Apnea
- Stress or Anxiety
- Family History of Arrhythmias or Sudden Cardiac Death
- Excessive Alcohol Consumption
- Smoking
- Illicit Drug Use

Workup and Diagnosis:
- <u>Medical History and Physical Examination:</u> assessment of symptoms and risk factors
- <u>ECG/EKG:</u> records the electrical activity of the heart and identify abnormalities.
- <u>Holter Monitor:</u> A portable device is worn for 24 to 48 hours (outpatient) to continuously record the heart rhythm.
- <u>Event Monitor:</u> similar to a Holter monitor but worn for longer periods to capture intermittent arrhythmias
- <u>Echocardiogram:</u> assess heart structure and function.
- <u>Electrophysiological Study (EPS):</u> invasive procedure to evaluate the electrical activity of the heart and induce arrhythmias for diagnosis, usually done by a cardiologist
- <u>Blood Tests:</u> assess electrolyte levels, thyroid function, and cardiac biomarkers.

Treatment:
- <u>Medications:</u>
  - Antiarrhythmic Drugs: help control heart rhythm.
  - Beta-Blockers: reduce heart rate and blood pressure.
  - Calcium Channel Blockers: control heart rate and rhythm.
  - Anticoagulants: reduce the risk of blood clots and stroke.
- <u>Cardioversion:</u> a procedure to restore normal heart rhythm using electrical shock or medications

- **Catheter Ablation:** a minimally invasive procedure to destroy abnormal heart tissue causing arrhythmias
- **Implantable Devices:**
    - Pacemaker: regulates heart rate in cases of bradycardia (slow heartbeat).
    - Implantable Cardioverter-Defibrillator (ICD): monitors heart rhythm and delivers shocks if life-threatening arrhythmias occur.
- **Lifestyle Modifications:**
    - Avoid Triggers: caffeine, alcohol, and stress
    - Healthy Diet: low in sodium, saturated fat, and cholesterol
    - Regular Exercise: as recommended by a healthcare provider
    - Smoking Cessation: if applicable
    - Stress Management: techniques like meditation or yoga
- **Surgery:** In certain cases, surgical procedures may be necessary to correct underlying heart conditions contributing to arrhythmias.

4.6. Atrial Fibrillation

> ➤ *Atrial fibrillation (Afib) is a common heart rhythm disorder characterized by irregular and often rapid heart rate, leading to increased risk of stroke, heart failure, and other cardiovascular complications.*
>
> ➤ *It's diagnosed primarily through an EKG showing an irregularly irregular rhythm and absent P waves.*
>
> ➤ *Treatment focuses on controlling heart rate, preventing stroke through anticoagulants, and restoring normal rhythm.*

Symptoms:
- Irregular Heartbeat: heart palpitations or irregular heartbeats
- Fatigue: tiredness and decreased ability to exercise
- Dizziness: feeling light-headed or experiencing fainting spells
- Shortness of Breath: especially during activity or lying down
- Chest Pain: a sign of heart attack or other serious conditions

Causes and Risk Factors:
- Age: The risk of developing Afib increases with age, particularly after 65.

- Heart Disease: existing heart conditions such as hypertension, coronary artery disease, heart valve problems, and previous heart surgery
- Chronic Conditions: diabetes, thyroid problems, sleep apnea, and other metabolic diseases
- Lifestyle Factors: obesity, smoking, high alcohol intake, and the use of stimulants
- Family History of Afib increases the risk.

Epidemiology:

Atrial fibrillation is the most common serious heart rhythm abnormality in people over the age of 65, affecting millions worldwide. Its prevalence increases with age and is slightly more common in men than in women. Due to the aging population, the number of individuals with Afib is expected to increase significantly in the coming decades.

Afib Score: Atrial fibrillation risk scores are tools used to assess the risk of stroke in patients with atrial fibrillation.

	CHA_2DS_2-VASc Score	
C	Congestive Heart Failure	1
H	Hypertension	1
A_2	Age ≥ 75 years	2
D	Diabetes Mellitus	1
S_2	Stroke/Transient Ischemic Attack/Thromboembolism	2
V	Vascular Disease (Prior Myocardial Infarction, Peripheral Artery Disease, or Aortic Plaque)	1
A	Age 65 - 74 years	1
Sc	Sex Category - Female	1

- ***Score of 0:*** Low risk: Anticoagulation therapy may not be necessary for stroke prevention.
- ***Score of 1:*** Low to moderate risk: Anticoagulation therapy may be considered, particularly in certain clinical scenarios.
- ***Score of 2 or more:*** Moderate to high risk: Anticoagulation therapy is generally recommended to reduce the risk of stroke.

Workup and Diagnosis:
- Electrocardiogram (EKG) findings:
  - Irregularly Irregular Rhythm: No predictable pattern in the heart's rhythm, distinguishing it from other forms of arrhythmia that may have a regular pattern.
  - Absent P Waves: In Afib, the atria do not contract in a coordinated manner, leading to the absence of P waves on the EKG. Instead of the normal P waves that precede each QRS complex, indicating atrial contraction, there are chaotic baseline undulations of varying amplitude and frequency.
  - Variable Ventricular Response: The QRS complexes (represent ventricular contraction) occur at irregular intervals.
  - Narrow QRS Complexes: Unless there is a coexisting bundle branch block or other condition affecting the ventricles, the QRS complexes in Afib are usually narrow.
- Holter Monitor: a portable EKG device worn for a day or more to record heart activity over time
- Event Monitor: similar to a Holter but used for longer periods to catch infrequent arrhythmias
- Echocardiogram: uses ultrasound waves to visualize the heart's structure and function, helping to identify underlying heart diseases.

Treatments:
- Medications:

  Anticoagulants to prevent clots, beta-blockers, and calcium channel blockers to control heart rate, and antiarrhythmic drugs to maintain normal heart rhythm.
- Cardioversion: either a procedure using medications or electric shock to reset the heart to its regular rhythm
- Catheter Ablation:

  The use of radiofrequency energy to destroy small areas of heart tissue that are causing irregular signals, usually done by an electrophysiologist, a subspecialist in cardiology.
- Surgery: In some cases, surgery may be recommended, such as the Maze procedure or implantation of a pacemaker or atrial defibrillator.

4.7. Bradycardia

> ➤ *Bradycardia refers to a slower than normal heart rate, typically defined as fewer than 60 beats per minute in adults.*
>
> ➤ *It can be a sign of strong cardiovascular fitness in some individuals, such as athletes, but may also indicate underlying health issues in others.*
>
> ➤ *Treatment depends on the underlying cause and the severity of symptoms, ranging from lifestyle changes and medication to the implantation of a pacemaker.*

Symptoms:
- Fatigue or feeling weak
- Dizziness or lightheadedness
- Fainting or near-fainting spells
- Shortness of breath
- Chest pain
- Confusion or memory problems
- Difficulty exercising

Causes and Risk Factors:
- Age: Older adults are at higher risk due to the natural aging of the heart and its electrical system.
- Heart Disease: Conditions such as coronary artery disease, myocardial infarction, and heart failure can lead to bradycardia.
- Hypothyroidism: Low levels of thyroid hormones can slow heart rate.
- Electrolyte Imbalances: can affect the heart's electrical system.
- Certain Medications: beta-blockers and other medications that treat high blood pressure or heart conditions
- Infections: such as Lyme disease that may affect the heart

Epidemiology:

Bradycardia is more common in older adults due to the natural aging process of the heart. The prevalence in the general population can vary widely, depending on factors such as age, underlying health conditions, and use of medications that can slow heart rate.

Diagnosis:
- Electrocardiogram:
  - Rate: The heart rate, calculated by the number of QRS complexes in a 10-second strip multiplied by 6, is **less than 60 beats per minute.**
  - Rhythm: can be regular or irregular, depending on the underlying cause of the bradycardia.
  - P Waves: Typically, each P wave is followed by a QRS complex, indicating normal sinus rhythm, but at a slower rate.
  - PR Interval: The PR interval may be normal or prolonged. If the cause of bradycardia is an AV block, the PR interval may be prolonged or the P wave may not always be followed by a QRS complex, depending on the type of block.
  - QRS Complex: usually normal in duration unless the bradycardia is associated with other conduction abnormalities.
- Holter Monitor: a portable EKG device worn for 24 hours or longer to capture heart rate variability over time
- Event Monitor: used for longer-term monitoring, especially if symptoms are infrequent
- Echocardiogram: assesses the heart's structure and function
- Blood Tests: check for underlying conditions like hypothyroidism or electrolyte imbalances

Treatment
- No Treatment: If bradycardia causes no symptoms and is not linked to an underlying disorder, treatment may not be necessary.
- Medication Changes: adjust or change medications that may be causing bradycardia.
- Pacemaker: For symptomatic bradycardia not due to reversible causes, a pacemaker may be implanted to regulate the heart's rhythm.
- Treating Underlying Conditions: address any underlying medical conditions that might be causing the slow heart rate.

4.8. Tachycardia

> ➢ *Tachycardia is an abnormally rapid heart rate, typically exceeding 100 beats per minute at rest. Symptoms include palpitations, chest discomfort, dizziness, shortness of breath, and fainting.*
>
> ➢ *Diagnosis involves medical history, physical examination, and diagnostic tests like electrocardiogram (ECG) to identify the underlying cause.*
>
> ➢ *Treatment varies based on the cause and severity, ranging from medication to procedures like ablation therapy or implantable devices.*

Symptoms:
- Rapid heartbeat, resting heart rate exceeding 100 beats per minute
- Symptoms can vary depending on the underlying cause and may include palpitations, chest discomfort, shortness of breath, dizziness, lightheadedness, fainting (syncope), and fatigue.

Causes and Risk Factors:
- Heart Conditions: coronary artery disease, heart failure, heart valve disorders, and congenital heart defects
- Electrolyte Imbalances: low potassium or magnesium levels
- Hormonal Imbalances: hyperthyroidism or adrenal gland disorders
- Medications and Substances: Certain medications, caffeine, nicotine, and illicit drugs can trigger tachycardia.
- Age: Tachycardia can affect individuals of any age but is more common in older adults with underlying heart conditions.

Epidemiology:

Tachycardia is a common condition with various causes. The prevalence depends on the specific type and underlying factors. For instance, supraventricular tachycardias (SVTs) are more prevalent in younger individuals, while atrial fibrillation is more common in older adults. Overall, tachycardia can affect people of all ages and backgrounds.

Diagnosis:
- Electrocardiogram:
    - Increased Heart Rate: higher than the normal range, often exceeding 100 beats per minute at rest
    - Narrow QRS Complex: In supraventricular tachycardias (SVTs), the QRS complex width is usually normal, indicating that the origin of the rapid heartbeat is above the ventricles.

- - Absence of P Waves: In certain types of tachycardia, such as atrial fibrillation, the P waves may be absent or irregularly spaced due to the chaotic electrical activity in the atria.
  - Regular or Irregular Rhythm: Depending on the underlying rhythm disturbance, the heartbeat may be regular or irregular.
- Holter Monitor: a portable device that continuously records the heart's rhythm over 24 to 48 hours
- Event Monitor: similar to a Holter monitor but worn for a longer duration and activated by the patient when symptoms occur
- Blood Tests: assess underlying conditions such as electrolyte imbalances or thyroid dysfunction.

Treatment:
- Medications: beta-blockers, calcium channel blockers, antiarrhythmic drugs, or medications to address underlying conditions.
- Cardioversion: a procedure to restore normal heart rhythm, often performed using electrical cardioversion or chemical cardioversion
- Ablation Therapy: a procedure to destroy abnormal heart tissue causing the arrhythmia
- Implantable Devices: pacemakers or implantable cardioverter-defibrillators (ICDs) to regulate heart rhythm and prevent life-threatening arrhythmias
- Lifestyle Modifications: reducing stress, avoiding triggers (such as caffeine or alcohol), maintaining a healthy weight, and managing underlying conditions such as hypertension or diabetes

4.9. Valvular Heart Disease

> *Valvular heart disease involves dysfunction or damage to one or more of the heart's valves—mitral, tricuspid, aortic, or pulmonary.*
>
> *Causes include congenital defects, age-related changes, infections, and other medical conditions. Symptoms may include chest pain, shortness of breath, fatigue, and palpitations.*
>
> *Treatment options range from medications to surgical repair or replacement of affected valves.*

Symptoms:
- Shortness of Breath: especially with exertion or when lying flat

- Fatigue: feeling tired or weak, even with minimal activity
- Palpitations: sensation of rapid or irregular heartbeat
- Chest Pain: especially during physical activity or when lying flat
- Dizziness or Fainting: especially with exertion or sudden changes in position
- Edema: typically in the legs, ankles, or abdomen
- Heart Murmur: unusual sound heard during a physical examination

Causes and Risk Factors:
- Age: Risk increases with age.
- Gender: Some types of valvular heart disease are more common in men or women.
- History of Rheumatic Fever: can lead to damage to heart valves.
- Congenital Heart Defects
- High Blood Pressure
- Coronary Artery Disease
- History of Heart Attack
- History of Endocarditis
- Other Heart Conditions: cardiomyopathy or heart failure.
- Radiation Therapy: previous radiation therapy to the chest area

Workup and Diagnosis:
- <u>Medical History and Physical Examination:</u> assessment of symptoms and risk factors, and listening for heart murmurs
- <u>Echocardiogram:</u> an ultrasound imaging to assess heart structure and function, including evaluation of the heart valves
- <u>Electrocardiogram (ECG/EKG):</u> evaluate heart rhythm and electrical activity.
- <u>Chest X-ray:</u> assess heart size and detect signs of fluid buildup in the lungs.
- <u>Transesophageal Echocardiogram (TEE):</u> invasive ultrasound imaging to obtain detailed images of the heart valves
- <u>Cardiac Catheterization:</u> invasive procedure to evaluate blood flow and pressure in the heart and coronary arteries
- <u>MRI or CT Scan:</u> further evaluate heart structure and function, and identify underlying causes.

Treatment:
- Medications:
  - Diuretics: reduce fluid buildup and relieve symptoms of congestion.
  - Anticoagulants: reduce the risk of blood clots and stroke in certain cases.
  - Medications to Control Heart Rate or Rhythm: beta-blockers or antiarrhythmic drugs
- Valve Repair or Replacement Surgery:
  - Valve Repair: surgical procedure to fix damaged heart valves
  - Valve Replacement: surgical procedure to replace damaged heart valves with artificial valves or biological tissue valves
- Transcatheter Valve Repair or Replacement (TAVR or TMVR): minimally invasive procedures to repair or replace heart valves using catheters inserted through blood vessels
- Balloon Valvuloplasty: minimally invasive procedure to open narrowed heart valves using a balloon catheter
- Endocarditis Prophylaxis: antibiotics before dental or surgical procedures to prevent infection of damaged heart valves

4.10. Mitral Valve Prolapse

> ➢ *Mitral valve prolapse is a common heart condition where the valve between the heart's left atrium and left ventricle does not close properly.*
> ➢ *Symptoms may include chest pain, palpitations, or shortness of breath.*
> ➢ *It often does not require treatment but can lead to complications like arrhythmias or valve regurgitation in severe cases.*

Symptoms:
- Asymptomatic: Many patients with MVP are asymptomatic and may not experience any symptoms.
- Palpitations: abnormal heartbeats or palpitations.
- Atypical Chest Pain: chest discomfort or atypical chest pain that mimic symptoms of angina
- Fatigue: excessive tiredness especially with physical exertion

- Dyspnea: shortness of breath, particularly during exertion or when lying flat.
- Episodes of dizziness or Lightheadedness: especially when standing up quickly or during exertion
- Syncope: rarely, patients with MVP may experience syncope (fainting) episodes, typically related to arrhythmias or autonomic dysfunction.

Causes and Risk Factors:
- Genetic Factors: MVP may have a familial or genetic predisposition, with a higher prevalence in patients with a family history of MVP or connective tissue disorders (e.g., Marfan syndrome, Ehlers-Danlos syndrome).
- Gender: MVP is more common in females than males, although the reasons for this gender disparity are not fully understood.
- Connective Tissue Disorders: Certain connective tissue disorders, such as Marfan syndrome or Ehlers-Danlos syndrome, are associated with an increased risk of MVP.
- Other Medical Conditions: MVP may occur in association with other medical conditions, such as mitral valve regurgitation, endocarditis, or hypertrophic cardiomyopathy.

Epidemiology:

MVP is one of the most common valvular abnormalities, with a prevalence estimated to be around 2-3% of the general population. MVP is more commonly diagnosed in younger patients, particularly adolescents and young adults, but may be detected at any age. The prevalence of MVP may vary depending on the population studied and the diagnostic criteria used.

Workup and Diagnosis:
- <u>Physical Examination:</u>

    Auscultation of the heart may reveal characteristic findings such as a mid-to-late systolic click and/or a late systolic murmur heard best at the apex.

- <u>Echocardiography:</u>

    Transthoracic Echocardiography (TTE) is the primary imaging modality used to diagnose MVP and assess its severity. TTE can visualize the prolapse of the mitral valve leaflets into the left atrium during systole and can quantify the degree of mitral regurgitation, if present.

- Electrocardiography (ECG): ECG may show nonspecific findings such as left atrial enlargement or repolarization abnormalities but is not specific for diagnosing MVP.
- Holter Monitor or Event Recorder: Ambulatory monitoring may be used to evaluate for arrhythmias or symptoms such as palpitations.
- Exercise Stress Test:

    Exercise stress testing may be performed in patients with symptoms suggestive of MVP to assess for exercise-induced arrhythmias or changes in symptoms.

Treatment:
- Asymptomatic MVP:

    Many patients with MVP are asymptomatic and do not require specific treatment. Regular follow-up with a cardiologist may be recommended to monitor for changes in symptoms or progression of valve disease.

- Symptomatic MVP:

    Symptomatic patients may benefit from treatment aimed at relieving symptoms, such as beta-blockers to reduce palpitations or chest discomfort.

- Mitral Valve Repair:

    In patients with severe mitral regurgitation or symptomatic MVP, mitral valve repair surgery may be indicated to correct the prolapse and restore valve function. Mitral valve repair is preferred over replacement whenever feasible, particularly in younger patients.

- Antibiotic Prophylaxis:

    Antibiotic prophylaxis to prevent infective endocarditis is generally not recommended for patients with isolated MVP without associated mitral regurgitation or other high-risk features.

4.11. Mitral Valve Regurgitation

> ➤ *Mitral valve regurgitation occurs when the mitral valve does not close tightly, allowing blood to flow backward into the heart chamber.*
> ➤ *Common symptoms are fatigue, shortness of breath, and heart palpitations.*
> ➤ *Treatment options include medication, surgery to repair or replace the valve, or minimally invasive procedures.*

Symptoms:

Symptoms of mitral valve regurgitation may vary depending on the severity and the rate at which the condition develops. They can include:

- Shortness of breath, especially with exertion or when lying down
- Fatigue, often due to the heart's decreased efficiency in pumping blood
- Heart palpitations or irregular heartbeats
- Swelling of the feet or ankles
- High-pitched "whooshing" or "swishing" heart murmur, heard through a stethoscope

Causes and Risk Factors:

- Mitral valve prolapse
- Heart diseases and conditions like endocarditis, rheumatic heart disease, or cardiomyopathy
- Congenital heart defects
- History of heart attack, which can damage the mitral valve
- Age-related wear and tear
- Use of certain medications

Epidemiology:

The prevalence of mitral valve regurgitation varies globally and can depend on underlying causes, such as age, prevalence of heart disease, and access to healthcare. It is more common in older populations due to the increased likelihood of degenerative diseases that affect the mitral valve.

Workup and Diagnosis:

- Symptoms:

    While some patients may be asymptomatic, especially in the early stages, others may experience symptoms such as shortness of breath, fatigue, palpitations, or swelling of the feet or legs.

- Physical Exam: The APh may detect a high-pitched heart murmur indicative of mitral regurgitation during auscultation with a stethoscope.
- Transthoracic Echocardiogram (TTE):

    This non-invasive ultrasound test is the primary tool for diagnosing MVR. It can visualize the mitral valve's structure and function, assess the severity of regurgitation, and evaluate its impact on heart size and the function of the left ventricle.

- Transesophageal Echocardiogram (TEE): If TTE results are inconclusive, TEE may be used for a closer look at the mitral valve and the degree of regurgitation.
- Chest X-ray: may show signs of heart enlargement or fluid buildup in the lungs.
- Cardiac MRI:

    This offers detailed images of the heart's structure and function to assess the severity of regurgitation and its effect on the heart.

- Electrocardiogram (EKG): An EKG can show atrial fibrillation, a common arrhythmia associated with MVR, and other changes indicating heart enlargement.

Treatment:

- Monitoring: regular check-ups and echocardiograms for those with mild symptoms or asymptomatic conditions
- Medications: drugs to reduce symptoms, such as diuretics to decrease fluid buildup, blood pressure medications to lower the heart's workload, and antiarrhythmics to control heart rhythm
- Surgical repair or replacement: In severe cases, surgery may be needed to repair the mitral valve or replace it with a mechanical or biological valve. Minimally invasive procedures, such as percutaneous mitral valve repair, are also an option for some patients.

4.12. Aortic Stenosis

> ➢ *Aortic stenosis is a heart condition characterized by narrowing of the aortic valve, obstructing blood flow from the heart to the body.*
> ➢ *Symptoms include chest pain, shortness of breath, and fainting, with severe cases leading to heart failure or sudden cardiac death.*
> ➢ *Treatment options range from medication to valve replacement surgery, depending on the severity of the condition.*

Symptoms:
- Chest pain or discomfort, especially during physical exertion or exercise
- Shortness of breath, particularly with exertion or when lying flat is common.
- Fatigue, unusually tired, even with minimal physical activity
- Dizziness or lightheadedness, fainting spells, or near-fainting episodes due to reduced blood flow to the brain
- Heart palpitations: irregular heartbeats, sensations of rapid or forceful heartbeats
- Chest tightness or pressure, particularly during exertion
- A characteristic heart murmur, known as an ejection systolic murmur, may be heard by a healthcare provider during a physical examination.

Causes and Risk Factors:
- Age: more common in patients over the age of 65
- Calcification of the aortic valve leaflets: most common cause of aortic stenosis in older adults
- Congenital heart defects: patients born with abnormalities of the aortic valve, such as bicuspid aortic valve
- Rheumatic fever history: particularly in childhood, can lead to scarring and thickening of the aortic valve leaflets.
- Other heart conditions: hypertrophic cardiomyopathy, aortic valve abnormalities, or previous heart surgery, etc.
- Hypertension: can contribute to the progression of aortic valve thickening and calcification.
- Hypercholesterolemia: High levels of cholesterol accelerate the development of aortic valve calcification and stenosis.

- Smoking: associated with an increased risk of atherosclerosis and cardiovascular disease
- A family history of aortic stenosis or other cardiovascular conditions

Epidemiology:

Aortic stenosis is the most common valvular heart disease in developed countries, with a prevalence that increases with age. The prevalence of aortic stenosis rises substantially in patients over the age of 65, affecting approximately 2-7% of this population. The incidence of aortic stenosis is expected to increase further as the population ages.

Workup and Diagnosis:
- Clinical evaluation:

    A healthcare provider will perform a thorough medical history and physical examination, including auscultation of the heart to detect characteristic murmurs associated with aortic stenosis.

- Echocardiography:

    Transthoracic Echocardiography (TTE) is the primary imaging modality used to diagnose aortic stenosis, assess the severity of valve narrowing, and evaluate cardiac structure and function.

- Electrocardiogram (ECG):

    An ECG may show evidence of left ventricular hypertrophy, arrhythmias, or other conduction abnormalities associated with aortic stenosis.

- Cardiac catheterization:

    Invasive hemodynamic assessment using cardiac catheterization may be performed to measure pressures within the heart chambers and assess the severity of aortic stenosis in patients with equivocal findings or complex cases.

Treatment:
- Medical management:

    Symptomatic relief and management of comorbidities such as hypertension, heart failure, or coronary artery disease may be initiated with medications such as diuretics, beta-blockers, ACE inhibitors, or statins.

- Valve replacement:

    For patients with severe symptomatic aortic stenosis, surgical aortic valve replacement (AVR) or transcatheter aortic valve

replacement (TAVR) may be recommended to relieve obstruction and improve symptoms.
- Monitoring:

    Patients with mild or moderate aortic stenosis may require regular monitoring with echocardiography and clinical evaluation to assess disease progression and determine the appropriate timing for intervention.

- Lifestyle modifications:

    Patients with aortic stenosis are advised to maintain a heart-healthy lifestyle, including regular exercise, a balanced diet low in saturated fats and cholesterol, smoking cessation, and management of cardiovascular risk factors.

4.13. Peripheral Artery Disease (PAD)

> ➢ *Narrowing or blockage of the arteries outside the heart, typically affecting the legs. Symptoms include leg pain, cramping, and decreased exercise tolerance.*
> ➢ *Risk factors include smoking, diabetes, hypertension, and high cholesterol.*
> ➢ *Treatment includes lifestyle changes, medication, and, in severe cases, procedures like angioplasty or bypass surgery to restore blood flow.*

Peripheral Artery Disease (PAD) occurs when narrowed arteries reduce blood flow to the limbs, typically the legs. It's often a result of atherosclerosis, a condition where plaque builds up in the arteries, limiting blood flow.

Symptoms:
- Leg Pain: cramping or aching in the calf, thigh, or buttock muscles during physical activity
- Leg Weakness or Numbness: especially during physical activity
- Coldness or Discoloration: of the legs or feet
- Slow Healing of Wounds or Sores: especially on the feet
- Weak Pulse: in the legs or feet
- Erectile Dysfunction: in men, due to impaired blood flow

Causes and Risk Factors:
- Smoking: the most significant risk factor
- Diabetes: increases the risk of atherosclerosis and vascular damage.

- High Blood Pressure
- High Cholesterol
- Obesity
- Older Age: Risk increases with age.
- Family History of PAD, Heart Disease, or Stroke
- Sedentary Lifestyle
- History of Heart Disease or Stroke
- Chronic Kidney Disease

Workup and Diagnosis:
- Medical History and Physical Examination: assessment of symptoms and risk factors, and checking pulses in the legs
- Ankle-Brachial Index (ABI): comparison of blood pressure in the ankle and arm to assess for PAD
- Doppler Ultrasound: non-invasive test to assess blood flow in the arteries
- Angiography: imaging test using dye and X-rays to visualize blood flow in the arteries
- Imaging Tests: magnetic Resonance Angiography (MRA) or Computed Tomography Angiography (CTA) to assess blood flow and detect arterial blockages
- Blood Tests: assess cholesterol levels, blood sugar, and kidney function.

Treatment:
- Lifestyle Modifications:
    - Smoking Cessation: most important for slowing disease progression.
    - Regular Exercise: walking program to improve circulation and relieve symptoms
    - Healthy Diet: low in saturated fats, cholesterol, and sodium
    - Weight Management: achieve and maintain a healthy weight.
- Medications:
    - Antiplatelet Agents: aspirin or clopidogrel reduces the risk of blood clots.

- Statins: lower cholesterol levels and reduce plaque buildup.
              - Medications for Symptom Relief: cilostazol to improve walking distance
      - Minimally Invasive Procedures:
              - Angioplasty and Stenting: open blocked arteries and restore blood flow.
              - Atherectomy: removal of plaque from the artery using specialized catheters
      - Surgery: Peripheral artery bypass surgery reroutes blood flow around blocked arteries using a graft.
      - Wound Care: for any wounds or ulcers, including cleaning, dressings, and possibly surgical debridement

4.14. Stroke and Transient Ischemic Attack

> - *Disruption of blood flow to the brain, resulting in neurological deficits. Ischemic stroke occurs due to blockage of a blood vessel, while hemorrhagic stroke involves bleeding into the brain.*
> - *Risk factors include hypertension, diabetes, smoking, atrial fibrillation, and obesity.*
> - *Immediate medical attention is crucial to minimize brain damage, and treatment may involve medication, surgery, or rehabilitation therapy.*

Stroke, also known as cerebrovascular accident (CVA), occurs when the blood supply to part of the brain is interrupted or reduced, depriving brain tissue of oxygen and nutrients.

Symptoms:
- Sudden Weakness or Numbness: typically on one side of the body, including the face, arm, or leg
- Sudden Confusion or Trouble Speaking: difficulty understanding or forming speech
- Sudden Vision Problems: blurred or double vision, or loss of vision in one or both eyes
- Sudden Trouble Walking: dizziness, loss of balance, or coordination
- Sudden Severe Headache: especially with no known cause (hemorrhagic stroke)

Causes and Risk Factors:
- High Blood Pressure: the most significant risk factor for stroke

- Smoking
- Diabetes
- High Cholesterol
- Atrial Fibrillation: irregular heart rhythm
- Obesity
- Physical Inactivity
- Family History of Stroke
- Age: Risk increases with age, especially over 55 years old.
- Race: African Americans, Hispanics, and Asian/Pacific Islanders are at higher risk.
- Gender: Men have a slightly higher risk than women.
- Previous Stroke or TIA

Transient Ischemic Attack (TIA)
- A TIA sometimes referred to as a "mini-stroke", is a brief episode of neurological dysfunction caused by the loss of blood flow to the brain, spinal cord, or retina, without acute infarction.
- TIAs present symptoms similar to a stroke, such as paralysis, speech difficulties, and sensory impairment, but these symptoms fully resolve within 24 hours.
- TIAs serve as important warnings and are risk factors for future strokes, highlighting the need for prompt medical evaluation and intervention to reduce stroke risk.

Workup and Diagnosis:
- <u>Medical History and Physical Examination:</u> Including assessment of symptoms and risk factors.
- <u>Neurological Examination:</u> Evaluation of deficits, strength, sensation, coordination, and reflexes.
- <u>Imaging Tests:</u>
    - CT Scan: To visualize brain structures and detect bleeding or ischemic changes.
    - MRI: Provides detailed images of the brain, useful for detecting ischemic strokes and assessing tissue damage.
- <u>Blood Tests:</u> To assess cholesterol levels, blood sugar, and clotting factors.
- <u>Electrocardiogram (ECG/EKG):</u> To evaluate heart rhythm and detect atrial fibrillation or other arrhythmias.

- Carotid Ultrasound: To assess for blockages in the carotid arteries supplying blood to the brain.
- Cerebral Angiography: Invasive procedure using dye and X-rays to visualize blood vessels in the brain.

Treatment:
- Acute Treatment:
    - Thrombolytics: Such as tissue plasminogen activator (tPA) given within a specific time window to dissolve blood clots causing ischemic strokes.
    - Mechanical Thrombectomy: Procedure to physically remove blood clots from blocked arteries, typically used for large vessel occlusions.
- Supportive Care:
    - Oxygen Therapy: ensures adequate oxygen supply to the brain.
    - Blood Pressure Management: maintains optimal blood flow to the brain.
    - Temperature Control: fever management to reduce metabolic demand
- Preventive Treatment:
    - Antiplatelet Medications: such as aspirin or clopidogrel to reduce the risk of recurrent strokes
    - Anticoagulants: for patients with atrial fibrillation or other cardiac sources of embolism
    - Statins: lower cholesterol levels and reduce the risk of atherosclerosis progression.
- Rehabilitation:
    - Physical Therapy: regains strength, mobility, and coordination.
    - Occupational Therapy: improves activities of daily living and independence.
    - Speech Therapy: addresses speech and language deficits.
    - Psychological Support: for coping with emotional and cognitive changes post-stroke

4.15. Deep Vein Thrombosis and Pulmonary Embolism

> ➤ *Formation of blood clots in the deep veins of the legs (DVT) that can break loose and travel to the lungs (PE). Symptoms of DVT include leg pain, swelling, and warmth, while PE can cause chest pain, shortness of breath, and coughing up blood.*
>
> ➤ *Risk factors include immobility, surgery, cancer, pregnancy, and certain medications.*
>
> ➤ *Treatment involves blood thinners, compression stockings, and sometimes procedures to remove or dissolve the clot.*

Deep Vein Thrombosis (DVT) occurs when a blood clot forms in a deep vein, typically in the legs. If a portion of the clot breaks loose and travels to the lungs, it can cause a Pulmonary Embolism (PE), which is a life-threatening condition.

Symptoms of DVT:

- Swelling: usually in one leg, sometimes accompanied by pain or tenderness
- Pain or Tenderness: often in the calf or thigh, sometimes described as cramping or soreness
- Red or Discolored Skin: warmth and discoloration over the affected area
- Visible Veins: swollen veins that are visible on the skin surface
- Leg Fatigue or Heaviness: feeling of tiredness or heaviness in the affected leg

Symptoms of PE:

- Shortness of Breath: sudden onset, often accompanied by rapid breathing
- Chest Pain: sharp, stabbing pain that may worsen with deep breaths or coughing
- Cough: often producing blood-streaked sputum
- Tachycardia: elevated heart rate, sometimes accompanied by lightheadedness or fainting
- Anxiety or Sweating

Causes and Risk Factors for DVT and PE:

- Prolonged Immobility: such as long flights or bed rest.
- Surgery: especially orthopedic or cancer surgery

- Hospitalization: especially for serious illness or injury
- Cancer: especially certain types and advanced stages
- Trauma or Injury: such as fractures or severe muscle injury
- Pregnancy and Postpartum Period: due to hormonal changes and increased pressure on veins
- Birth Control Pills or Hormone Replacement Therapy
- Previous History of DVT or PE: increases risk of recurrence.
- Family History of DVT or PE: genetic predisposition
- Obesity
- Smoking
- Age: Risk increases with age.

Workup and Diagnosis:
- Medical History and Physical Examination: assessment of symptoms and risk factors
- D-dimer Test: a blood test to detect a substance released when a blood clot dissolves
- Ultrasound Imaging: Doppler ultrasound to visualize blood flow and detect clots in the legs
- Venography: imaging test using dye and X-rays to visualize blood flow and detect clots in the veins
- CT Pulmonary Angiography (CTPA): imaging test using contrast dye and CT scan to visualize blood flow in the lungs and detect pulmonary embolism
- MRI Venography: magnetic resonance imaging to visualize blood flow and detect clots in the veins, especially in cases where ultrasound is inconclusive

Treatment:
- Anticoagulant Medications:
    - Heparin: given initially to prevent clot propagation.
    - Warfarin (Coumadin): oral anticoagulant for long-term management
    - Direct Oral Anticoagulants (DOACs): such as apixaban, rivaroxaban, or dabigatran, are increasingly used as alternatives to warfarin.
- Thrombolytic Therapy: clot-dissolving medication used in cases of massive or life-threatening PE

- Inferior Vena Cava (IVC) Filter: a device inserted into the inferior vena cava to catch blood clots and prevent them from reaching the lungs in high-risk cases
- Compression Stockings: graduated compression stockings to improve blood flow and reduce the risk of post-thrombotic syndrome in DVT cases

4.16. Aortic Aneurysm

> ➢ An aortic aneurysm is a localized dilation of the aorta, the body's largest artery, which can lead to a life-threatening rupture if left untreated.
> ➢ Risk factors include hypertension, smoking, atherosclerosis, and genetic predisposition.
> ➢ Treatment may involve surveillance, lifestyle modifications, medication, or surgical intervention to prevent rupture.

Symptoms:

Thoracic Aortic Aneurysm (TAA) Symptoms:
- Chest or back pain: dull, sharp, or throbbing
- Hoarseness or difficulty swallowing due to compression of the trachea or esophagus.
- Shortness of breath or difficulty breathing (if the aneurysm presses on the lungs)
- Coughing or wheezing
- Pulsating sensation in the abdomen, chest, or neck

Abdominal Aortic Aneurysm (AAA) Symptoms:
- Most AAAs are asymptomatic and are incidentally discovered during routine imaging studies.
- In some cases, patients may experience abdominal or back pain, which can be severe and sudden if the aneurysm ruptures.
- A pulsating mass in the abdomen may be palpable on physical examination.

Causes and Risk Factors:
- Age: Aortic aneurysms are more common in older adults, particularly those over 65 years of age.
- Gender: Men are more likely than women to develop aortic aneurysms.

- Tobacco Use: Smoking is a significant risk factor for the development and progression of aortic aneurysms.
- Hypertension: can weaken the walls of the aorta and increase the risk of aneurysm formation.
- Atherosclerosis: A buildup of plaque in the arteries can contribute to the development of aortic aneurysms.
- Family History of Aortic Aneurysms: increases a patient's risk of developing the condition.
- Genetic Conditions: Certain genetic disorders, such as Marfan syndrome, Ehlers-Danlos syndrome, and familial thoracic aortic aneurysm and dissection (TAAD), predispose patients to aortic aneurysms.
- Trauma: A history of blunt or penetrating trauma to the chest or abdomen can increase the risk of aortic injury and subsequent aneurysm formation.
- Infections: such as syphilis or tuberculosis can cause inflammation and weakening of the aortic wall, leading to aneurysm formation.

Epidemiology:
- Aortic aneurysms are relatively common, with abdominal aortic aneurysms being more prevalent than thoracic aortic aneurysms.
- The prevalence of abdominal aortic aneurysms increases with age, peaking in patients aged 65 years and older.
- Thoracic aortic aneurysms are less common but are associated with a higher risk of rupture and mortality.
- Aortic aneurysms are a significant cause of morbidity and mortality, particularly when ruptured, and are responsible for thousands of deaths each year worldwide.

Workup and Diagnosis:
- <u>Abdominal Ultrasound:</u> primarily screens for abdominal aortic aneurysms.
- <u>CT Scan:</u> provides detailed images of the aorta and can help assess the aneurysm's size, shape, and location, as well as the involvement of nearby structures. Contrast material may be used to enhance visualization.
- <u>MRI:</u> offers detailed images of the aorta and is particularly useful in planning treatment for an aortic aneurysm by showing its exact location and size.

- Echocardiography: less frequently used for diagnosing abdominal aortic aneurysms but can be helpful for thoracic aortic aneurysms.

Treatment:

- Monitoring and Surveillance:

    Small, asymptomatic aortic aneurysms may be monitored regularly with imaging studies, such as ultrasound, CT scan, or MRI, to assess for growth and the risk of rupture.

- Medical Management:

    Control of risk factors, such as blood pressure management and smoking cessation, is important in preventing the progression of aortic aneurysms.

- Surgical Intervention:

    Large or symptomatic aortic aneurysms, or those at risk of rupture, may require surgical repair or endovascular intervention to prevent complications. Procedures include open surgical repair, endovascular aneurysm repair (EVAR), or thoracic endovascular aneurysm repair (TEVAR).

- Ruptured Aneurysm Management:

    A ruptured aortic aneurysm is a medical emergency and requires immediate surgical intervention to repair the aneurysm and prevent life-threatening bleeding. Treatment may involve open surgical repair or endovascular techniques, depending on the patient's condition and anatomical factors.

4.17. Myocardial Infarction

> ➤ *Myocardial infarction, commonly known as a heart attack, occurs when blood flow to a part of the heart is blocked, leading to tissue damage or death.*
>
> ➤ *Symptoms include chest pain, shortness of breath, nausea, and sweating.*
>
> ➤ *Prompt medical intervention is crucial to prevent complications and minimize damage to the heart muscle.*

Symptoms:

- Chest pain or discomfort: pressure, squeezing, heaviness, or tightness in the chest
- Pain or discomfort in the arms, back, neck, jaw, or stomach

- Shortness of breath: with or without chest discomfort
- Nausea, vomiting, or indigestion
- Sweating
- Lightheadedness or dizziness
- Fatigue or weakness
- Anxiety or a sense of impending doom

Causes and Risk Factors:
- Age: The risk of myocardial infarction increases with age.
- Gender: Men are generally at higher risk of myocardial infarction than premenopausal women. However, women's risk increases after menopause.
- Family History of Heart Disease: especially if it occurred at a young age, increases the risk of myocardial infarction.
- Smoking: significantly increases the risk of myocardial infarction due to its damaging effects on blood vessels and the cardiovascular system.
- Hypertension: can damage blood vessels and increase the risk of plaque rupture and myocardial infarction.
- Cholesterol Levels: Elevated levels of LDL cholesterol and low levels of HDL cholesterol increase the risk of plaque buildup in the arteries.
- Obesity: particularly abdominal obesity, is associated with an increased risk of myocardial infarction.
- Diabetes: Diabetes mellitus, especially if poorly controlled, is a significant risk factor for myocardial infarction due to its effects on blood vessels and metabolism.
- Physical Inactivity: Lack of regular physical activity or exercise is associated with an increased risk of myocardial infarction.
- Unhealthy Diet: Diets high in saturated fats, trans fats, sodium, and processed foods increase the risk of myocardial infarction.
- Chronic stress or excessive stress: can contribute to the development of myocardial infarction through various physiological mechanisms.

Epidemiology:

Myocardial infarction is a leading cause of morbidity and mortality worldwide. The incidence of myocardial infarction varies by age, gender, and geographic region. Men generally have a higher incidence of myocardial infarction than women, but the gap narrows with increasing age. The risk of myocardial infarction increases with age, with the highest incidence observed in patients over 65 years old. Certain populations, such as those with diabetes, hypertension, or a family history of heart disease, have an elevated risk of myocardial infarction.

Workup and Diagnosis:
- Electrocardiogram (EKG) finding in acute myocardial infarction:

    ST-segment elevation (STEMI), ST-segment depression, or T-wave inversions, may suggest acute MI or ongoing myocardial ischemia.

- Cardiac Biomarkers:
    - Troponins (cTnI and cTnT): Elevated troponin levels are a key marker of MI. Troponins are highly sensitive and specific for myocardial injury and remain elevated for days after an MI.
    - Creatine Kinase-MB (CK-MB): can provide useful information about the extent of heart muscle damage and the timing of MI.

- Imaging Tests:
    - Echocardiography: can assess the heart's function and structures, identifying areas of poor blood flow or muscle damage.
    - Coronary Angiography: often performed in the setting of acute MI to visualize blockages in the coronary arteries.

Treatment:
- Reperfusion Therapy:

    Thrombolytic therapy or percutaneous coronary intervention (PCI), aims at restoring blood flow to the affected area of the heart and minimizing myocardial damage.

- Medications:

    Antiplatelet agents (such as aspirin and clopidogrel), beta-blockers, angiotensin-converting enzyme (ACE) inhibitors or angiotensin receptor blockers (ARBs), statins, and nitroglycerin

- Oxygen Therapy: Supplemental oxygen may be administered to improve oxygenation and relieve symptoms of hypoxemia.
- Pain Management: Analgesics, such as morphine, may be given to alleviate chest pain and discomfort.
- Cardiac Rehabilitation:

    Exercise training, education, and counseling, are recommended to improve cardiovascular health and reduce the risk of recurrent myocardial infarction.

- Lifestyle Modifications:

    Smoking cessation, adoption of a heart-healthy diet, regular physical activity, weight management, and stress reduction techniques, are essential components of myocardial infarction management and secondary prevention.

4.18. Cardiomyopathy

> ➢ *Cardiomyopathy refers to diseases of the heart muscle, impairing its ability to pump blood effectively. Types include dilated, hypertrophic, and restrictive cardiomyopathy, each with distinct causes and presentations.*
> ➢ *Symptoms may include shortness of breath, fatigue, swelling, and arrhythmias.*
> ➢ *Treatment aims at managing symptoms and addressing underlying causes.*

Symptoms:
- Dyspnea: especially during exertion or lying flat
- Fatigue and weakness
- Swelling of the legs, ankles, feet, or abdomen
- Irregular heartbeat or palpitations
- Chest pain or discomfort
- Dizziness or lightheadedness
- Fainting or syncope
- Persistent cough or wheezing, particularly when lying down
- Difficulty breathing while lying down or sudden awakening with shortness of breath

Causes and Risk Factors:
- Genetic Factors: family history of cardiomyopathy or sudden cardiac death
- Infections: Viral infections, such as myocarditis, can damage the heart muscle and lead to cardiomyopathy.
- Toxins and Drugs: Exposure to toxins (e.g., alcohol, cocaine, certain chemotherapy drugs) or long-term use of certain medications (e.g., chemotherapy drugs, antipsychotics) can contribute to cardiomyopathy.

- Autoimmune Disorders: such as lupus or rheumatoid arthritis, can cause inflammation and damage to the heart muscle.
- Hypertension: can lead to hypertrophic cardiomyopathy.
- Coronary Artery Disease: Reduced blood flow to the heart muscle can result in ischemic cardiomyopathy.
- Valvular Heart Disease: Malfunctioning heart valves can lead to dilated or hypertrophic cardiomyopathy.
- Pregnancy: Peripartum cardiomyopathy can occur in the late stages of pregnancy or shortly after giving birth.
- Metabolic Disorders: Diabetes, thyroid disease, and obesity are associated with an increased risk of cardiomyopathy.
- Age: While cardiomyopathy can affect patients of all ages, certain types (e.g., hypertrophic cardiomyopathy) often present in young adulthood.
- Heavy Alcohol Use: Chronic alcohol abuse can weaken the heart muscle and lead to alcoholic cardiomyopathy.

Epidemiology:

Cardiomyopathy is a leading cause of heart failure and sudden cardiac death. The prevalence and incidence of cardiomyopathy vary depending on the type and geographic region. Dilated cardiomyopathy is the most common type, followed by hypertrophic and restrictive cardiomyopathy. Cardiomyopathy can affect patients of all ages, from infants to the elderly, and can be inherited or acquired. The prognosis and outcomes of cardiomyopathy depend on various factors, including the underlying cause, severity of symptoms, and response to treatment.

Diagnosis:
- Echocardiogram: shows abnormalities in the heart's structure and function.
- EKG: identifies irregularities in heart rhythm or structure.
- Cardiac MRI: provides detailed images of the heart, helping to assess the extent of damage or abnormality.
- Blood Tests: markers of heart stress, damage, or genetic markers associated with specific types of cardiomyopathy
- Cardiac Catheterization and Biopsy: invasive tests where a small sample of heart tissue may be examined for signs of cardiomyopathy

Treatment:
- Medications:

  Angiotensin-converting enzyme (ACE) inhibitors, beta-blockers, diuretics, and antiarrhythmic drugs help manage symptoms, control blood pressure, reduce fluid buildup, regulate heart rhythm, and improve heart function.

- Lifestyle Modifications:

  Limiting alcohol intake, quitting smoking, maintaining a healthy weight, and exercising regularly

- Implantable Devices:

  In some cases, pacemakers, implantable cardioverter-defibrillators (ICDs), or cardiac resynchronization therapy (CRT) devices may be recommended to regulate heart rhythm and prevent sudden cardiac death.

- Surgical Interventions:

  Septal myectomy or alcohol septal ablation for hypertrophic cardiomyopathy, or heart transplant for end-stage heart failure, may be considered in select cases.

- Genetic Counseling:

  For patients with a family history of cardiomyopathy to assess the risk of inherited forms of the disease and provide guidance on family planning and screening

4.19. Rheumatic Heart Disease

> ➤ *Rheumatic heart disease results from complications of rheumatic fever, causing scarring and damage to the heart valves.*
> ➤ *Commonly affecting children in developing countries, it can lead to valve dysfunction, heart failure, and other cardiovascular complications.*
> ➤ *Prevention involves timely treatment of streptococcal infections and long-term antibiotic prophylaxis.*

Symptoms:
- Heart Murmur
- Shortness of Breath especially during physical activity or when lying flat (orthopnea)
- Feeling tired or weak, even with minimal exertion

- Chest Pain: dull ache or pressure in the chest
- Palpitations: abnormal heartbeats, irregular heart rhythm, or fluttering sensations
- Swollen Joints: particularly in acute rheumatic fever, commonly affecting the knees, elbows, ankles, and wrists
- Acute rheumatic fever: along with other symptoms such as rash and swollen lymph nodes

Causes and Risk Factors:
- Group A *Streptococcal* Infection: RHD is primarily caused by untreated or inadequately treated streptococcal throat infections, particularly with group A *Streptococcus* bacteria.
- Young Age: RHD typically affects children and young adults, with the majority of cases occurring between the ages of 5 and 15 years.
- Geographic Location: RHD is more prevalent in low- and middle-income countries, particularly in areas with limited access to healthcare and inadequate antibiotic treatment for streptococcal infections.
- Socioeconomic Factors: Poor living conditions, overcrowding, and limited access to healthcare services increase the risk of streptococcal infections and subsequent RHD.
- Genetic Factors: Some patients may be genetically predisposed to developing RHD, although specific genetic factors have not been fully elucidated.

Epidemiology:

Rheumatic heart disease remains a significant cause of cardiovascular morbidity and mortality in many parts of the world, particularly in developing countries. The global burden of RHD is estimated to affect millions of patients, with the highest prevalence observed in regions with limited healthcare resources and poor socioeconomic conditions.

RHD disproportionately affects children and young adults in endemic regions, with a peak incidence in patients aged 5 to 15 years. While the incidence of RHD has declined in many high-income countries due to improved living conditions, access to healthcare, and antibiotic treatment of streptococcal infections, it remains a public health concern in resource-limited settings.

Workup and Diagnosis:
- Clinical Evaluation:
    - A thorough medical history is obtained, focusing on past episodes of acute rheumatic fever (ARF), symptoms suggestive

of RHD (e.g., dyspnea, chest pain, palpitations), and risk factors such as previous streptococcal infections or living in an endemic region.
    - Physical examination includes auscultation of the heart for characteristic murmurs (e.g., mitral regurgitation, aortic regurgitation), assessment for signs of heart failure (e.g., elevated jugular venous pressure, peripheral edema), and examination for extra-cardiac manifestations of rheumatic fever (e.g., joint swelling, skin rash).
- Laboratory Tests:
    - Serological tests: Antistreptolysin O (ASO) titer and anti-DNase B titers may be elevated in patients with recent streptococcal infections, providing evidence of preceding streptococcal pharyngitis or skin infections.
    - Inflammatory markers: Erythrocyte sedimentation rate (ESR) and C-reactive protein (CRP) may be elevated, indicating ongoing inflammation.
    - Complete blood count (CBC): CBC may reveal leukocytosis, anemia, or thrombocytosis.
- Imaging Studies:
    - Echocardiography: Transthoracic Echocardiography (TTE) is the primary imaging modality used to evaluate cardiac structure and function in patients suspected of having RHD. TTE can detect valvular abnormalities such as leaflet thickening, regurgitation, or stenosis, and assess the severity of valve lesions.
    - Transesophageal echocardiography (TEE) may be performed in cases where TTE findings are inconclusive or when higher-resolution imaging is needed.
- Electrocardiography (ECG):

    ECG may show evidence of atrial enlargement, conduction abnormalities, or arrhythmias secondary to RHD. Common findings include atrial fibrillation, atrial flutter, or evidence of previous myocarditis.
- Other Tests:
    - Chest X-ray: may show cardiomegaly, pulmonary congestion, or signs of pulmonary hypertension in patients with advanced RHD.

- Cardiac MRI or CT scan: used in selected cases to provide additional information about cardiac structure and function, particularly in patients with complex RHD lesions.
- <u>Diagnostic Challenges:</u>
  - Diagnosing RHD can be challenging due to its variable clinical presentation and the absence of specific diagnostic tests.
  - The diagnosis of RHD is often based on a combination of clinical findings, laboratory tests, and imaging studies, rather than a single diagnostic test.
  - RHD may coexist with other cardiac conditions or may be masked by other comorbidities, making diagnosis more difficult.

Treatment:
- <u>Antibiotic Prophylaxis:</u>

    Antibiotic treatment of streptococcal throat infections (such as penicillin or other antibiotics) is crucial in preventing the development of acute rheumatic fever and subsequent RHD.

- <u>Anti-inflammatory Medications:</u>

    In cases of acute rheumatic fever, anti-inflammatory drugs (such as aspirin or corticosteroids) may be prescribed to reduce inflammation and alleviate symptoms.

- <u>Symptomatic Treatment:</u>

    Treatment of symptoms associated with RHD, such as heart failure, arrhythmias, or valve dysfunction, may include medications to manage heart function, control blood pressure, and prevent blood clots.

- <u>Surgical Intervention:</u>

    In severe cases of RHD with significant valve damage or heart failure, surgical repair or replacement of affected heart valves may be necessary to restore normal function and alleviate symptoms.

- <u>Secondary Prevention:</u>

    Long-term management of RHD involves regular monitoring, adherence to antibiotic prophylaxis, and ongoing surveillance for complications to prevent disease progression and optimize outcomes.

4.20. Congenital Heart Defects

> ➤ *Congenital heart defects are structural abnormalities present at birth, affecting the heart's chambers, valves, or major blood vessels.*
> ➤ *They vary in severity, with symptoms ranging from mild to life-threatening, and may require surgical intervention or medical management to improve cardiac function and quality of life.*
> ➤ *Treatment aims to alleviate symptoms, prevent complications, and optimize long-term outcomes.*

Symptoms:
- Cyanosis: bluish discoloration of the skin, lips, or nails due to decreased oxygen levels in the blood
- Difficulty Breathing: rapid breathing, shortness of breath, or difficulty feeding, especially during exertion
- Poor Weight Gain: difficulty gaining weight or failure to thrive in infants.
- Fatigue: tiring easily during physical activity or feeding
- Irregular Heartbeat: abnormal heart rhythms or palpitations
- Swelling of the legs, abdomen, or other areas due to fluid retention
- Clubbing: abnormal enlargement or rounding of the fingertips or toes.

Causes and Risk Factors:
- Genetic Factors: Certain genetic syndromes or chromosomal abnormalities, such as Down syndrome (Trisomy 21) or DiGeorge syndrome (22q11.2 deletion syndrome), increase the risk of CHD.
- Family History: Having a parent or sibling with a congenital heart defect increases the risk of CHD in offspring.
- Maternal Factors: Maternal factors during pregnancy, such as maternal age, exposure to certain medications or substances (e.g., alcohol, tobacco, medications that affect fetal development), and maternal health conditions (e.g., diabetes, obesity), can increase the risk of CHD in the fetus.
- Environmental Factors: Exposure to certain environmental toxins or radiation during pregnancy may increase the risk of CHD.
- Assisted Reproductive Technologies: Some studies suggest a higher incidence of CHD in infants conceived through assisted reproductive technologies.

- Infections: Maternal infections during pregnancy, such as rubella or certain viral infections, can increase the risk of CHD in the fetus.

Epidemiology:

Congenital heart defects are the most common type of birth defect, affecting approximately 1% of live births worldwide. The prevalence of CHD varies by type and severity, with some defects being more common than others.

Advances in prenatal screening and diagnostic techniques have led to earlier detection of CHD, resulting in improved outcomes and survival rates. The overall prognosis and outcomes for patients with CHD have improved significantly over the past few decades due to advances in medical and surgical management. While many patients with CHD survive into adulthood, they may require lifelong cardiac monitoring and medical care to manage symptoms and prevent complications.

Workup and Diagnosis:

- Clinical Evaluation:
    - A comprehensive medical history is obtained, including prenatal history, family history of CHDs or genetic syndromes, and any symptoms or signs suggestive of heart disease.
    - Physical examination includes assessment of vital signs, inspection for signs of cyanosis (bluish discoloration of the skin or mucous membranes), clubbing of the fingers or toes, abnormal heart sounds (e.g., murmurs), and signs of heart failure (e.g., tachypnea, hepatomegaly).
    - Newborns are routinely screened for congenital heart defects using pulse oximetry to detect hypoxemia. Abnormal results may prompt further evaluation.
- Imaging Studies:
    - Echocardiography is the primary imaging modality used to diagnose and characterize CHDs. Both transthoracic echocardiography (TTE) and transesophageal echocardiography (TEE) may be used, depending on the age of the patient and the complexity of the defect.
    - Fetal echocardiography may be performed during pregnancy if there are concerns about fetal heart development or if there is a family history of CHDs.
    - Cardiac catheterization may be indicated for certain complex CHDs to assess hemodynamics, obtain pressure measurements, and guide interventions or surgical planning.

- Electrocardiography (ECG):

    ECG may reveal abnormalities such as arrhythmias, conduction defects, or evidence of right or left ventricular hypertrophy. However, ECG findings alone may not definitively diagnose CHDs and are often used in conjunction with other diagnostic tests.

- Chest X-ray:

    Chest X-ray may show cardiomegaly, pulmonary congestion, or other signs of heart disease, but it is not specific for diagnosing CHDs and is usually performed as part of the initial evaluation.

- Genetic Testing:

    Genetic testing may be considered in certain cases, particularly if there is a family history of genetic syndromes associated with CHDs (e.g., Down syndrome, DiGeorge syndrome). Chromosomal microarray analysis (CMA) and targeted gene sequencing may be used to identify genetic abnormalities.

- Other Tests:

    Additional tests may be performed based on the specific clinical presentation and suspected diagnosis. These may include cardiac MRI, CT angiography, or perfusion scans.

- Diagnostic Challenges:
    - Some CHDs may have subtle or nonspecific symptoms, making diagnosis challenging.
    - The spectrum of CHDs is broad, ranging from simple defects with minimal symptoms to complex defects with significant hemodynamic consequences.
    - Diagnosis may be delayed in some cases, particularly if the defect is not detected until later in life or if the presentation is atypical.

Treatment:
- Lifestyle Modifications: Regular exercise, a heart-healthy diet, smoking cessation, and weight management optimize overall cardiovascular health.
- Monitoring and Surveillance: Close monitoring of infants with CHD is essential to assess cardiac function, growth and development, and to detect any complications early.
- Medications: Some CHDs may require medications to help the heart function more efficiently, control symptoms such as heart failure or arrhythmias, or prevent blood clots.

- Surgical Intervention: Surgical procedures including open-heart surgery, cardiac catheterization, or minimally invasive procedures help improve cardiac function and alleviate symptoms.
- Interventional Cardiology: Some CHDs can be treated using techniques like balloon valvuloplasty or transcatheter closure of septal defects.

4.21. Endocarditis

> ➤ *Endocarditis is an infection of the inner lining of the heart chambers and valves, often caused by bacteria entering the bloodstream.*
>
> ➤ *Symptoms include fever, fatigue, and abnormal heart rhythms, with complications including heart valve damage and septic emboli.*
>
> ➤ *Diagnosis involves blood cultures and echocardiography, while treatment typically requires antibiotics and, in severe cases, surgical intervention.*

Symptoms:
- Fever: Persistent fever is a common symptom of endocarditis, often accompanied by chills and sweating.
- Heart Murmur: New or changing heart murmurs may be detected during physical examination.
- Fatigue: Generalized weakness or fatigue may be present.
- Malaise: a general feeling of being unwell or "out of sorts"
- Shortness of Breath: especially with physical exertion
- Chest Pain: particularly if there is involvement of the heart valves or heart muscle
- Joint Pain: Arthralgia may occur, especially in larger joints.
- Nail Bed Hemorrhages: Petechiae or purpura may appear under the nails or on the skin.
- Osler's Nodes: painful, raised lesions on the fingers or toes.
- Janeway Lesions: non-tender, red or purple spots on the palms or soles

Causes and Risk Factors:
- Previous Heart Valve Disease: Patients with pre-existing heart valve abnormalities, congenital heart defects, or prosthetic heart valves are at higher risk.

- Intravenous Drug Use: particularly with contaminated needles or equipment, increases the risk of endocarditis.
- Invasive Medical Procedures: such as dental procedures, surgeries, or invasive diagnostic tests, can introduce bacteria into the bloodstream and increase the risk of endocarditis.
- Poor Dental Hygiene: increases the risk of bacteria entering the bloodstream during routine activities such as brushing or flossing.
- Age: Endocarditis can affect patients of any age, but older adults are at higher risk.
- Underlying Health Conditions: such as rheumatic fever, diabetes, or immunodeficiency disorders, may increase susceptibility to endocarditis.
- Intravascular Catheters: such as central venous catheters or pacemaker leads, can provide a portal of entry for bacteria.
- Structural Heart Abnormalities: such as ventricular septal defects or patent ductus arteriosus, increase the risk of endocarditis.
- Prosthetic Devices: Prosthetic heart valves, ventricular assist devices, or other implanted devices increase the risk of endocarditis due to the potential for bacterial colonization.

Epidemiology:

Endocarditis is relatively rare but can be life-threatening if not promptly diagnosed and treated. The incidence of endocarditis varies depending on factors such as age, underlying health conditions, and risk factors.

Endocarditis is more common in certain populations, such as patients with pre-existing heart valve disease, congenital heart defects, or intravenous drug use. The overall incidence of endocarditis has been increasing in recent years, possibly due to factors such as aging populations, increased use of invasive medical procedures, and the emergence of antibiotic-resistant bacteria.

Workup and Diagnosis:

Diagnosing endocarditis typically involves a combination of clinical evaluation, laboratory tests, imaging studies, and microbiological analysis.

- <u>Clinical Evaluation:</u>
    - A thorough medical history is obtained, focusing on symptoms such as fever, new or changing heart murmurs, signs of systemic embolization (e.g., petechiae, splinter hemorrhages), and risk factors for endocarditis (e.g., pre-existing heart valve disease, intravenous drug use).

- Physical examination includes auscultation of the heart for abnormal heart sounds (e.g., murmurs), assessment for signs of systemic embolization (e.g., Janeway lesions, Osler's nodes), and evaluation for signs of heart failure or other complications.
- Laboratory Tests:
  - Blood cultures are obtained to identify the causative organism. Multiple blood cultures are typically drawn over a 24-hour period to increase the sensitivity of detection.
  - CBC may reveal leukocytosis or leukopenia, anemia, or thrombocytopenia.
  - Inflammatory markers ESR/CRP are often elevated in endocarditis.
- Imaging Studies:
  - Transthoracic Echocardiography (TTE): the initial imaging modality used to evaluate for the presence of valvular abnormalities, vegetations, and other structural abnormalities of the heart. TTE is non-invasive but has limitations in detecting small vegetations or lesions on certain valves.
  - Transesophageal Echocardiography (TEE): provides higher-resolution imaging and is more sensitive for detecting smaller vegetations, especially those located on the mitral valve or within the left atrium. TEE is considered the gold standard for diagnosing endocarditis and is often performed if TTE results are inconclusive or if high clinical suspicion remains despite negative TTE findings.
- Microbiological Analysis:
  - Identification of the causative organism through blood cultures is essential for confirming the diagnosis and guiding antibiotic therapy.
  - Additional microbiological testing may include serological tests, polymerase chain reaction (PCR) assays, or culture of other body fluids or tissues (e.g., cerebrospinal fluid, joint fluid) if endocarditis-related complications are suspected.

Duke Criteria: a clinical criteria used to establish the likelihood of Infective Endocarditis (IE)

I. Major Criteria
   1. Positive Blood Cultures
      - Typical microorganisms are consistent with IE from two separate blood cultures, such as *Streptococcus viridans*,

Streptococcus bovis, HACEK group, *Staphylococcus aureus*, or community-acquired enterococci.
- Microorganisms are consistent with IE from persistently positive blood cultures, defined as at least 2 positive cultures of blood samples drawn >12 hours apart.

2. Evidence of Endocardial Involvement

    Positive echocardiogram for IE (oscillating intracardiac mass on valve or supporting structures, in the path of regurgitant jets, or on implanted material in the absence of an alternative anatomical explanation; abscess; new partial dehiscence of prosthetic valve; or new valvular regurgitation)

II. Minor Criteria
    1. Predisposition: predisposing heart condition or intravenous drug use
    2. Temperature >38°C
    3. Vascular Phenomena: major arterial emboli, septic pulmonary infarcts, mycotic aneurysm, intracranial hemorrhage, conjunctival hemorrhages, and Janeway lesions
    4. Immunologic Phenomena: Glomerulonephritis, Osler nodes, Roth spots, and rheumatoid factor
    5. Microbiological Evidence: Positive blood culture but does not meet a major criterion as noted above or serological evidence of active infection with organisms consistent with IE.
    6. Echocardiographic Findings: Findings consistent with IE but do not meet a major criterion as noted above.

Diagnosis IE based on Duke criteria
- Definite IE: 2 majors/ 1 major + 3 minors/ 5 minors
- Possible IE: 1 major + 1 minor/ 3 minors
- Rejected:

    Firm alternative diagnosis explaining evidence of IE; or resolution of IE syndrome with antibiotic therapy for ≤4 days; pathological evidence of IE at surgery or autopsy, with antibiotic therapy for ≤4 days; or does not meet any of the above criteria.

Treatment:
- Antibiotic Therapy:

    Treatment typically involves intravenous antibiotics, often for several weeks, based on the specific type of bacteria causing the infection and antibiotic susceptibility testing.

- Surgical Intervention: In some cases, surgical procedures may be necessary to repair or replace damaged heart valves, drain abscesses, or remove infected tissue.
- Supportive Care: Fluid resuscitation, pain management, and monitoring for complications are essential during treatment.
- Management of Underlying Conditions: such as intravenous drug use or poor dental hygiene should be addressed.
- Prevention: Prophylactic antibiotic therapy may be recommended for patients at high risk of developing endocarditis before certain invasive dental or medical procedures.

4.22. Pericarditis

> ➢ *Pericarditis is the inflammation of the pericardium, the fibrous sac surrounding the heart, often presenting with sharp chest pain, pericardial friction rub, and changes in the ECG*
>
> ➢ *Causes range from viral infections to systemic autoimmune diseases, with treatment typically involving NSAIDs, colchicine, and addressing any underlying condition.*
>
> ➢ *While most cases resolve with appropriate management, complications can include cardiac tamponade and chronic constrictive pericarditis.*

Symptoms:
- Chest Pain: typically sharp and worsened by lying down or taking a deep breath; improved by sitting up and leaning forward
- Pericardial Friction Rub: a scratchy or squeaky sound heard with a stethoscope, caused by the pericardial layers rubbing against each other
- Other Symptoms: fever, shortness of breath, especially when reclining, and general malaise

Causes and Risk Factors:
- Infectious Causes: viral (e.g., coxsackievirus, echovirus, adenovirus, influenza), bacterial (e.g., tuberculosis, especially in developing countries), fungal, and parasitic infections

- Non-infectious Causes: autoimmune diseases (e.g., lupus, rheumatoid arthritis), cancer (metastasis to the pericardium), uremia, myocardial infarction (Dressler syndrome), trauma, and radiation therapy
- Idiopathic: In many cases, the cause remains unknown despite thorough investigation.

Epidemiology:

Pericarditis is a relatively common cardiac condition. Viral pericarditis is the most frequent cause in the developed world, while tuberculosis remains a significant cause in developing countries. The incidence is difficult to ascertain accurately due to varied diagnostic criteria and practices, but it is a relatively frequent cause of chest pain and hospital admission for cardiac reasons.

Diagnosis:

- Clinical Presentation: Combination of chest pain, pericardial friction rub, and suggestive EKG changes are highly suggestive of pericarditis.
- EKG: characteristic diffuse ST elevation and PR depression in the acute phase
- Echocardiography: detects pericardial effusion and cardiac tamponade.
- Blood Tests: elevated markers of inflammation (CRP, ESR) and troponins
- Imaging: chest X-ray, CT, and MRI to assess the extent of inflammation

Treatment:

- Medications:
    - Nonsteroidal anti-inflammatory drugs (NSAIDs): mainstay of treatment for viral or idiopathic pericarditis
    - Colchicine: often added to reduce the risk of recurrence
    - Corticosteroids: reserved for cases where NSAIDs are contraindicated, ineffective, or for specific causes such as autoimmune diseases
- Treating Underlying Causes: antibiotics for bacterial causes, antituberculous therapy for tuberculosis, and appropriate management for other specific causes
- Pericardiocentesis: drainage of excess fluid if there is cardiac tamponade or significant effusion causing hemodynamic instability

- Pericardiectomy: Surgical removal of part or all of the pericardium may be necessary in recurrent or constrictive pericarditis.

4.23. Atrial Septal Defect

> ➤ *Atrial septal defect (ASD) is a congenital heart defect characterized by a hole in the atrial septum, allowing blood to flow between the heart's upper chambers.*
> ➤ *It can lead to symptoms such as shortness of breath, fatigue, and palpitations.*
> ➤ *Treatment may involve observation, medication, or surgical closure to prevent complications and improve heart function.*

Symptoms:
- Asymptomatic: Many patients with small ASDs may not experience any symptoms and may only be diagnosed incidentally during routine physical examination or diagnostic testing.
- Fatigue: Some patients with larger ASDs may experience fatigue or tiredness, especially with physical exertion.
- Shortness of Breath: dyspnea or difficulty breathing, particularly during exertion or when lying flat
- Heart Murmur: characteristic "flow murmur" or "systolic ejection murmur"
- Recurrent Respiratory Infections: Children with untreated ASDs may be at increased risk of recurrent respiratory infections, such as pneumonia or bronchitis.

Causes and Risk Factors:
- Congenital Heart Disease: may be associated with other congenital anomalies or genetic syndromes (e.g. Down syndrome).
- Family History: a parent or sibling with a congenital heart defect.
- Maternal Factors: such as maternal age, exposure to certain medications or substances (e.g., alcohol, tobacco), or maternal health conditions (e.g., diabetes), may increase the risk of ASD in the fetus.
- Genetic Factors: certain genetic mutations or chromosomal abnormalities
- Environmental Factors: exposure to certain environmental toxins or radiation during pregnancy

Epidemiology:

ASDs are one of the most common types of congenital heart defects, accounting for approximately 10-15% of all congenital heart defects. The prevalence of ASDs varies depending on factors such as the size and location of the defect, with small ASDs being more common than larger defects. ASDs are often detected incidentally during routine physical examination or diagnostic testing in asymptomatic patients.

Workup and Diagnosis:

- Physical Examination: Characteristic heart murmurs or abnormal findings on physical examination may raise suspicion for ASD.
- Echocardiography: Transthoracic echocardiography (TTE) is the primary imaging modality used to diagnose ASD and assess its size, location, and hemodynamic significance.
- Electrocardiography (ECG): ECG may reveal characteristic findings such as right axis deviation, right bundle branch block, or evidence of right atrial enlargement.
- Chest X-ray: Chest X-ray may demonstrate enlargement of the right heart chambers or increased pulmonary vascularity in patients with significant shunting.

Treatment:

- Observation:

    Small ASDs that are asymptomatic and have minimal shunting may not require immediate intervention and may be managed with observation and regular follow-up.

- Surgical Repair:

    Surgical closure of ASD may be recommended for larger defects or symptomatic patients to prevent complications such as pulmonary hypertension, heart failure, or arrhythmias. Surgical repair is typically performed using open-heart surgery (cardiopulmonary bypass) or minimally invasive techniques.

- Transcatheter Closure:

    Transcatheter closure of ASD is an alternative to surgical repair in selected cases, particularly for secundum ASDs with suitable anatomy and favorable characteristics. Transcatheter closure involves inserting a closure device through a catheter inserted into the heart via a vein in the groin.

- Medical Management:

    Symptomatic patients may require medical management of associated symptoms such as heart failure, arrhythmias, or pulmonary hypertension. Medications may include diuretics, ACE inhibitors, beta-blockers, or anticoagulants as indicated.

4.24. Cardiac Arrest

> ➤ *Cardiac arrest is a sudden loss of heart function, typically caused by an electrical disturbance in the heart that stops it from beating effectively.*
>
> ➤ *It leads to the cessation of blood flow to vital organs, resulting in unconsciousness and death if not treated immediately.*
>
> ➤ *Immediate CPR and defibrillation are critical for survival, along with identifying and addressing underlying causes such as heart disease or electrolyte imbalances.*

Symptoms:

- Loss of Consciousness: Patients suddenly collapse and become unresponsive.
- Absence of Pulse: In cardiac arrest, there is no detectable pulse, and the patient may not be breathing.
- No Response to Stimuli: The patient does not respond to verbal commands, tactile stimuli, or painful stimuli.
- Gasping or Agonal Breathing: Some patients may exhibit gasping or agonal breathing, which is irregular, labored breathing that may occur briefly after cardiac arrest.

Causes and Risk Factors:

- Coronary Artery Disease (CAD) is a major risk factor for cardiac arrest, particularly in patients with a history of myocardial infarction or significant coronary artery stenosis.
- Heart Failure: at increased risk of cardiac arrest due to impaired cardiac function and electrical instability
- Arrhythmias, such as ventricular fibrillation (VF) or ventricular tachycardia (VT), can precipitate cardiac arrest.
- Electrolyte Imbalances (e.g., potassium, magnesium): can disrupt cardiac electrical activity and increase the risk of arrhythmias and cardiac arrest.
- Drug Toxicity: Certain medications or drug overdoses can predispose to cardiac arrhythmias and sudden cardiac arrest.
- Family History: A family history of sudden cardiac death or inherited cardiac conditions may increase the risk of cardiac arrest.

- Structural Heart Disease: such as hypertrophic cardiomyopathy or congenital heart defects, can predispose to arrhythmias and sudden cardiac arrest.

Epidemiology:

Cardiac arrest is a leading cause of death worldwide, accounting for a significant proportion of out-of-hospital and in-hospital deaths. The incidence of cardiac arrest varies depending on the population studied, with higher rates observed in older adults and patients with underlying cardiovascular disease. In the United States, it is estimated that approximately 356,000 cases of out-of-hospital cardiac arrest occur annually.

Workup and Diagnosis:

- Clinical Evaluation: The diagnosis of cardiac arrest is primarily clinical, based on the absence of a pulse, unresponsiveness, and lack of spontaneous breathing.
- Electrocardiography (ECG): ECG may be performed to identify the underlying arrhythmia responsible for cardiac arrest, such as ventricular fibrillation, ventricular tachycardia, or asystole.
- Laboratory Tests: Assess for electrolyte imbalances, cardiac biomarkers (e.g., troponin), and other markers of cardiac injury or dysfunction.
- Imaging Studies: Echocardiography or cardiac MRI may be performed to evaluate for structural heart disease or assess cardiac function in survivors of cardiac arrest.

Treatment:

- Cardiopulmonary Resuscitation (CPR): Immediate initiation of high-quality CPR is essential to support circulation and maintain oxygenation during cardiac arrest.
- Defibrillation:

    If the underlying rhythm is ventricular fibrillation or pulseless ventricular tachycardia, prompt defibrillation with an automated external defibrillator (AED) or manual defibrillator is indicated to restore normal cardiac rhythm.

- Advanced Cardiac Life Support (ACLS):

    ACLS protocols are followed to manage cardiac arrest, including administration of medications (e.g., epinephrine, amiodarone), airway management, and continued assessment and monitoring.

- Post-Resuscitation Care:

    Survivors of cardiac arrest require intensive care management, including targeted temperature management (hypothermia therapy), hemodynamic support, and evaluation for the underlying cause of cardiac arrest.

- Secondary Prevention:

    Patients who have experienced cardiac arrest are at increased risk of recurrent events and require comprehensive secondary prevention measures, including lifestyle modifications, medications (e.g., antiarrhythmics, beta-blockers), implantable cardioverter-defibrillator (ICD) placement, and cardiac rehabilitation.

4.25. Thrombophlebitis

> *Thrombophlebitis is the inflammation of a vein, often accompanied by the formation of a blood clot within the affected vein.*
>
> *It commonly occurs in the legs and can cause pain, swelling, and redness along the affected vein.*
>
> *Treatment typically involves medications to alleviate symptoms and prevent clot propagation, along with measures to reduce the risk of complications such as pulmonary embolism.*

Symptoms:

- Localized pain or tenderness along the affected vein, aching or throbbing
- Redness or erythema over the area of the affected vein
- Edema can occur along the course of the affected vein
- Increased warmth or heat over the area of inflammation
- Palpable Cord: firm, tender lump may be felt under the skin along the affected vein
- Fever: if the inflammation is severe or there is an associated infection

Causes and Risk Factors:

- Venous Stasis: Conditions that impair venous blood flow, such as prolonged immobility (bed rest, long flights or car rides), obesity, or pregnancy, increase the risk of thrombophlebitis.

- **Venous Injury:** Trauma or injury to the vein, such as from intravenous catheter insertion, surgery, or physical trauma, can predispose to thrombophlebitis.
- **Hypercoagulable States:** Conditions associated with increased blood clotting risk, such as inherited thrombophilias (Factor V Leiden mutation), malignancy, or use of estrogen-containing medications (oral contraceptives, hormone replacement therapy), increase the risk of thrombophlebitis.
- **Infection:** Superficial thrombophlebitis may occur secondary to local infection of the vein, particularly in patients with venous catheters or intravenous drug use.
- **Smoking:** Smoking is a risk factor for venous thromboembolism, which includes thrombophlebitis, due to its effects on vascular endothelium and blood coagulation.
- **Varicose Veins:** resulting from impaired venous valve function and increased venous pressure, are associated with an increased risk of thrombophlebitis.

Epidemiology:

Thrombophlebitis can occur in patients of any age but is more common in adults, particularly those with underlying risk factors. The incidence of superficial thrombophlebitis is higher than that of deep vein thrombosis (DVT) and pulmonary embolism (PE), which are more severe forms of venous thromboembolism. Superficial thrombophlebitis is more common than deep vein thrombophlebitis, with estimates suggesting an incidence of 1 to 2 cases per 1000 patients per year.

Workup and Diagnosis:
- <u>Clinical Evaluation:</u> clinical assessment, including history and physical examination.
- <u>Duplex Ultrasonography:</u> imaging modality of choice for diagnosing thrombophlebitis and evaluating the extent and severity of venous thrombosis
- <u>D-dimer Test:</u> screening test to rule out thromboembolic events, but it is less specific for superficial thrombophlebitis
- <u>Venography:</u>
    - An invasive imaging procedure is rarely used for diagnosing thrombophlebitis but may be considered in cases where ultrasound findings are inconclusive or when evaluating for deep vein involvement.

Treatment:

- Conservative Measures: rest, elevation of the affected limb, and application of warm compresses to alleviate pain and inflammation
- Nonsteroidal Anti-Inflammatory Drugs (NSAIDs): such as ibuprofen or naproxen to relieve pain and inflammation associated with superficial thrombophlebitis
- Compression Therapy: compression stockings or bandages to improve venous blood flow and reduce swelling
- Anticoagulation: generally not indicated for isolated superficial thrombophlebitis but may be considered in cases of extensive involvement or high risk of progression to DVT or PE.
- Surgical Intervention: rarely needed for superficial thrombophlebitis but may be considered in cases of extensive or recurrent thrombophlebitis, particularly if associated with underlying venous insufficiency or varicose veins.

4.26. Varicose Vein

> ➤ *Varicose veins are enlarged, twisted veins, usually in the legs, resulting from weakened or damaged valves. They can cause discomfort, pain, and aesthetic concerns.*
>
> ➤ *Risk factors include genetics, age, pregnancy, and prolonged standing or sitting.*
>
> ➤ *Treatment ranges from self-care measures like compression stockings to medical procedures such as sclerotherapy or surgery. Seeking medical advice is crucial for proper diagnosis and tailored treatment.*

Symptoms:

- Visible and Enlarged Veins: twisted, bulging, or rope-like veins that are visible on the surface of the skin, typically in the legs.
- Aching or Throbbing Sensations: in the affected legs, particularly after prolonged standing or sitting
- Edema: in the ankles and lower legs, especially at the end of the day or after prolonged standing
- Fatigue or Restlessness: in leg, particularly at night
- Itching or Burning: over the affected veins, particularly in warm weather or after prolonged periods of standing
- Discoloration, dryness, or thickening of the skin may occur overlying varicose veins, particularly in advanced cases.

- Complications of varicose veins may include superficial thrombophlebitis, bleeding from ruptured veins, or the development of venous ulcers in severe cases.

Causes and Risk Factors:
- Family History: Genetic factors play a significant role in the development of varicose veins, with a family history of venous insufficiency or varicose veins increasing the risk.
- Age: The prevalence of varicose veins increases with age.
- Gender: Women are more likely to develop varicose veins than men, possibly due to hormonal influences (e.g., pregnancy, hormone therapy).
- Pregnancy: a risk factor for varicose veins due to hormonal changes, increased blood volume, and pressure on the veins from the growing uterus
- Excess Body Weight: increases the pressure on the veins in the legs, contributing to the development of varicose veins.
- Prolonged Standing or Sitting: Occupations or activities that involve prolonged periods of standing or sitting may increase the risk of varicose veins by impairing venous blood flow.
- History of Deep Vein Thrombosis (DVT) or Other Venous Thromboembolic Events: are at increased risk of developing varicose veins,
- Prior Leg Trauma: such as fractures or surgery, may damage the veins and increase the risk of varicose vein development.

Epidemiology:

Varicose veins are a common vascular condition, with a reported prevalence of approximately 25% in the general population. The prevalence of varicose veins increases with age, with estimates suggesting that up to 40% of adults may develop varicose veins by age 70. Varicose veins are more common in women than men, with studies reporting a higher prevalence in women of reproductive age and older women.

Workup and Diagnosis:
- <u>Clinical Evaluation:</u> clinical assessment, including history and physical examination
- <u>Duplex Ultrasonography:</u>
    The preferred imaging modality for evaluating varicose veins and assessing venous insufficiency. It can identify the location, extent, and severity of venous reflux and assess for associated

complications such as deep vein thrombosis (DVT) or venous ulcers.
- <u>Venous Imaging Studies:</u> such as venography or magnetic resonance venography (MRV) may be used in selected cases to further evaluate venous anatomy and function.

Treatment:
- <u>Conservative Measures:</u> lifestyle modifications and symptomatic relief measures such as:
    - Leg elevation
    - Compression stockings
    - Regular exercise
    - Weight management
    - Avoidance of prolonged sitting or standing
- <u>Minimally Invasive Procedures:</u> Endovenous ablation techniques (e.g., laser ablation, radiofrequency ablation) or sclerotherapy may be recommended to treat varicose veins and address venous reflux.
- <u>Surgical Interventions:</u> Vein stripping or ligation may be considered in cases of severe varicose veins or when minimally invasive treatments are not suitable.
- <u>Complications Management:</u>
    Complications such as superficial thrombophlebitis or venous ulcers, may require specific management strategies, including anticoagulation, wound care, or surgical intervention.

4.27. EKG Findings in Common Cardiac Conditions

> ➤ *An electrocardiogram (EKG or ECG) is a non-invasive test that records the electrical activity of the heart to detect cardiac abnormalities.*
>
> ➤ *It provides vital information on heart rate, rhythm, and can indicate the presence of conditions such as atrial fibrillation, myocardial infarction, and structural heart disease.*

Please refer to chapter 17 for a basic EKG interpretation.

Item	Description
Atrial Fibrillation	○ Rhythm: Irregularly irregular. ○ P Waves: Absent, replaced by fine fibrillatory waves.

	o QRS Complexes: Normal but irregularly timed.
Atrial Flutter	o Rhythm: Regular or variable due to varying conduction ratios. o P Waves: Absent, replaced by "flutter waves" with a sawtooth pattern in leads II, III, and aVF. o Conduction: Fixed or variable AV block, often 2:1, leading to a ventricular rate that is a fraction of the atrial rate.
Ventricular Tachycardia	o Rhythm: Regular, rapid. o P Waves: Absent or independent of QRS complexes. o QRS Complexes: Wide and abnormal shape.
Myocardial Infarction (MI)	o Rhythm: Regular, rapid. o P Waves: Absent or independent of QRS complexes. o QRS Complexes: Wide and abnormal shape.
Ischemia	o ST Segment: Horizontal or downsloping ST depression. o T Waves: T wave inversion in leads overlying the ischemic area.
Pericarditis	o ST Segment: Diffuse ST elevation with upward concavity across multiple leads. o PR Segment: PR depression in multiple leads.
Left Ventricular Hypertrophy (LVH)	o Increased Voltage: High R wave amplitude in left-sided leads. o ST and T Wave Changes: Secondary repolarization abnormalities opposite the QRS direction.
Right Ventricular Hypertrophy (RVH)	o R Wave Progression: Prominent R waves in right precordial leads (V1-V2). o S Wave Depth: Deep S waves in left precordial leads (V5-V6). o Right Axis Deviation: Axis > +90 degrees.

1. Bundle Branch Blocks
2. Atrial Fibrillation (Afib)
    - Rhythm: Irregularly irregular.
    - P Waves: Absent, replaced by fine fibrillatory waves.
    - QRS Complexes: Normal but irregularly timed.
3. Atrial Flutter
    - Rhythm: Regular or variable due to varying conduction ratios.
    - P Waves: Absent, replaced by "flutter waves" with a sawtooth pattern in leads II, III, and aVF.
    - Conduction: Fixed or variable AV block, often 2:1, leading to a ventricular rate that is a fraction of the atrial rate.
4. Ventricular Tachycardia
    - Rhythm: Regular, rapid.
    - P Waves: Absent or independent of QRS complexes.
    - QRS Complexes: Wide and abnormal shape.
5. Myocardial Infarction (MI)
    - ST Elevation: In leads overlying the infarcted area for STEMI.
    - Q Waves: Pathological Q waves indicating necrosis.
    - T Wave Changes: Inversion in the acute phase, normalization over time.
6. Ischemia
    - ST Segment: Horizontal or downsloping ST depression.
    - T Waves: T wave inversion in leads overlying the ischemic area.
7. Pericarditis
    - ST Segment: Diffuse ST elevation with upward concavity across multiple leads.
    - PR Segment: PR depression in multiple leads.
8. Left Ventricular Hypertrophy (LVH)
    - Increased Voltage: High R wave amplitude in left-sided leads.
    - ST and T Wave Changes: Secondary repolarization abnormalities opposite the QRS direction.

9. Right Ventricular Hypertrophy (RVH)
    - R Wave Progression: Prominent R waves in right precordial leads (V1-V2).
    - S Wave Depth: Deep S waves in left precordial leads (V5-V6).
    - Right Axis Deviation: Axis > +90 degrees.
10. Bundle Branch Blocks
    - Right Bundle Branch Block (RBBB): Wide QRS, R' wave in V1-V2, deep S wave in V5-V6.
    - Left Bundle Branch Block (LBBB): Wide QRS, broad R wave in I, aVL, V5-V6, absent Q waves in these leads.
11. First-Degree AV Block
    - PR Interval: Prolonged (>0.20 seconds), constant across all beats.
12. Second-Degree AV Block (Type 1, Wenckebach)
    - PR Interval: Progressive lengthening until a QRS complex is dropped.
13. Second-Degree AV Block (Type 2)
    - PR Interval: Constant for conducted beats, but some P waves not followed by QRS complexes.
14. Third-Degree AV Block (Complete Heart Block)
    - Atrioventricular Dissociation: P waves and QRS complexes independent of each other.
15. Premature Ventricular Contractions (PVCs)
    - QRS Complexes: Wide (>0.12 seconds), bizarre QRS occurring prematurely; T wave usually in opposite direction of QRS.
16. Wolff-Parkinson-White Syndrome (WPW)
    - PR Interval: Short (<0.12 seconds).
    - Delta Wave: Slurred upstroke of the QRS complex.
    - QRS Duration: Slightly widened due to the delta wave.
17. Hyperkalemia
    - T Waves: Peaked T waves are a classic sign of hyperkalemia.
    - QRS Duration: Severe hyperkalemia may also cause widening of the QRS complex.

References

- James, P. A., Oparil, S., Carter, B. L., et al. (2014). 2014 evidence-based guideline for the management of high blood pressure in adults: Report from the panel members appointed to the Eighth Joint National Committee (JNC 8). JAMA, 311(5), 507-520.

- Whelton, P. K., Carey, R. M., Aronow, W. S., et al. (2018). 2017 ACC/AHA/AAPA/ABC/ACPM/AGS/APhA/ASH/ASPC/NMA/PCNA guideline for the prevention, detection, evaluation, and management of high blood pressure in adults: A report of the American College of Cardiology/American Heart Association Task Force on Clinical Practice Guidelines. Journal of the American College of Cardiology, 71(19), e127-e248.

- Fihn, S. D., Blankenship, J. C., Alexander, K. P., et al. (2014). 2014 ACC/AHA/AATS/PCNA/SCAI/STS focused update of the guideline for the diagnosis and management of patients with stable ischemic heart disease: A report of the American College of Cardiology/American Heart Association Task Force on Practice Guidelines, and the American Association for Thoracic Surgery, Preventive Cardiovascular Nurses Association, Society for Cardiovascular Angiography and Interventions, and Society of Thoracic Surgeons. Circulation, 130(19), 1749-1767.

- Yancy, C. W., Jessup, M., Bozkurt, B., et al. (2017). 2017 ACC/AHA/HFSA focused update of the 2013 ACCF/AHA guideline for the management of heart failure: A report of the American College of Cardiology/American Heart Association Task Force on Clinical Practice Guidelines and the Heart Failure Society of America. Circulation, 136(6), e137-e161.

- January, C. T., Wann, L. S., Calkins, H., et al. (2019). 2019 AHA/ACC/HRS focused update of the 2014 AHA/ACC/HRS guideline for the management of patients with atrial fibrillation: A report of the American College of Cardiology/American Heart Association Task Force on Clinical Practice Guidelines and the Heart Rhythm Society. Circulation, 140(2), e125-e151.

- Nishimura, R. A., Otto, C. M., Bonow, R. O., et al. (2014). 2014 AHA/ACC guideline for the management of patients with valvular heart disease: A report of the American College of Cardiology/American Heart Association Task Force on Practice Guidelines. Journal of the American College of Cardiology, 63(22), e57-e185.

- Gerhard-Herman, M. D., Gornik, H. L., Barrett, C., et al. (2017). 2016 AHA/ACC guideline on the management of patients with lower extremity peripheral artery disease: A report of the American College of Cardiology/American Heart Association Task Force on Clinical Practice Guidelines. Circulation, 135(12), e726-e779.

- Powers, W. J., Rabinstein, A. A., Ackerson, T., et al. (2018). 2018 guidelines for the early management of patients with acute ischemic stroke: A guideline for healthcare professionals from the American Heart Association/American Stroke Association. Stroke, 49(3), e46-e110.

- Kearon, C., Akl, E. A., Ornelas, J., et al. (2016). Antithrombotic therapy for VTE disease: CHEST guideline and expert panel report. Chest, 149(2), 315-352.
- Hiratzka, L. F., Bakris, G. L., Beckman, J. A., et al. (2010). 2010 ACCF/AHA/AATS/ACR/ASA/SCA/SCAI/SIR/STS/SVM guidelines for the diagnosis and management of patients with Thoracic Aortic Disease: A report of the American College of Cardiology Foundation/American Heart Association Task Force on Practice Guidelines, American Association for Thoracic Surgery, American College of Radiology, American Stroke Association, Society of Cardiovascular Anesthesiologists, Society for Cardiovascular Angiography and Interventions, Society of Interventional Radiology, Society of Thoracic Surgeons, and Society for Vascular Medicine. Circulation, 121(13), e266-e369.
- Amsterdam, E. A., Wenger, N. K., Brindis, R. G., et al. (2014). 2014 AHA/ACC guideline for the management of patients with non–ST-elevation acute coronary syndromes: A report of the American College of Cardiology/American Heart Association Task Force on Practice Guidelines. Journal of the American College of Cardiology, 64(24), e139-e228.
- Yancy, C. W., Jessup, M., Bozkurt, B., et al. (2017). 2017 ACC/AHA/HFSA focused update of the 2013 ACCF/AHA guideline for the management of heart failure: A report of the American College of Cardiology/American Heart Association Task Force on Clinical Practice Guidelines and the Heart Failure Society of America. Circulation, 136(6), e137-e161.
- Gewitz, M. H., Baltimore, R. S., Tani, L. Y., et al. (2015). Revision of the Jones Criteria for the diagnosis of acute rheumatic fever in the era of Doppler echocardiography: A scientific statement from the American Heart Association. Circulation, 131(20), 1806-1818.
- Warnes, C. A., Williams, R. G., Bashore, T. M., et al. (2008). ACC/AHA 2008 guidelines for the management of adults with congenital heart disease: Executive summary: A report of the American College of Cardiology/American Heart Association Task Force on Practice Guidelines (writing committee to develop guidelines for the management of adults with congenital heart disease). Circulation, 118(23), 2395-2451
- Baddour, L. M., Wilson, W. R., Bayer, A. S., et al. (2015). Infective endocarditis in adults: Diagnosis, antimicrobial therapy, and management of complications: A scientific statement for healthcare professionals from the American Heart Association. Circulation, 132(15), 1435-1486.
- Baumgartner, H., De Backer, J., Babu-Narayan, S. V., et al. (2020). 2020 ESC guidelines for the management of adult congenital heart disease: The Task Force for the Management of Adult Congenital Heart Disease of the European Society of Cardiology (ESC). European Heart Journal, 42(6), 563-645.
- Nishimura, R. A., Otto, C. M., Bonow, R. O., et al. (2014). 2014 AHA/ACC guideline for the management of patients with valvular heart disease: A report of the American College of Cardiology/American Heart Association

Task Force on Practice Guidelines. Journal of the American College of Cardiology, 63(22), e57-e185.

- Nishimura, R. A., Otto, C. M., Bonow, R. O., et al. (2014). 2014 AHA/ACC guideline for the management of patients with valvular heart disease: A report of the American College of Cardiology/American Heart Association Task Force on Practice Guidelines. Journal of the American College of Cardiology, 63(22), e57-e185.

- Link, M. S., Berkow, L. C., Kudenchuk, P. J., et al. (2015). Part 7: Adult advanced cardiovascular life support: 2015 American Heart Association guidelines update for cardiopulmonary resuscitation and emergency cardiovascular care. Circulation, 132(18 Suppl 2), S444-S464.

- Kearon, C., Akl, E. A., Ornelas, J., et al. (2016). Antithrombotic therapy for VTE disease: CHEST guideline and expert panel report. Chest, 149(2), 315-352.

- Gloviczki, P., Comerota, A. J., Dalsing, M. C., et al. (2011). The care of patients with varicose veins and associated chronic venous diseases: Clinical practice guidelines of the Society for Vascular Surgery and the American Venous Forum. Journal of Vascular Surgery, 53(5 Suppl), 2S-48S.

Chapter 5. Respiratory Disorders

Reviewed by
Loan Thi Vo, MD, RRT

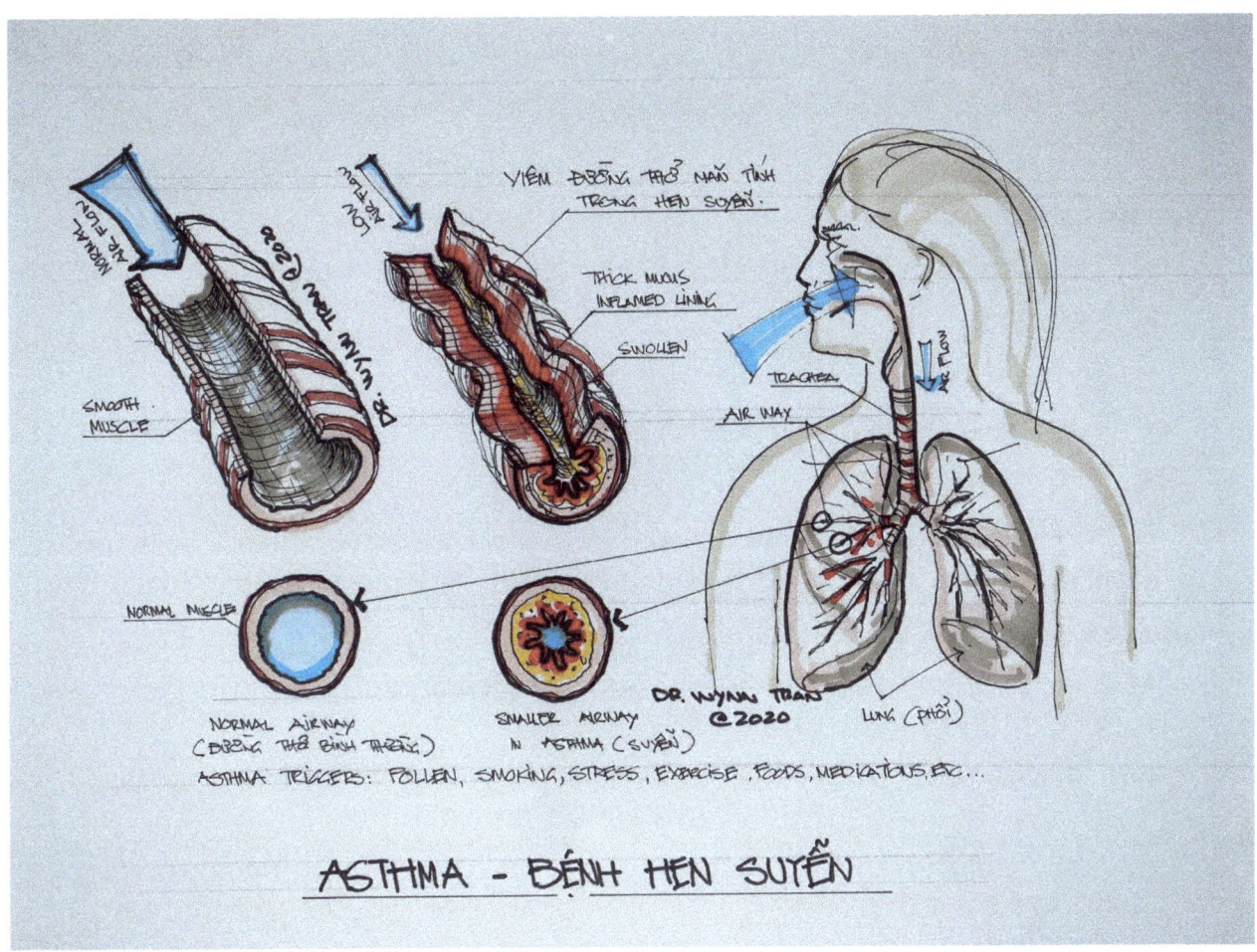

The APh should be familiar with the presentation, diagnosis, and management of these common lung disorders to provide appropriate care and referral to the pulmonologist when necessary.

5.1. Common Cold

> *Viral rhinitis, commonly known as the common cold, is a viral infection of the upper respiratory tract that primarily affects the nose and throat.*
>
> *It is typically caused by rhinoviruses, but other viruses such as adenoviruses, coronaviruses, and enteroviruses can also be responsible.*
>
> *Treatment focuses on relieving symptoms with rest, hydration, over-the-counter medications, and sometimes antiviral drugs in severe cases.*

Symptoms:

- Runny or Stuffy Nose: Nasal congestion or discharge.
- Sneezing
- Sore Throat
- Cough: Typically mild and dry.
- Mild Headache
- Mild Fatigue
- Mild Fever: Low-grade fever, if present, is usually mild.

Causes and Risk Factors:

- Exposure to Respiratory Viruses: Direct contact with infected patients or contaminated surfaces.
- Time of Year: Viral rhinitis is more prevalent in colder months, especially during the fall and winter seasons.
- Age: Children under 6 years old are at higher risk due to developing immune systems and frequent exposure to viruses in school or daycare.
- Weakened Immune System: Due to underlying medical conditions, such as HIV/AIDS, cancer treatments, or certain medications.
- Smoking or Secondhand Smoke Exposure: Smoking can impair immune function and increase susceptibility to respiratory infections.
- Stress: Chronic stress can weaken the immune system and increase vulnerability to infections.
- Chronic Conditions: Such as allergies or asthma, which can predispose patients to frequent respiratory infections.

- Certain Occupations: Such as healthcare workers or teachers, who may have increased exposure to infected patients.

Workup and Diagnosis:
- Medical History and Physical Examination: Including assessment of symptoms and risk factors.
- Clinical Diagnosis: Typically based on the presence of characteristic symptoms and absence of more severe signs suggestive of other respiratory infections such as influenza or pneumonia.
- Laboratory Testing: Generally not required for routine cases of viral rhinitis unless complications or severe symptoms are present.

Treatment:
- Symptomatic Relief:
    - Rest: Get plenty of rest to aid recovery.
    - Fluids: Drink plenty of fluids, such as water, herbal tea, or broth, to stay hydrated.
    - Saline Nasal Sprays or Drops: To relieve nasal congestion and moisturize nasal passages.
    - Humidifiers: Use a humidifier to add moisture to the air and ease nasal congestion.
    - Over-the-Counter (OTC) Medications: Such as pain relievers (acetaminophen, ibuprofen) for headache or fever, and cough suppressants or expectorants for cough relief.
- Avoidance of Irritants: Such as cigarette smoke or allergens, which can exacerbate symptoms.
- Antiviral Medications: Generally not recommended for routine cases of viral rhinitis as they are not effective against cold viruses.

5.2. Influenza

> ➢ *Influenza, commonly known as the flu, is a contagious respiratory illness caused by influenza viruses.*
> ➢ *It can range from mild to severe and can lead to complications, especially in vulnerable populations.*
> ➢ *Influenza treatment typically involves antiviral medications such as oseltamivir (Tamiflu) and symptomatic treatment to shorten the duration and severity of symptoms.*

Symptoms:
- Fever: Often high, typically above 100.4°F (38°C).
- Cough: Usually dry and persistent.
- Sore Throat
- Runny or Stuffy Nose
- Muscle or Body Aches
- Headache
- Fatigue: Often severe and debilitating.
- Chills
- Nausea, Vomiting, or Diarrhea: More common in children than adults.

Causes and Risk Factors:
- Age: Infants, young children, elderly adults, and patients with weakened immune systems are at higher risk of severe complications.
- Chronic Medical Conditions: Such as asthma, chronic obstructive pulmonary disease (COPD), diabetes, heart disease, or obesity.
- Pregnancy: Pregnant women are at higher risk of flu-related complications.
- Weakened Immune System: Due to HIV/AIDS, cancer treatments, or certain medications.
- Living or Working Conditions: Such as residing in long-term care facilities, crowded environments, or healthcare settings.
- Smoking
- Malnutrition
- Travel: Increased exposure to influenza viruses during travel, especially in confined spaces like airplanes.

Workup and Diagnosis:
- <u>Medical History and Physical Examination:</u> Including assessment of symptoms and risk factors.
- <u>Rapid Influenza Diagnostic Tests (RIDTs):</u> Nasal or throat swab tests to detect influenza viruses within minutes, though sensitivity can vary.
- <u>Reverse Transcription Polymerase Chain Reaction (RT-PCR):</u> More sensitive laboratory tests to confirm influenza virus infection, typically used in hospital settings.

- Complete Blood Count (CBC): To assess white blood cell count, which may be elevated in cases of influenza infection.
- Chest X-ray: To evaluate for complications such as pneumonia in severe cases or patients with underlying conditions.

Treatment:
- Antiviral Medications:
  - Oseltamivir (Tamiflu)
  - Zanamivir (Relenza)
  - Peramivir (Rapivab)
  - Baloxavir (Xofluza)
  - These medications are most effective when started within the first 48 hours of symptom onset and can help reduce the severity and duration of symptoms.
- Supportive Care:
  - Rest: Get plenty of rest to aid recovery.
  - Fluids: Drink plenty of fluids to stay hydrated, especially water, herbal tea, or broth.
  - Pain Relievers: Such as acetaminophen (Tylenol) or ibuprofen (Advil, Motrin) for fever, headache, and muscle aches.
  - Cough Suppressants or Expectorants: To relieve cough symptoms.
- Influenza Vaccination: Annual vaccination is recommended for everyone 6 months and older to prevent influenza infection and reduce the severity of illness if infection occurs.

5.3. Sinusitis

> *Sinusitis is inflammation of the sinuses, often triggered by viral, bacterial, or fungal infections.*
>
> *Symptoms include facial pain, nasal congestion, and nasal discharge.*
>
> *Treatment usually involves antibiotics, decongestants, or nasal corticosteroids depending on the cause and severity. Chronic sinusitis may require prolonged therapy or surgical intervention to alleviate symptoms.*

Symptoms:
- Nasal Congestion: Difficulty breathing through the nose.

- Facial Pain or Pressure: Especially around the eyes, forehead, or cheeks.
- Nasal Discharge: Thick, yellow or green mucus from the nose.
- Reduced Sense of Smell and Taste
- Postnasal Drip: Mucus dripping down the back of the throat.
- Cough: Often worse at night.
- Fatigue
- Headache: Especially worsened by bending forward or lying down.
- Sore Throat: Often caused by postnasal drip.
- Bad Breath

Causes and Risk Factors:
- Upper Respiratory Tract Infections: Especially viral infections such as the common cold.
- Allergies: Allergic rhinitis or hay fever.
- Nasal Polyps: Noncancerous growths in the nasal passages.
- Structural Abnormalities: Such as a deviated septum.
- Smoking or Secondhand Smoke Exposure
- Immune System Disorders: Such as HIV/AIDS or autoimmune diseases.
- Chronic Rhinosinusitis: Persistent inflammation of the sinuses lasting more than 12 weeks.
- Cystic Fibrosis
- Gastroesophageal Reflux Disease (GERD): Acid reflux can irritate the sinuses.
- Dental Infections: Such as infected teeth or gum disease.
- Air Travel: Changes in air pressure can affect sinus function.

Workup and Diagnosis:
- <u>Medical History and Physical Examination:</u> Including assessment of symptoms and risk factors.
- <u>Nasal Endoscopy:</u> Procedure using a thin, flexible tube with a camera to visualize the nasal passages and sinuses.
- <u>Imaging Studies:</u>
    - CT Scan (Computed Tomography): Provides detailed images of the sinuses to identify inflammation, polyps, or structural abnormalities.

- MRI (Magnetic Resonance Imaging): Less commonly used than CT, but may be preferred in certain cases such as evaluating allergic fungal sinusitis.
- Nasal Culture: To identify bacterial or fungal infections in cases of chronic or recurrent sinusitis.
- Allergy Testing: To identify potential allergens triggering sinus inflammation.

Treatment:
- Medications:
  - Decongestants: To reduce nasal congestion and swelling.
  - Nasal Steroid Sprays: Anti-inflammatory medications to reduce sinus inflammation.
  - Antibiotics: If bacterial infection is suspected or confirmed.
  - Antihistamines: To relieve symptoms of allergic sinusitis.
  - Pain Relievers: Such as acetaminophen or ibuprofen for pain relief.
- Nasal Irrigation: Using saline solution to flush out mucus and allergens from the nasal passages.
- Steam Inhalation: Breathing in steam to help loosen mucus and relieve congestion.
- Warm Compresses: Applied to the face to relieve facial pain and pressure.
- Sinus Surgery:

    In cases of chronic or severe sinusitis that do not respond to conservative treatments, procedures such as endoscopic sinus surgery or functional endoscopic sinus surgery (FESS) may be recommended to improve drainage and ventilation of the sinuses.

5.4. Pharyngitis

> ➢ *Pharyngitis is inflammation of the throat, typically caused by viral or bacterial infections.*
>
> ➢ *Symptoms include sore throat, difficulty swallowing, and swollen tonsils, with treatment often involving rest, hydration, and over-the-counter pain relievers.*
>
> ➢ *Bacterial pharyngitis may require antibiotics to prevent complications such as tonsillitis or strep throat.*

Symptoms:

- Sore Throat: Pain or discomfort in the throat, which may worsen with swallowing.
- Difficulty Swallowing: Especially with solid foods or liquids.
- Redness and Swelling: In the back of the throat.
- Swollen Tonsils: Tonsillitis may accompany pharyngitis.
- Hoarseness: Changes in voice quality or loss of voice.
- Cough: Dry or productive cough may be present.
- Fever: Low-grade fever may occur, especially with bacterial infections.
- Enlarged Lymph Nodes: Swollen glands in the neck.

Causes and Risk Factors:

- Viral Infections: Common cold viruses, influenza viruses, or Epstein-Barr virus (causing infectious mononucleosis) are common causes of viral pharyngitis.
- Bacterial Infections: Streptococcus pyogenes (group A streptococcus) is the most common bacterial cause of pharyngitis, leading to strep throat.
- Age: Children and adolescents are at higher risk, particularly for viral pharyngitis.
- Season: Pharyngitis is more common during colder months when viral infections are more prevalent.
- Close Contact: Exposure to patients with viral or bacterial infections, especially in crowded or confined spaces.
- Environmental Irritants: Such as tobacco smoke, air pollution, or dry air.

- Allergies: Allergic reactions to pollen, mold, dust, or pet dander can cause pharyngeal inflammation.
- Weakened Immune System: Due to underlying medical conditions or medications.

Workup and Diagnosis

1. Histories: The patient typically presents with a sore throat, pain with swallowing, and may also have fever, headache, or swollen lymph nodes in the neck.
2. Physical Examination: The APh examines the throat for redness, swelling, pus on the tonsils, and enlarged lymph nodes. The presence of cough, nasal congestion, and hoarseness may suggest a viral cause.

+ Laboratory Tests

- Rapid Antigen Detection Test (RADT): This test can detect group A streptococcus directly from a throat swab within minutes. If positive, it confirms strep throat. However, a negative test might be followed by a confirmatory throat culture in certain cases, especially in children, due to higher rates of group A strep infections and potential complications.
- Throat Culture: Considered the gold standard for diagnosing streptococcal pharyngitis. A swab from the throat is cultured in a laboratory for 24-48 hours to see if group A streptococcus bacteria grow. It's more accurate than the RADT but takes longer to get results.

+ Other Tests

- Monospot Test: Used if there's suspicion of infectious mononucleosis (mono), typically caused by the Epstein-Barr virus.
- Complete Blood Count (CBC): May help in identifying viral vs. bacterial infections indirectly through the white blood cell count and differential.
- Allergy Tests: If an allergic reaction is suspected as the cause of the pharyngitis.

Diagnosis Criteria

For streptococcal pharyngitis, the Centor Criteria or the modified Centor criteria are often used to estimate the probability of a streptococcal infection:
- Presence of tonsillar exudates (1 point)
- Tender anterior cervical adenopathy (1 point)

- Fever by history (1 point)
- Absence of cough (1 point)

The more points present, the higher the likelihood of a streptococcal infection, which may influence the decision to perform rapid testing or start empirical antibiotic treatment.

Treatment:
- Symptomatic Relief:
  - Pain Relievers: Over-the-counter medications such as acetaminophen (Tylenol) or ibuprofen (Advil, Motrin) for pain and fever relief.
  - Throat Lozenges or Sprays: To soothe throat irritation.
  - Warm Saltwater Gargles: Helps relieve throat discomfort.
- Antibiotics:

  Only prescribed for bacterial pharyngitis (e.g., strep throat) confirmed by testing to reduce the duration of symptoms, prevent complications, and minimize transmission to others.
- Rest and Hydration: Get plenty of rest and drink fluids to stay hydrated.
- Avoidance of Irritants: Such as tobacco smoke or allergens, which can exacerbate throat symptoms.

5.5. Tonsillitis

> ➢ *Tonsillitis is inflammation of the tonsils, commonly caused by viral or bacterial infections.*
> ➢ *Symptoms include sore throat, swollen tonsils, and difficulty swallowing, often accompanied by fever and fatigue.*
> ➢ *Treatment may involve rest, fluids, pain relievers, and antibiotics for bacterial infections or recurrent cases.*

Symptoms:
- Sore Throat: Pain or discomfort in the throat, which may be severe.
- Difficulty Swallowing: Especially with solid foods or liquids.
- Red, Swollen Tonsils: Tonsils may appear swollen and may have white or yellow spots indicating pus.

- Painful Swallowing: Pain or discomfort when swallowing, particularly with solid foods or fluids.
- Fever: Low-grade fever is common, especially with bacterial tonsillitis.
- Enlarged Lymph Nodes: Swollen glands in the neck.
- Bad Breath: Foul-smelling breath due to bacterial infection.
- Headache
- Ear Pain: Pain radiating to the ears due to shared nerve pathways.

Causes and Risk Factors:
- Viral Infections: Common cold viruses, influenza viruses, or Epstein-Barr virus (causing infectious mononucleosis) are common causes of viral tonsillitis.
- Bacterial Infections: Streptococcus pyogenes (group A streptococcus) is the most common bacterial cause of tonsillitis, leading to strep throat.
- Age: Tonsillitis is more common in children and adolescents, especially between the ages of 5 and 15.
- Close Contact: Exposure to patients with viral or bacterial infections, especially in crowded or confined spaces.
- Weakened Immune System: Due to underlying medical conditions or medications.
- Allergies: Allergic reactions to pollen, mold, dust, or pet dander can cause tonsillar inflammation.

Workup and Diagnosis:
- Medical History and Physical Examination: Including assessment of symptoms and risk factors.
- Throat Culture: A throat swab may be taken to identify the presence of group A streptococcus bacteria, especially if strep throat is suspected.
- Rapid Antigen Test: Provides quick results for the presence of group A streptococcus antigens, though sensitivity can vary.
- Complete Blood Count (CBC): To assess white blood cell count, which may be elevated in cases of bacterial infection.

Treatment:

- <u>Symptomatic Relief</u>:
    - Pain Relievers: Over-the-counter medications such as acetaminophen (Tylenol) or ibuprofen (Advil, Motrin) for pain and fever relief.
    - Throat Lozenges or Sprays: To soothe throat irritation.
    - Warm Saltwater Gargles: Helps relieve throat discomfort.
- <u>Antibiotics:</u>

    Only prescribed for bacterial tonsillitis (e.g., strep throat) confirmed by testing to reduce the duration of symptoms, prevent complications, and minimize transmission to others.
- <u>Rest and Hydration:</u> Get plenty of rest and drink fluids to stay hydrated.
- <u>Surgical Removal of Tonsils (Tonsillectomy):</u> In cases of recurrent or chronic tonsillitis that do not respond to conservative treatments.

5.6. Community Acquired Pneumonia

> ➤ *Community-acquired pneumonia (CAP) is a lung infection acquired outside of healthcare settings, often caused by bacteria like Streptococcus pneumoniae or viruses like influenza.*
>
> ➤ *Symptoms include fever, cough, chest pain, and difficulty breathing, with treatment typically involving antibiotics for bacterial infections and supportive care to alleviate symptoms. Vaccination against common pathogens can help prevent CAP.*

Symptoms:

- Cough: May produce phlegm or pus, which can be green, yellow, or blood-tinged.
- Fever: High fever is common, often accompanied by chills and sweating.
- Shortness of Breath: Especially with exertion or deep breathing.
- Chest Pain: Sharp or stabbing pain that may worsen with coughing or deep breathing.
- Fatigue: Feeling tired or weak.
- Nausea, Vomiting, or Diarrhea: Especially in bacterial pneumonia.
- Confusion or Delirium: Particularly in older adults or patients with weakened immune systems.

Causes and Risk Factors:
- Age: Infants, young children, and older adults are at higher risk of developing community-acquired pneumonia.
- Weakened Immune System: Due to underlying medical conditions such as HIV/AIDS, cancer, organ transplantation, or medications that suppress the immune system.
- Chronic Medical Conditions: Such as chronic obstructive pulmonary disease (COPD), asthma, heart disease, or diabetes.
- Smoking: Tobacco smoke damages the lungs and impairs immune function, increasing the risk of pneumonia.
- Recent Respiratory Infections: Such as influenza or the common cold, which can weaken the immune system and make patients more susceptible to pneumonia.
- Hospitalization: Especially for patients on mechanical ventilation or with compromised immunity.
- Living Conditions: Crowded living spaces, such as nursing homes or prisons, increase the risk of pneumonia transmission.
- Aspiration: Inhaling food, drink, saliva, or vomit into the lungs, especially in patients with swallowing difficulties or altered consciousness.
- Alcoholism: Chronic alcohol abuse weakens the immune system and impairs lung function, increasing susceptibility to pneumonia.
- Exposure to Environmental Factors: Such as air pollution, indoor smoke from cooking or heating fuels, or occupational exposures to dust, chemicals, or fumes.

Workup and Diagnosis:
- <u>Medical History and Physical Examination:</u> Including assessment of symptoms and risk factors.
- <u>Chest X-ray:</u> Imaging test to visualize the lungs and detect areas of inflammation or consolidation characteristic of pneumonia.
- <u>Blood Tests:</u>
    - Complete Blood Count (CBC): To assess white blood cell count, which may be elevated in cases of bacterial pneumonia.
    - Blood Cultures: To identify the specific microorganism causing pneumonia, especially in severe cases or patients with risk factors for complicated pneumonia.
- <u>Sputum Culture and Gram Stain:</u> To identify bacteria or fungi in cases where bacterial or fungal pneumonia is suspected.

- **Pulse Oximetry:** Measures oxygen saturation in the blood, which may be decreased in cases of pneumonia-related respiratory failure.

Treatment:

- **Antibiotics:** If bacterial pneumonia is suspected or confirmed, appropriate antibiotics are prescribed based on the specific pathogen and antibiotic susceptibility testing.
- **Antiviral Medications:** If viral pneumonia is suspected or confirmed, antiviral medications may be prescribed for specific viral pathogens such as influenza or respiratory syncytial virus (RSV).
- **Supportive Care:**
  - Fluids: Adequate hydration to prevent dehydration.
  - Rest: Get plenty of rest to aid recovery.
  - Pain Relievers: Over-the-counter medications such as acetaminophen (Tylenol) or ibuprofen (Advil, Motrin) for pain and fever relief.
  - Oxygen Therapy: Supplemental oxygen may be provided for patients with severe pneumonia-related respiratory failure.
- **Hospitalization:** For patients with severe pneumonia, especially those with risk factors for complications or compromised immunity, hospitalization may be necessary for close monitoring and intravenous administration of antibiotics or supportive therapies.
- **Vaccination:** Annual influenza vaccination and pneumococcal vaccination are recommended to prevent pneumonia, especially in high-risk populations.

5.7. Healthcare-Associated Pneumonia

> ➤ *Healthcare-associated pneumonia (HCAP) refers to pneumonia that develops in patients who have recently received healthcare services, such as hospitalization, nursing home residence, or outpatient procedures.*
>
> ➤ *It is typically caused by multidrug-resistant organisms and is associated with higher rates of morbidity and mortality compared to community-acquired pneumonia.*
>
> ➤ *Management involves prompt diagnosis, appropriate antibiotic therapy, and infection control measures to prevent transmission in healthcare settings.*

Symptoms:

Symptoms of HCAP are similar to those of community-acquired pneumonia and may include:

- Cough: May produce phlegm or pus, which can be green, yellow, or blood-tinged.
- Fever: High fever is common, often accompanied by chills and sweating.
- Shortness of Breath: Especially with exertion or deep breathing.
- Chest Pain: Sharp or stabbing pain that may worsen with coughing or deep breathing.
- Fatigue: Feeling tired or weak.
- Nausea, Vomiting, or Diarrhea: Especially in bacterial pneumonia.
- Confusion or Delirium: Particularly in older adults or patients with weakened immune systems.

Causes and Risk Factors:

- Hospitalization: Recent hospitalization or admission to a long-term care facility within the past 90 days.
- Residence in Long-Term Care Facilities: Such as nursing homes or rehabilitation centers, where multidrug-resistant organisms are more prevalent.
- Recent Antibiotic Therapy: Especially broad-spectrum antibiotics, which can disrupt normal flora and promote the growth of multidrug-resistant organisms.
- Underlying Medical Conditions: Such as chronic obstructive pulmonary disease (COPD), heart failure, diabetes, or chronic kidney disease.
- Immunosuppression: Due to underlying medical conditions (e.g., HIV/AIDS, cancer) or medications (e.g., corticosteroids, chemotherapy).
- Advanced Age: Older adults are at higher risk of developing healthcare-associated pneumonia due to weakened immune function and higher rates of comorbidities.
- Invasive Devices or Procedures: Such as mechanical ventilation, endotracheal intubation, or placement of urinary catheters or feeding tubes, which increase the risk of nosocomial infections.
- Exposure to Healthcare Environments: Healthcare workers or patients who frequently visit healthcare facilities may be at increased risk of exposure to multidrug-resistant organisms.

Workup and Diagnosis:
- Medical History and Physical Examination: Including assessment of symptoms and risk factors.
- Chest X-ray: Imaging test to visualize the lungs and detect areas of inflammation or consolidation characteristic of pneumonia.
- Blood Tests:
    - Complete Blood Count (CBC): To assess white blood cell count, which may be elevated in cases of bacterial pneumonia.
    - Blood Cultures: To identify the specific microorganism causing pneumonia, especially in severe cases or patients with risk factors for complicated pneumonia.
- Sputum Culture and Gram Stain: To identify bacteria or fungi in cases where bacterial or fungal pneumonia is suspected.
- Pulse Oximetry: Measures oxygen saturation in the blood, which may be decreased in cases of pneumonia-related respiratory failure.

Treatment:
- Antibiotics:

    Empirical antibiotic therapy is initiated promptly, often with broad-spectrum antibiotics targeting multidrug-resistant organisms, until the specific pathogen and antibiotic susceptibility testing are available.

- Antimicrobial Stewardship:

    Healthcare facilities should have protocols in place to optimize antibiotic use, minimize unnecessary antibiotic exposure, and prevent the emergence of antibiotic resistance.

- Supportive Care:
    - Fluids: Adequate hydration to prevent dehydration.
    - Rest: Get plenty of rest to aid recovery.
    - Pain Relievers: Over-the-counter medications such as acetaminophen (Tylenol) or ibuprofen (Advil, Motrin) for pain and fever relief.
    - Oxygen Therapy: Supplemental oxygen may be provided for patients with severe pneumonia-related respiratory failure.
- Hospitalization:

    Most cases of healthcare-associated pneumonia require hospitalization for close monitoring and intravenous administration of antibiotics or supportive therapies.

5.8. Bronchitis

> ➢ *Bronchitis is inflammation of the bronchial tubes, commonly caused by viral infections or irritants like smoking.*
> ➢ *Symptoms include coughing, chest discomfort, and production of mucus, typically lasting for several weeks.*
> ➢ *Treatment involves rest, hydration, and symptom management with over-the-counter medications, while antibiotics may be prescribed for bacterial bronchitis in some cases.*

Symptoms:
- Cough: Initially dry and irritating, may progress to produce mucus (phlegm).
- Fatigue: Feeling tired or weak.
- Shortness of Breath: Especially with exertion.
- Chest Discomfort: Mild chest discomfort or tightness.
- Sore Throat: Due to postnasal drip from coughing.
- Mild Fever: Low-grade fever may be present, especially with acute bronchitis.

Causes and Risk Factors:
- Viral Infections: Acute bronchitis is commonly caused by viral infections, particularly respiratory syncytial virus (RSV), influenza viruses, or rhinoviruses.
- Smoking: Tobacco smoke irritates the bronchial tubes and increases the risk of both acute and chronic bronchitis.
- Exposure to Irritants: Such as air pollution, dust, or fumes from chemicals or industrial pollutants.
- Occupational Hazards: Certain occupations, such as coal mining, grain handling, or working with textiles or chemicals, involve exposure to respiratory irritants and increase the risk of bronchitis.
- Weakened Immune System: Due to underlying medical conditions (e.g., HIV/AIDS, chronic illness) or medications that suppress the immune system.
- Gastric Reflux: Acid reflux from the stomach can irritate the bronchial tubes and contribute to chronic bronchitis.

Workup and Diagnosis:
- <u>Medical History and Physical Examination:</u> Including assessment of symptoms, risk factors, and duration of symptoms.

- <u>Chest X-ray:</u> Imaging test to rule out other lung conditions such as pneumonia or chronic obstructive pulmonary disease (COPD).
- <u>Pulmonary Function Tests:</u> To assess lung function and rule out underlying conditions such as asthma or COPD.
- <u>Sputum Culture:</u> If bacterial infection is suspected, a sputum sample may be tested to identify the specific pathogen causing bronchitis.

Treatment:
- <u>Symptomatic Relief:</u>
    - Rest: Get plenty of rest to aid recovery.
    - Fluids: Drink plenty of fluids to stay hydrated and help loosen mucus.
    - Humidifiers: Use a humidifier to add moisture to the air and ease coughing.
    - Cough Suppressants or Expectorants: Over-the-counter medications may help relieve cough symptoms, though they should be used with caution, especially in children.
- <u>Pain Relievers:</u> Over-the-counter medications such as acetaminophen (Tylenol) or ibuprofen (Advil, Motrin) for pain and fever relief.
- <u>Avoidance of Irritants:</u> Such as cigarette smoke or air pollution, which can exacerbate bronchitis symptoms.
- <u>Antibiotics:</u> Only prescribed for bacterial bronchitis if symptoms are severe or prolonged, or if there is evidence of bacterial infection.
- <u>Bronchodilators:</u> Inhaled medications may be prescribed for patients with underlying lung conditions such as asthma or COPD to help open the airways and improve breathing.
- <u>Steroids:</u> Oral or inhaled corticosteroids may be prescribed for patients with severe or chronic bronchitis to reduce inflammation and improve symptoms.

5.9. Bronchiolitis

> ➢ *Bronchiolitis is a viral respiratory infection affecting the smallest air passages in the lungs, primarily in infants and young children.*
> ➢ *It commonly presents with symptoms like coughing, wheezing, and difficulty breathing, often triggered by respiratory syncytial virus (RSV).*
> ➢ *Treatment focuses on supportive care, such as hydration and monitoring, with severe cases sometimes requiring hospitalization for oxygen support.*

Symptoms:
- Cough: Initially dry, may progress to become productive.
- Runny Nose: Nasal congestion and discharge.
- Wheezing: High-pitched whistling sound when breathing, especially on exhaling.
- Rapid or Difficult Breathing: Respiratory distress, characterized by rapid breathing, flaring nostrils, and chest retractions.
- Fever: Low-grade fever is common, but some infants may have high fever.
- Irritability or Restlessness: Difficulty feeding or sleeping due to respiratory discomfort.
- Decreased Appetite: Reluctance to feed due to difficulty breathing.
- Fatigue: Excessive tiredness or weakness.

Causes and Risk Factors:
- Age: Bronchiolitis primarily affects infants and young children under the age of 2, with the highest incidence in infants aged 3-6 months.
- Season: Bronchiolitis is more common during the fall and winter months, coinciding with the peak season for respiratory syncytial virus (RSV) infections.
- Premature Birth: Preterm infants are at higher risk of developing severe bronchiolitis due to immature immune systems and underdeveloped airways.
- Underlying Health Conditions: Infants with underlying medical conditions such as congenital heart disease, chronic lung disease, or immunodeficiency are at increased risk of severe bronchiolitis.
- Exposure to Tobacco Smoke: Infants exposed to secondhand smoke are at higher risk of respiratory infections, including bronchiolitis.

- Crowded Living Conditions: Infants in crowded households or daycare settings are at increased risk of exposure to respiratory viruses.

Workup and Diagnosis:

- Medical History and Physical Examination: Including assessment of symptoms, age, and risk factors.
- Nasal Swab Test: Nasopharyngeal swab may be collected to test for respiratory viruses, particularly respiratory syncytial virus (RSV), which is the most common cause of bronchiolitis.
- Chest X-ray: May be performed in severe cases or if there is uncertainty about the diagnosis, though findings are typically nonspecific in bronchiolitis.

Treatment:

- Supportive Care:
    - Hydration: Ensuring adequate fluid intake to prevent dehydration, especially if feeding is affected.
    - Nasal Saline Drops: To help clear nasal congestion and improve breathing.
    - Humidified Air: Using a humidifier to add moisture to the air and ease respiratory symptoms.
- Monitoring:

    Close observation of respiratory status, hydration, and overall condition, especially in infants with severe symptoms or underlying health conditions.

- Oxygen Therapy: Supplemental oxygen may be provided for infants with severe respiratory distress or low oxygen levels.
- Inhaled Bronchodilators: May be considered in some cases, though evidence supporting their effectiveness in bronchiolitis is limited.
- Antiviral Medications:

    Palivizumab, a monoclonal antibody, may be recommended for certain high-risk infants to prevent severe RSV infections, though it is not routinely used for the treatment of bronchiolitis.

- Hospitalization:

    Infants with severe bronchiolitis, respiratory distress, dehydration, or underlying medical conditions may require hospitalization for close monitoring and supportive care.

5.10. Tuberculosis

> ➢ *Tuberculosis (TB) is a bacterial infection caused by Mycobacterium tuberculosis, primarily affecting the lungs but can involve other organs.*
>
> ➢ *Symptoms include persistent cough, weight loss, fever, and night sweats, with transmission occurring through airborne particles.*
>
> ➢ *Treatment involves a combination of antibiotics taken for several months to cure the infection and prevent transmission.*

Symptoms:
- Cough: Persistent cough lasting more than three weeks, often with blood-tinged sputum.
- Fever: Low-grade fever, particularly in the afternoon or evening.
- Night Sweats: Profuse sweating, especially during sleep.
- Fatigue: Feeling tired or weak, often accompanied by decreased appetite and weight loss.
- Chills: Especially in the early stages of infection.
- Shortness of Breath: Especially with exertion or advanced disease.
- Chest Pain: Pain or discomfort in the chest, particularly with deep breathing or coughing.
- Loss of Appetite: Decreased appetite and unintended weight loss.
- Swollen Lymph Nodes: Particularly in the neck.

Causes and Risk Factors:
- Close Contact with an Infected Person: patients who live or work in close proximity to someone with active TB are at higher risk of infection.
- Immune System Compromise: patients with weakened immune systems, such as those with HIV/AIDS, diabetes, or undergoing immunosuppressive therapy, are at increased risk of developing active TB disease.
- Healthcare Settings: Healthcare workers and patients receiving medical care in facilities where TB patients are treated are at higher risk of exposure.
- Substance Abuse: Injection drug use increases the risk of TB infection.

- Crowded Living Conditions: Homeless shelters, prisons, and refugee camps with overcrowded and poorly ventilated environments increase the risk of TB transmission.
- Travel to High-Incidence Areas: Travel to or residence in regions with high rates of TB increases the risk of exposure and infection.
- Age: Infants, young children, and the elderly are at higher risk of developing active TB disease.
- Malnutrition: Poor nutrition weakens the immune system and increases susceptibility to TB infection.
- Tobacco Use: Smoking damages the lungs and increases the risk of TB disease.

Workup and Diagnosis:
- Medical History and Physical Examination: Including assessment of symptoms and risk factors.
- Tuberculin Skin Test (TST) or Interferon-Gamma Release Assays (IGRAs): Blood tests to detect immune response to TB infection.
- Chest X-ray: Imaging test to visualize the lungs and detect abnormalities suggestive of TB infection or disease.
- Sputum Culture: Collection and testing of sputum samples to identify the presence of Mycobacterium tuberculosis bacteria.
- Molecular Testing: Polymerase chain reaction (PCR) tests to detect TB DNA in sputum samples, providing rapid diagnosis.

Treatment:
- Drug Therapy: Treatment for active TB disease typically involves a combination of antibiotics taken for several months to kill the bacteria and prevent the development of drug resistance.
    - First-Line Drugs: Isoniazid, rifampin, ethambutol, and pyrazinamide are commonly used as first-line drugs for TB treatment.
    - Directly Observed Therapy (DOT): the APP or trained personnel may directly observe patients taking their medications to ensure adherence and treatment completion.
- Preventive Therapy:

    Patients with latent TB infection (positive TST or IGRA without active disease) may receive preventive therapy with isoniazid to reduce the risk of developing active TB disease.
- Contact Investigation:

Identifying and testing patients who have had close contact with a person with active TB disease to detect and treat latent TB infection or active disease.
- Supportive Care:

    Adequate nutrition, rest, and symptom management to support recovery and minimize complications associated with TB disease and treatment.

5.11. Chronic Obstructive Pulmonary Disease

> ➢ *Chronic Obstructive Pulmonary Disease (COPD) is a progressive lung condition characterized by airflow limitation and breathing difficulties.*
> ➢ *It's commonly caused by long-term exposure to irritants like cigarette smoke and presents with symptoms such as coughing, wheezing, and shortness of breath.*
> ➢ *Treatment aims to alleviate symptoms, improve lung function, and prevent exacerbations through medications, pulmonary rehabilitation, and lifestyle changes.*

Symptoms:
- Chronic Cough: Persistent cough that produces mucus (sputum).
- Shortness of Breath: Especially with physical activity, progressively worsening over time.
- Wheezing: High-pitched whistling sound when breathing, particularly during exhalation.
- Chest Tightness: Feeling of constriction or pressure in the chest.
- Fatigue: Feeling tired or lacking energy, especially during exertion.
- Frequent Respiratory Infections: Increased susceptibility to respiratory infections, such as colds, flu, or pneumonia.

Causes and Risk Factors:
- Smoking: Tobacco smoke is the primary cause of COPD, accounting for the majority of cases.
- Environmental Exposures: Long-term exposure to pollutants or irritants, such as secondhand smoke, air pollution, chemical fumes, or dust, increases the risk of COPD.
- Genetic Factors: A rare genetic disorder called alpha-1 antitrypsin deficiency predisposes patients to early-onset COPD, particularly in non-smokers.

- Age: COPD is more common in older adults, with the risk increasing with age.
- Occupational Exposures: Certain occupations with exposure to dust, chemicals, or fumes, such as coal mining, construction, or manufacturing, increase the risk of COPD.
- Asthma: patients with poorly controlled or longstanding asthma are at higher risk of developing COPD.
- Respiratory Infections: Severe or frequent respiratory infections, particularly in childhood, may increase the risk of developing COPD later in life.
- Poor Lung Growth and Development: Factors such as low birth weight, childhood respiratory infections, or maternal smoking during pregnancy can impair lung growth and increase susceptibility to COPD later in life.

Workup and Diagnosis:
- Medical History and Physical Examination: Including assessment of symptoms, risk factors, and lung function.
- Spirometry: Lung function test to measure airflow obstruction and assess the severity of COPD.
- Chest X-ray: Imaging test to visualize the lungs and detect signs of COPD, such as hyperinflation or flattening of the diaphragm.
- Blood Tests: Arterial blood gas analysis to assess oxygen and carbon dioxide levels in the blood, which may be abnormal in advanced COPD.

Treatment:
- Smoking Cessation:

    The most important intervention in managing COPD is quitting smoking to slow disease progression and reduce symptoms.

- Medications:
    - Bronchodilators: Inhaled medications such as short-acting or long-acting bronchodilators (beta-agonists or anticholinergics) to relax the muscles around the airways and improve airflow.
    - Inhaled Corticosteroids: Used in combination with bronchodilators to reduce airway inflammation and prevent exacerbations in some patients.
- Pulmonary Rehabilitation:

    Comprehensive program including exercise training, education, and support to improve quality of life and reduce symptoms.

- Oxygen Therapy:

    Supplemental oxygen may be prescribed for patients with severe COPD and low blood oxygen levels, particularly during exertion or sleep.

- Surgery:

    In some cases, surgical interventions such as lung volume reduction surgery or lung transplantation may be considered for severe COPD.

- Vaccinations:

    Annual influenza vaccination and pneumococcal vaccination to prevent respiratory infections and exacerbations of COPD.

- Lifestyle Modifications:

    Avoiding exposure to irritants or pollutants, maintaining a healthy diet, staying physically active within limits, and managing comorbid conditions such as obesity or heart disease.

5.12. Bronchiectasis

> ➤ *Bronchiectasis is a chronic lung condition characterized by abnormal widening and scarring of the bronchial tubes, leading to mucus buildup and recurrent infections.*
>
> ➤ *Symptoms include chronic cough, excessive mucus production, and recurrent respiratory infections.*
>
> ➤ *Treatment focuses on clearing mucus, managing infections, and improving lung function through medications, airway clearance techniques, and sometimes surgery.*

Symptoms:

- Chronic Cough: Persistent cough that produces large amounts of mucus (sputum).
- Recurrent Respiratory Infections: Frequent episodes of bronchitis, pneumonia, or other respiratory infections.
- Shortness of Breath: Especially with physical activity, coughing, or exertion.
- Wheezing: High-pitched whistling sound when breathing, particularly during exhalation.

- Chest Pain: Discomfort or tightness in the chest, especially with coughing or deep breathing.
- Fatigue: Feeling tired or lacking energy, especially during respiratory exacerbations.

Causes and Risk Factors:
- Chronic Respiratory Infections: Severe or recurrent respiratory infections, especially in childhood, can lead to bronchiectasis.
- Cystic Fibrosis: Bronchiectasis is a common complication of cystic fibrosis, a genetic disorder affecting the lungs and digestive system.
- Immunodeficiency: Conditions that weaken the immune system, such as HIV/AIDS or immunosuppressive therapy, increase the risk of bronchiectasis.
- Autoimmune Disorders: Certain autoimmune conditions, such as rheumatoid arthritis or Sjögren's syndrome, are associated with bronchiectasis.
- Obstructive Lung Diseases: Conditions that obstruct the airways, such as chronic obstructive pulmonary disease (COPD) or asthma, can predispose patients to bronchiectasis.
- Aspiration: Inhalation of foreign substances, such as food or gastric contents, into the lungs can cause chronic inflammation and bronchiectasis.
- Smoking: Tobacco smoke irritates the airways and increases the risk of respiratory infections and bronchiectasis.
- Environmental Exposures: Long-term exposure to pollutants, such as air pollution, chemical fumes, or dust, can contribute to bronchiectasis.

Workup and Diagnosis:
- <u>Medical History and Physical Examination:</u> Including assessment of symptoms, risk factors, and previous respiratory infections.
- <u>Chest Imaging:</u>
    Chest X-ray or computed tomography (CT) scan to visualize the lungs and detect characteristic signs of bronchiectasis, such as dilated bronchi and thickened airway walls.
- <u>Sputum Culture:</u> Collection and testing of sputum samples to identify the presence of bacteria or other pathogens causing respiratory infections.
- <u>Pulmonary Function Tests:</u> Lung function tests to assess airflow obstruction and lung capacity.

- Bronchoscopy:

    Procedure to visualize the airways and collect samples for further evaluation, particularly in cases of suspected aspiration or underlying airway abnormalities.

Treatment:

- Antibiotics: Treatment of respiratory infections with appropriate antibiotics to control bacterial overgrowth and prevent exacerbations.

- Airway Clearance Techniques:

    Methods such as chest physiotherapy, postural drainage, percussion, and vibration to help clear mucus from the airways and improve lung function.

- Bronchodilators:

    Inhaled medications to relax the muscles around the airways and improve airflow, particularly in patients with underlying obstructive lung diseases.

- Mucus-Thinning Medications:

    Oral or inhaled medications such as mucolytics or hypertonic saline to help thin mucus and make it easier to clear from the airways.

- Pulmonary Rehabilitation:

    Comprehensive program including exercise training, education, and support to improve quality of life and reduce symptoms.

- Oxygen Therapy:

    Supplemental oxygen may be prescribed for patients with severe bronchiectasis and low blood oxygen levels, particularly during exertion or sleep.

- Surgery:

    In some cases, surgical interventions such as lung resection or lung transplantation may be considered for severe, localized bronchiectasis that does not respond to conservative treatment.

5.13. Asthma

> ➤ Asthma is a chronic lung condition characterized by inflammation and narrowing of the airways, leading to recurrent episodes of wheezing, coughing, chest tightness, and shortness of breath.
>
> ➤ Triggers include allergens, irritants, and respiratory infections, with treatment involving medications like bronchodilators and corticosteroids to control symptoms and prevent exacerbations, along with avoidance of triggers and proper management plans.

Symptoms:

- Wheezing: High-pitched whistling sound when breathing, particularly during exhalation.
- Shortness of Breath: Difficulty breathing, especially with physical activity or during asthma attacks.
- Chest Tightness: Feeling of constriction or pressure in the chest.
- Coughing: Persistent cough, particularly at night or early in the morning, may be the only symptom in some patients.
- Respiratory Distress: Rapid breathing, flaring nostrils, and chest retractions during severe asthma attacks.
- Fatigue: Feeling tired or lacking energy, especially during or after asthma exacerbations.

Causes and Risk Factors:

- Family History: patients with a family history of asthma or allergic conditions are at higher risk of developing asthma.
- Allergies: Sensitivity to allergens such as pollen, dust mites, pet dander, or mold increases the risk of asthma.
- Environmental Exposures: Exposure to tobacco smoke, air pollution, chemical irritants, or occupational triggers (e.g., dust, fumes) can trigger or exacerbate asthma symptoms.
- Respiratory Infections: Viral respiratory infections, particularly during childhood, can increase the risk of developing asthma.
- Obesity: Obesity is associated with an increased risk of asthma and may worsen asthma symptoms.
- Exercise: Exercise-induced asthma is common in some patients, particularly in cold, dry air or during intense physical activity.

- Occupational Exposures: Certain occupations with exposure to irritants or allergens, such as agriculture, manufacturing, or healthcare, may increase the risk of asthma.
- Childhood Factors: Factors such as low birth weight, maternal smoking during pregnancy, or early exposure to tobacco smoke increase the risk of childhood asthma.
- Gastroesophageal Reflux Disease (GERD): Acid reflux from the stomach can worsen asthma symptoms in some patients.

Workup and Diagnosis:
- <u>Medical History and Physical Examination:</u> Including assessment of symptoms, triggers, and family history of asthma or allergic conditions.
- <u>Lung Function Tests:</u> Spirometry or peak flow meter measurements to assess airflow obstruction and lung function.
- <u>Allergy Testing:</u> Skin prick tests or blood tests to identify specific allergens that may trigger asthma symptoms.
- <u>Bronchial Provocation Tests:</u> Inhalation tests to assess airway responsiveness to various stimuli, such as methacholine or exercise.
- <u>Chest X-ray or CT Scan:</u> Imaging tests to rule out other lung conditions or complications of asthma, particularly in severe or atypical cases.

Treatment:
- <u>Medications:</u>
  - Bronchodilators: Quick-relief medications such as short-acting beta-agonists (e.g., albuterol) to relieve acute asthma symptoms and open the airways during attacks.
  - Inhaled Corticosteroids: Long-term control medications to reduce airway inflammation and prevent asthma exacerbations.
  - Combination Inhalers: Medications containing both a bronchodilator and a corticosteroid for convenience and improved asthma control.
  - Leukotriene Modifiers: Oral medications to reduce inflammation and improve asthma control, particularly in patients with allergic asthma.
- <u>Allergen Avoidance:</u>

  Minimizing exposure to known allergens or triggers, such as dust mites, pollen, pet dander, or mold, to prevent asthma exacerbations.

- **Trigger Management:** Identifying and avoiding asthma triggers such as tobacco smoke, air pollution, cold air, exercise, or respiratory infections.
- **Immunotherapy:**

    Allergy shots or sublingual immunotherapy to desensitize patients to specific allergens and reduce asthma symptoms in allergic asthma.
- **Pulmonary Rehabilitation:**

    Comprehensive program including education, exercise training, and support to improve asthma management and quality of life.
- **Biologic Therapies:**

    Targeted therapies for severe asthma, such as monoclonal antibodies targeting specific inflammatory pathways (e.g., anti-IgE, anti-IL-5), may be considered in some cases.
- **Emergency Treatment:**

    Prompt administration of bronchodilators and systemic corticosteroids during severe asthma exacerbations or attacks, followed by close monitoring and evaluation in a healthcare setting.

5.14. Interstitial Lung Diseases

> *Interstitial lung diseases (ILD) encompass a group of disorders characterized by inflammation and scarring of the lung tissue between the air sacs.*
>
> *Symptoms include shortness of breath, cough, and fatigue, often progressing to irreversible fibrosis.*
>
> *Treatment involves managing symptoms, addressing underlying causes, and in some cases, lung transplantation for advanced disease.*

Symptoms:

- Dry Cough: Persistent cough that may worsen over time.
- Shortness of Breath: Especially with exertion, progressively worsening over time.
- Fatigue: Feeling tired or lacking energy, often due to decreased oxygen levels in the blood.
- Weakness: Reduced physical stamina and strength.

- Clubbing of Fingers or Toes: Enlargement and rounding of the fingertips or toes, a sign of chronic oxygen deficiency.
- Chest Discomfort: Chest pain or discomfort, particularly with breathing or coughing.
- Unintended Weight Loss: Loss of appetite and weight loss, particularly in advanced stages of ILD.

Causes and Risk Factors:
- Occupational Exposures: Exposure to occupational hazards such as asbestos, silica dust, coal dust, or agricultural dust increases the risk of developing ILD.
- Environmental Exposures: Exposure to environmental pollutants, such as air pollution, mold, or bird droppings, can contribute to ILD.
- Smoking: Tobacco smoke is a known risk factor for several types of ILD, including idiopathic pulmonary fibrosis (IPF).
- Age: ILD is more common in older adults, with the risk increasing with age.
- Genetic Factors: Some forms of ILD, such as familial pulmonary fibrosis, have a genetic component.
- Connective Tissue Diseases: Certain autoimmune diseases, such as rheumatoid arthritis, scleroderma, or systemic lupus erythematosus (SLE), are associated with ILD.
- Medications: Some medications, such as certain chemotherapy drugs, antibiotics, or anti-inflammatory agents, can cause drug-induced ILD.
- Radiation Therapy: Previous radiation therapy to the chest or lungs increases the risk of developing ILD.
- Gastroesophageal Reflux Disease (GERD): Chronic acid reflux from the stomach can worsen ILD symptoms in some patients.

Workup and Diagnosis:
- <u>Medical History and Physical Examination:</u> Including assessment of symptoms, risk factors, and family history of ILD or autoimmune diseases.
- <u>Pulmonary Function Tests (PFTs):</u> Lung function tests to assess airflow obstruction, lung volumes, and gas exchange.
- <u>High-Resolution Computed Tomography (HRCT):</u>
    - Imaging test to visualize the lungs in detail and detect characteristic signs of ILD, such as fibrosis, honeycombing, or ground-glass opacities.

- Bronchoscopy:

    Procedure to examine the airways and collect samples (biopsies) for further evaluation, particularly in cases of suspected infection or malignancy.

- Blood Tests:

    Including autoimmune antibodies (e.g., antinuclear antibodies, rheumatoid factor) and markers of inflammation (e.g., C-reactive protein, erythrocyte sedimentation rate) to assess for underlying autoimmune diseases or inflammation.

- Pulmonary Exercise Testing: Exercise testing to evaluate exercise capacity and oxygen uptake during physical exertion.

- Lung Biopsy:

    Surgical or minimally invasive procedure to obtain a tissue sample for pathological examination and confirmation of ILD diagnosis, particularly in cases of uncertain diagnosis or suspected underlying conditions.

Treatment:

- Medications:
    - Corticosteroids: Oral or inhaled corticosteroids to reduce inflammation and slow disease progression in some forms of ILD.
    - Immunosuppressive Agents: Medications such as azathioprine, mycophenolate, or cyclophosphamide to suppress the immune system and reduce inflammation in autoimmune-related ILD.
    - Antifibrotic Agents: Pirfenidone and nintedanib are FDA-approved medications for idiopathic pulmonary fibrosis (IPF) that can slow disease progression and reduce decline in lung function.

- Oxygen Therapy: Supplemental oxygen may be prescribed for patients with ILD and low blood oxygen levels, particularly during exertion or sleep.

- Pulmonary Rehabilitation: Comprehensive program including exercise training, education, and support to improve quality of life and reduce symptoms.

- Supportive Care: Adequate nutrition, rest, and symptom management to support overall health and well-being.

- Lung Transplantation: Considered for patients with advanced ILD and severe respiratory impairment who do not respond to other treatments.

- Clinical Trials: Participation in clinical research studies or trials investigating new treatments or interventions for ILD.

5.15. Sarcoidosis

> ➤ *Sarcoidosis is a multisystem inflammatory disease characterized by the formation of granulomas, affecting various organs, most commonly the lungs and lymph nodes.*
> ➤ *Symptoms include cough, shortness of breath, fatigue, and skin lesions, with treatment focusing on managing symptoms and inflammation using corticosteroids or other immunosuppressive medications.*
> ➤ *The cause of sarcoidosis is unclear, but it's believed to involve immune system dysfunction.*

Symptoms:
- Respiratory Symptoms: Persistent dry cough, shortness of breath, chest pain, and wheezing.
- Lymph Node Enlargement: Swelling of lymph nodes, particularly in the neck, armpits, or groin.
- Fatigue: Feeling tired or lacking energy, often due to inflammation and immune activation.
- Fever: Low-grade fever, particularly in the early stages of sarcoidosis.
- Skin Lesions: Skin rash, nodules, or discoloration, often on the face, arms, or legs.
- Eye Symptoms: Eye redness, pain, dryness, or blurred vision, due to inflammation of the eyes (uveitis).
- Joint Pain: Arthritis-like symptoms, including joint pain, stiffness, and swelling.
- Neurological Symptoms: Headaches, dizziness, weakness, or numbness, due to involvement of the nervous system.
- Cardiac Symptoms: Palpitations, chest pain, or shortness of breath due to cardiac involvement (cardiac sarcoidosis).

Causes and Risk Factors:
- Age and Gender: Sarcoidosis can occur at any age but is most common in adults aged 20 to 40 years, and it is slightly more common in women than men.

- Ethnicity: Sarcoidosis is more common in certain ethnic groups, including African Americans, Northern Europeans, and patients of Scandinavian descent.
- Family History: patients with a family history of sarcoidosis are at higher risk of developing the condition, suggesting a genetic predisposition.
- Environmental Exposures: Exposure to certain environmental factors or occupational hazards may trigger sarcoidosis in susceptible patients, though specific triggers are not well-understood.
- Occupational Exposures: Some studies have suggested an increased risk of sarcoidosis in occupations with exposure to organic dust, gases, or chemicals, though the evidence is limited.

Workup and Diagnosis:
- Medical History and Physical Examination: Including assessment of symptoms, risk factors, and family history of sarcoidosis or autoimmune diseases.
- Chest X-ray or CT Scan:

    Imaging tests to visualize the lungs and detect characteristic signs of sarcoidosis, such as bilateral hilar lymphadenopathy and pulmonary infiltrates.
- Pulmonary Function Tests (PFTs): Lung function tests to assess airflow obstruction, lung volumes, and gas exchange.
- Biopsy: Sampling of affected tissues (e.g., lung, skin, lymph nodes) to confirm the presence of granulomas and rule out other conditions.
- Blood Tests:

    Including tests for inflammatory markers (e.g., C-reactive protein, erythrocyte sedimentation rate) and markers of organ function (e.g., liver enzymes, kidney function tests).
- Eye Examination:

    Evaluation by an ophthalmologist to assess for eye involvement (uveitis) and monitor for complications such as glaucoma or cataracts.

Treatment:
- Observation: In many cases, sarcoidosis may resolve on its own without specific treatment, especially in mild cases with minimal symptoms.
- Corticosteroids:

Oral or inhaled corticosteroids are commonly used to reduce inflammation and suppress the immune response in moderate to severe cases of sarcoidosis.

- Immunosuppressive Agents:

    Medications such as methotrexate, azathioprine, or mycophenolate may be used as steroid-sparing agents or in combination with corticosteroids for refractory or severe cases.

- Biologic Therapies:

    Targeted therapies such as tumor necrosis factor (TNF) inhibitors (e.g., infliximab, adalimumab) or interleukin-1 (IL-1) inhibitors (e.g., anakinra) may be considered for patients with severe, refractory sarcoidosis.

- Symptom Management: Treatment of specific symptoms or complications such as skin lesions, joint pain, eye inflammation, or cardiac involvement.

- Pulmonary Rehabilitation:

    Comprehensive program including exercise training, education, and support to improve quality of life and manage respiratory symptoms.

- Monitoring and Follow-up:

    Regular monitoring of symptoms, lung function, and organ function, with adjustments to treatment as needed to optimize disease management.

5.16. Hypersensitivity Pneumonitis

> ➤ *Hypersensitivity pneumonitis is an inflammatory lung disease caused by repeated inhalation of allergens or irritants, triggering an immune response in the lungs.*
>
> ➤ *Symptoms include cough, shortness of breath, and fatigue, often developing gradually and worsening with continued exposure.*
>
> ➤ *Treatment involves avoiding triggers and, in severe cases, using corticosteroids or other immunosuppressive medications to reduce inflammation.*

Symptoms:

- Respiratory Symptoms: Persistent cough, shortness of breath, chest tightness, and wheezing.

- Flu-like Symptoms: Fever, chills, fatigue, and muscle aches, particularly after exposure to triggering allergens.
- Dyspnea: Difficulty breathing, especially with exertion or during acute exacerbations.
- Malaise: General feeling of discomfort, weakness, or ill health.
- Weight Loss: Unintended weight loss due to decreased appetite and energy expenditure.
- Clubbing of Fingers or Toes: Enlargement and rounding of the fingertips or toes, a sign of chronic oxygen deficiency in advanced cases.

Causes and Risk Factors:
- Exposure to Allergens: Regular exposure to organic dust, mold, bird droppings, or other environmental allergens or irritants is the primary risk factor for developing HP.
- Occupational Exposures: Certain occupations with exposure to specific allergens or irritants, such as farming, bird handling, woodworking, or working in textile factories, increase the risk of HP.
- Environmental Exposures: Living in or near environments with high levels of mold, bird droppings, or other organic dust can increase the risk of HP.
- Genetic Factors: Some patients may have a genetic predisposition to developing HP, though specific genetic factors are not well-understood.
- Smoking: Smoking may increase the risk of developing HP or exacerbate existing symptoms in susceptible patients.
- Age: HP can occur at any age but is more common in adults, with the risk increasing with age.

Workup and Diagnosis:
- <u>Medical History and Physical Examination:</u> Including assessment of symptoms, occupational or environmental exposures, and risk factors for HP.
- <u>Pulmonary Function Tests (PFTs):</u> Lung function tests to assess airflow obstruction, lung volumes, and gas exchange.
- <u>High-Resolution Computed Tomography (HRCT):</u>
    Imaging test to visualize the lungs and detect characteristic signs of HP, such as ground-glass opacities, nodular infiltrates, or mosaic attenuation patterns.
- <u>Serological Testing:</u>

> Blood tests to measure levels of specific antibodies (e.g., precipitating antibodies) against common HP antigens, though serological testing alone is not diagnostic.

- Bronchoalveolar Lavage (BAL):

    Procedure to collect samples of fluid from the lungs for analysis, including cell counts, differential, and examination for inflammatory markers or organisms.

- Lung Biopsy:

    Surgical or minimally invasive procedure to obtain a tissue sample for pathological examination and confirmation of HP diagnosis, particularly in cases of uncertain diagnosis or atypical presentation.

Treatment:

- Avoidance of Triggering Allergens: The most important aspect of managing HP is avoiding exposure to known allergens or irritants that trigger symptoms.
- Corticosteroids:

    Oral or inhaled corticosteroids are commonly used to reduce inflammation and suppress the immune response during acute exacerbations of HP.

- Immunosuppressive Agents:

    Medications such as azathioprine, mycophenolate, or cyclophosphamide may be used as steroid-sparing agents or in combination with corticosteroids for refractory or severe cases of HP.

- Symptom Management: Treatment of specific symptoms or complications such as respiratory infections, cough, shortness of breath, or fever.
- Pulmonary Rehabilitation:

    Comprehensive program including exercise training, education, and support to improve quality of life and manage respiratory symptoms.

- Oxygen Therapy: Supplemental oxygen may be prescribed for patients with HP and low blood oxygen levels, particularly during exertion or sleep.
- Monitoring and Follow-up: Regular monitoring of symptoms, lung function, and disease progression, with adjustments to treatment as needed to optimize disease management.

5.17. Obstructive Sleep Apnea

> ➤ *Obstructive sleep apnea (OSA) is a sleep disorder characterized by repeated episodes of partial or complete blockage of the upper airway during sleep, leading to breathing pauses and disrupted sleep patterns.*
>
> ➤ *Symptoms include loud snoring, daytime sleepiness, and morning headaches, with risk factors including obesity and anatomical abnormalities.*
>
> ➤ *Treatment options include continuous positive airway pressure (CPAP) therapy, oral appliances, lifestyle changes, and in some cases, surgery to alleviate airway obstruction.*

Symptoms:

- Loud Snoring: Persistent, loud snoring, often accompanied by gasping or choking sounds during sleep.
- Breathing Pauses: Episodes of breathing cessation (apneas) or shallow breathing (hypopneas) during sleep, observed by a bed partner.
- Excessive Daytime Sleepiness: Feeling tired, fatigued, or sleepy during the day, despite adequate time spent in bed.
- Morning Headaches: Headaches upon waking in the morning, often due to altered oxygen levels and disrupted sleep.
- Difficulty Concentrating: Impaired concentration, memory problems, or decreased cognitive function.
- Irritability: Mood changes, irritability, or difficulty coping with stress.
- Frequent Nighttime Urination: Nocturia, or waking up multiple times during the night to urinate.
- Dry Mouth or Sore Throat: Dry mouth, sore throat, or hoarseness upon waking, due to mouth breathing or snoring.
- Witnessed Pauses in Breathing: Family members or bed partners may observe pauses in breathing during sleep.

Causes and Risk Factors:

- Obesity: Excess body weight, particularly fat deposits around the neck, increases the risk of airway obstruction during sleep.
- Neck Circumference: Large neck circumference (>17 inches in men, >16 inches in women) is associated with an increased risk of OSA.

- Male Gender: Men are at higher risk of OSA compared to premenopausal women, though the risk equalizes after menopause.
- Age: OSA becomes more common with age, particularly after age 40.
- Family History: Having a family history of OSA or sleep disorders increases the risk of developing OSA.
- Anatomical Factors: Structural abnormalities of the upper airway, such as enlarged tonsils, deviated septum, or recessed chin, increase the risk of airway obstruction.
- Smoking: Tobacco smoke irritates the airways and increases inflammation, contributing to airway narrowing and OSA.
- Alcohol and Sedative Use: Alcohol and sedatives relax the muscles of the upper airway, increasing the risk of airway collapse during sleep.
- Medical Conditions: Certain medical conditions such as hypertension, diabetes, heart failure, and hormonal disorders (e.g., hypothyroidism, acromegaly) increase the risk of OSA.
- Ethnicity: OSA is more common in certain ethnic groups, including African Americans, Hispanics, and Pacific Islanders.

Workup and Diagnosis:
- <u>Medical History and Physical Examination:</u> Including assessment of symptoms, risk factors, and comorbidities associated with OSA.
- <u>Sleep Questionnaires:</u>
    - Screening tools such as the Epworth Sleepiness Scale (ESS) or STOP-BANG questionnaire to assess daytime sleepiness and risk of OSA.
- <u>Polysomnography (Sleep Study):</u>
    - Overnight sleep study conducted in a sleep laboratory or home setting to monitor physiological parameters including airflow, respiratory effort, oxygen saturation, and sleep stages.
- <u>Home Sleep Apnea Testing (HSAT):</u>
    - Portable sleep monitoring device used for screening and diagnosis of OSA in select patients with high pretest probability and no significant comorbidities.
- <u>Physical Examination:</u> Evaluation of the upper airway, neck circumference, tonsil size, and signs of nasal obstruction or craniofacial abnormalities.

- Imaging Studies:

    Imaging tests such as lateral neck X-ray, CT scan, or MRI may be performed to evaluate the upper airway anatomy and identify structural abnormalities.

Treatment:
- Continuous Positive Airway Pressure (CPAP):
    - CPAP therapy is the first-line treatment for OSA and involves wearing a mask connected to a machine that delivers a continuous stream of air to keep the airway open during sleep.
    - CPAP is highly effective in reducing symptoms, improving sleep quality, and preventing complications associated with OSA.
- Oral Appliance Therapy:
    - Dental devices or oral appliances may be prescribed for patients with mild to moderate OSA or those who cannot tolerate CPAP therapy.
    - These devices work by repositioning the lower jaw or tongue to prevent airway collapse during sleep.
- Lifestyle Modifications:
    - Weight loss: Achieving and maintaining a healthy weight through diet and exercise can significantly improve OSA symptoms, particularly in overweight or obese patients.
    - Avoiding alcohol and sedatives: Limiting alcohol consumption and avoiding sedative medications can reduce the risk of airway collapse during sleep.
    - Positional therapy: Avoiding sleeping on the back (supine position) may help reduce airway obstruction in some patients with positional OSA.
- Surgery:

    Surgical interventions such as uvulopalatopharyngoplasty (UPPP), tonsillectomy, septoplasty, or maxillomandibular advancement may be considered for select patients with anatomical abnormalities or severe OSA refractory to conservative treatment.
- Adaptive Servo-Ventilation (ASV):

    ASV therapy is a type of positive airway pressure therapy that adjusts pressure levels based on respiratory patterns, particularly for patients with complex sleep apnea syndrome or central sleep apnea with Cheyne-Stokes respiration.

- Bilevel Positive Airway Pressure (BiPAP):
    BiPAP therapy delivers two levels of positive airway pressure (higher pressure during inhalation, lower pressure during exhalation) and may be used for patients who cannot tolerate CPAP therapy.

5.18. Cystic Fibrosis

> ➢ Cystic fibrosis (CF) is a genetic disorder that primarily affects the lungs and digestive system, leading to thick and sticky mucus production.
> ➢ Symptoms include chronic cough, recurrent lung infections, poor growth, and digestive problems.
> ➢ Treatment involves airway clearance techniques, medications to improve lung function, nutritional support, and specialized care to manage complications.

Symptoms:

Respiratory Symptoms:
- Persistent cough, often with thick mucus.
- Wheezing or shortness of breath, especially with exertion.
- Frequent respiratory infections, such as pneumonia or bronchitis.
- Nasal congestion or sinusitis.
- Digital clubbing (enlarged fingertips).

Gastrointestinal Symptoms:
- Pancreatic insufficiency leading to malabsorption of nutrients, resulting in:
    - Poor weight gain or failure to thrive in infants.
    - Greasy, foul-smelling stools (steatorrhea).
    - Abdominal pain or discomfort.
    - Nutritional deficiencies, including fat-soluble vitamins (A, D, E, K).
- Meconium ileus in newborns, a blockage of the intestine.

Other Symptoms:
- Salt loss in sweat, leading to salty-tasting skin.
- Dehydration and electrolyte imbalances.

- Delayed puberty or infertility in males due to congenital absence of the vas deferens.
- Increased susceptibility to heat-related illness.

Causes and Risk Factors:
- Genetic Factors: CF is an autosomal recessive genetic disorder caused by mutations in the CFTR gene. patients must inherit two copies of the defective CFTR gene (one from each parent) to develop CF.
- Family History: Having a family history of CF increases the risk of inheriting the disease.
- Ethnicity: CF occurs in patients of all ethnicities, but it is more common in Caucasians of northern European descent.
- Carrier Status: Parents who are carriers of the CF gene have a 1 in 4 chance of having a child with CF with each pregnancy.
- Consanguinity: Offspring of consanguineous couples (related by blood) have an increased risk of inheriting autosomal recessive disorders, including CF.

Workup and Diagnosis:
- <u>Newborn Screening:</u>

    CF is routinely screened for in newborns using a blood test to detect elevated levels of immunoreactive trypsinogen (IRT). Positive screening results are followed by additional diagnostic tests.

- <u>Sweat Chloride Test:</u>

    The gold standard diagnostic test for CF measures the concentration of chloride in sweat. Elevated sweat chloride levels (>60 mEq/L) confirm the diagnosis of CF.

- <u>Genetic Testing:</u> Molecular genetic testing can identify mutations in the CFTR gene, confirming the diagnosis of CF and identifying specific mutations.

- <u>Pulmonary Function Tests (PFTs):</u>

    Lung function tests such as spirometry or forced expiratory volume in 1 second (FEV1) measure lung function and assess the severity of respiratory impairment.

- <u>Imaging Studies:</u>

    Chest X-ray or CT scan may be performed to assess lung structure, identify complications (e.g., bronchiectasis), and monitor disease progression.

- Stool Analysis: Stool tests may be performed to assess pancreatic function and detect fat malabsorption.

Treatment:
- Airway Clearance Techniques:

    Chest physiotherapy, percussion, vibration, or high-frequency chest wall oscillation devices help mobilize and clear thick mucus from the airways.

- Bronchodilators: Inhaled medications such as albuterol or ipratropium help relax the muscles around the airways, making breathing easier.
- Mucolytics: Medications such as dornase alfa (Pulmozyme) help thin and loosen thick mucus in the airways.
- Pancreatic Enzyme Replacement Therapy (PERT): Oral enzymes (e.g., pancrelipase) are taken with meals and snacks to aid digestion and nutrient absorption.
- Nutritional Support:

    High-calorie, high-protein diet and fat-soluble vitamin supplementation (A, D, E, K) help maintain adequate nutrition and prevent malnutrition.

- Antibiotics: Oral, inhaled, or intravenous antibiotics are used to treat respiratory infections and prevent exacerbations.
- Lung Transplantation: In severe cases of CF with advanced lung disease, lung transplantation may be considered as a treatment option.
- Multidisciplinary Care:

    Comprehensive care provided by a team of healthcare professionals including pulmonologists, gastroenterologists, dietitians, respiratory therapists, and social workers to optimize treatment and manage complications.

5.19. Pleural Effusion

> ➤ *Pleural effusion is an accumulation of fluid in the space between the lungs and the chest wall (pleural space), often caused by conditions such as heart failure, pneumonia, or cancer.*
>
> ➤ *Symptoms include chest pain, cough, shortness of breath, and decreased breath sounds on examination.*
>
> ➤ *Treatment involves addressing the underlying cause and may include draining the fluid with a needle or tube, along with managing symptoms and complications.*

Symptoms:

- Dyspnea: particularly with exertion or lying flat.
- Chest Pain: worsens with deep breathing or coughing.
- Cough: Persistent, dry, often nonproductive.
- Orthopnea: Difficulty breathing while lying flat, relieved by sitting or standing upright.
- Pleuritic Chest Pain: worsens with inspiration or coughing, localized to the chest or back.
- Decreased breath sounds or absent breath sounds on auscultation
- Dullness to Percussion or decreased resonance on percussion
- Tachypnea: often due to decreased lung expansion and impaired gas exchange.
- Hypoxemia: particularly in advanced cases of pleural effusion.

Causes and Risk Factors:

- Pulmonary Conditions: diseases such as pneumonia, tuberculosis, lung cancer, or pulmonary embolism increase the risk of developing pleural effusion.
- Cardiac Conditions: Congestive heart failure, pericarditis, or myocardial infarction can lead to fluid in the pleural cavity.
- Liver Disease: Liver cirrhosis or hepatic hydrothorax can cause pleural effusion due to impaired fluid regulation and portal hypertension.
- Kidney Disease: Nephrotic syndrome or renal failure can result in pleural effusion due to fluid retention and imbalances in electrolytes.
- Cancer: Malignant pleural effusion, often due to metastatic spread from lung cancer, breast cancer, or lymphoma, is a common cause of pleural effusion in adults.

- Pulmonary Embolism: Blood clots in the pulmonary vasculature can lead to pleural effusion, particularly if associated with infarction or pulmonary hypertension.
- Infection: Bacterial, viral, or fungal infections of the lungs (pneumonia), pleura (pleurisy), or other organs can cause inflammation and fluid accumulation in the pleural space.
- Autoimmune Disorders: Rheumatoid arthritis, systemic lupus erythematosus (SLE), or other autoimmune diseases can result in pleural effusion due to inflammation and immune-mediated processes.

Workup and Diagnosis:
- <u>Medical History and Physical Examination:</u> Including assessment of symptoms, history, risk factors, and clinical findings may suggest the cause of pleural effusion.
- <u>Upright Chest X-ray:</u>

    Initial imaging test to visualize the lungs and pleural cavity, often showing blunting of the costophrenic angles or meniscus sign indicative of pleural effusion.
- <u>Ultrasound:</u>

    Ultrasonography of the chest can confirm the presence of pleural effusion, guide thoracentesis, and assess for loculated or complex effusions.
- <u>CT Scan:</u>

    Computed tomography (CT) imaging may be performed to evaluate the extent of pleural effusion, assess underlying lung or pleural abnormalities, and guide further management.
- <u>Thoracentesis:</u>

    Procedure to sample fluid from the pleural space for analysis, including cell count, protein, glucose, lactate dehydrogenase (LDH), pH, and microbiological cultures.
- <u>Laboratory Tests:</u>

    Analysis of pleural fluid to determine its composition and characteristics, helping to differentiate transudate from exudative effusions and identify underlying causes.
- <u>Pleural Biopsy:</u>

    Surgical or image-guided biopsy of the pleura may be performed to obtain tissue samples for pathological examination, particularly in cases of suspected malignancy or granulomatous disease.

Treatment:

- Underlying Cause Management:

    Treatment of the underlying condition causing pleural effusion, such as antibiotics for pneumonia, diuretics for heart failure, or chemotherapy for cancer.

- Thoracentesis:

    Therapeutic removal of excess pleural fluid via thoracentesis can provide symptomatic relief and improve respiratory function, particularly in cases of large or symptomatic effusions.

- Pleurodesis:

    Chemical or mechanical pleurodesis may be performed to induce adhesion of the pleural layers and prevent recurrent pleural effusion, often using agents such as talc or doxycycline.

- Pleural Drainage:

    Placement of a chest tube or indwelling pleural catheter (pleuRX catheter) may be necessary for continuous drainage of pleural fluid in refractory cases or recurrent effusions.

- Medications:

    Analgesics for pain management, bronchodilators for respiratory symptoms, and antibiotics for infectious causes of pleural effusion may be prescribed as adjunctive therapy.

- Thoracic Surgery:

    Surgical interventions such as pleurectomy, decortication, or thoracoscopy may be considered for definitive management of pleural effusion in select cases, particularly for loculated or complex effusions.

5.20. Pulmonary Hypertension

> ➤ *Pulmonary hypertension is a progressive condition characterized by high blood pressure in the arteries of the lungs, leading to strain on the heart and reduced blood oxygen levels.*
>
> ➤ *Symptoms include shortness of breath, fatigue, chest pain, and fainting, with causes ranging from underlying heart or lung diseases to genetic factors.*
>
> ➤ *Treatment aims to alleviate symptoms, improve quality of life, and slow disease progression through medication, oxygen therapy, and lifestyle adjustments.*

Symptoms:
- Dyspnea: particularly with exertion or at rest, is the most common symptom of pulmonary hypertension.
- Fatigue: Persistent tiredness or weakness, often due to decreased oxygen delivery to the body tissues.
- Chest Pain: Sharp or dull chest pain, discomfort, or pressure, especially during physical activity or exertion.
- Syncope: Fainting or lightheadedness, particularly with exertion or during episodes of low blood pressure.
- Edema: Swelling in the legs, ankles, or abdomen due to fluid retention.
- Cyanosis: Bluish discoloration of the lips, skin, or nail beds due to reduced oxygen levels in the blood.
- Palpitations: Irregular or rapid heartbeat, often due to underlying heart rhythm disturbances.
- Decreased Exercise Tolerance: Reduced ability to perform physical activities or exercise due to shortness of breath and fatigue.

Causes and Risk Factors:

Primary Pulmonary Hypertension:
- Genetics: Family history of pulmonary hypertension or hereditary predisposition.
- Gender: More common in females, particularly during childbearing years.
- Age: Most commonly diagnosed in young to middle-aged adults, but can occur at any age.

Secondary Pulmonary Hypertension:

- Connective Tissue Disorders: Systemic lupus erythematosus (SLE), scleroderma, rheumatoid arthritis.
- Heart Conditions: Congenital heart disease, left heart failure, valvular heart disease.
- Lung Diseases: Chronic obstructive pulmonary disease (COPD), interstitial lung disease (ILD), pulmonary embolism.
- Sleep Apnea: Obstructive sleep apnea (OSA) or central sleep apnea with Cheyne-Stokes respiration.
- Liver Disease: Cirrhosis, portal hypertension, or hepatic veno-occlusive disease.
- HIV Infection: Human immunodeficiency virus (HIV) infection or AIDS-related pulmonary hypertension.
- Chronic Kidney Disease: Renal artery stenosis, nephrotic syndrome, or end-stage renal disease (ESRD).
- High Altitude: Exposure to high altitude or chronic hypoxia (e.g., living at high altitude, chronic lung disease).

   Medications and Toxins: Certain medications or environmental exposures may increase the risk of developing pulmonary hypertension, including:
- Appetite suppressants: Fenfluramine-phentermine (Fen-Phen), dexfenfluramine (Redux).
- Recreational Drugs: Cocaine, methamphetamine, or amphetamine derivatives.
- Toxins: Exposure to asbestos, silica, or other occupational hazards.

Workup and Diagnosis:
- <u>Medical History and Physical Examination:</u> Including assessment of symptoms, risk factors, and signs of heart or lung disease.
- <u>Echocardiography:</u>

    Ultrasound imaging of the heart to assess cardiac structure and function, estimate pulmonary artery pressures, and detect signs of pulmonary hypertension.
- <u>Electrocardiography (ECG):</u>

    Recording of the heart's electrical activity to detect abnormal rhythms, signs of right ventricular hypertrophy, or strain patterns suggestive of pulmonary hypertension.

- Chest X-ray:

    Imaging test to evaluate lung and heart structure, detect signs of pulmonary congestion, and assess for underlying lung or heart disease.

- Pulmonary Function Tests (PFTs):

    Lung function tests to assess airflow obstruction, lung volumes, and gas exchange, particularly in cases of suspected lung disease contributing to pulmonary hypertension.

- High-Resolution Computed Tomography (HRCT):

    CT imaging of the chest to assess lung structure, detect interstitial lung disease, or identify pulmonary embolism as underlying causes of pulmonary hypertension.

- Ventilation-Perfusion (V/Q) Scan:

    Nuclear medicine imaging to evaluate for pulmonary embolism in suspected cases of acute or chronic thromboembolic pulmonary hypertension (CTEPH).

- Cardiac Catheterization:

    Invasive procedure to measure pulmonary artery pressures directly, assess cardiac function, and confirm the diagnosis of pulmonary hypertension.

Treatment:

- Medications:
    - Pulmonary Vasodilators: prostacyclin analogs (epoprostenol, treprostinil), endothelin receptor antagonists (bosentan, ambrisentan), and phosphodiesterase-5 inhibitors (sildenafil, tadalafil) help dilate pulmonary arteries and improve blood flow.
    - Diuretics: furosemide (Lasix), hydrochlorothiazide (HCTZ), spironolactone (Aldactone), and bumetanide (Bumex) to reduce fluid retention and relieve symptoms of right heart failure.
    - Anticoagulants: Blood thinners may be prescribed to prevent clot formation in cases of pulmonary embolism or chronic thromboembolic pulmonary hypertension (CTEPH).
- Oxygen Therapy: Supplemental oxygen may be prescribed to improve oxygenation and alleviate symptoms of hypoxemia.
- Exercise and Rehabilitation: Pulmonary rehabilitation programs including exercise and physical therapy.

References

- Eccles, R. (2005). Understanding the symptoms of the common cold and influenza. The Lancet Infectious Diseases, 5(11), 718-725.
- Fiore, A. E., Fry, A., Shay, D., et al. (2010). Antiviral agents for the treatment and chemoprophylaxis of influenza: Recommendations of the Advisory Committee on Immunization Practices (ACIP). MMWR Recommendations and Reports, 59(RR-8), 1-62.
- Rosenfeld, R. M., Piccirillo, J. F., Chandrasekhar, S. S., et al. (2015). Clinical practice guideline (update): Adult sinusitis. Otolaryngology-Head and Neck Surgery, 152(2 Suppl), S1-S39.
- Scottish Intercollegiate Guidelines Network (SIGN). (2010). Management of sore throat and indications for tonsillectomy: A national clinical guideline. Retrieved from: https://www.sign.ac.uk/media/1071/sign117.pdf
- Mandell, L. A., Wunderink, R. G., Anzueto, A., et al. (2007). Infectious Diseases Society of America/American Thoracic Society consensus guidelines on the management of community-acquired pneumonia in adults. Clinical Infectious Diseases, 44(Suppl 2), S27-S72.
- American Thoracic Society, & Infectious Diseases Society of America. (2005). Guidelines for the management of adults with hospital-acquired, ventilator-associated, and healthcare-associated pneumonia. American Journal of Respiratory and Critical Care Medicine, 171(4), 388-416.
- Albert, R. H. (2010). Diagnosis and treatment of acute bronchitis. American Family Physician, 82(11), 1345-1350.
- Ralston, S. L., Lieberthal, A. S., Meissner, H. C., et al. (2014). Clinical practice guideline: The diagnosis, management, and prevention of bronchiolitis. Pediatrics, 134(5), e1474-e1502.
- Nahid, P., Dorman, S. E., Alipanah, N., et al. (2016). Official American Thoracic Society/Centers for Disease Control and Prevention/Infectious Diseases Society of America clinical practice guidelines: Treatment of drug-susceptible tuberculosis. Clinical Infectious Diseases, 63(7), e147-e195.
- Global Initiative for Chronic Obstructive Lung Disease (GOLD). (2021). Global strategy for the diagnosis, management, and prevention of chronic obstructive pulmonary disease: 2021 report. Retrieved from: https://goldcopd.org/wp-content/uploads/2020/11/GOLD-REPORT-2021-v1.1-25Nov20_WMV.pdf
- Polverino, E., Goeminne, P. C., McDonnell, M. J., et al. (2017). European Respiratory Society guidelines for the management of adult bronchiectasis. European Respiratory Journal, 50(3), 1700629.
- Global Initiative for Asthma (GINA). (2021). Global strategy for asthma management and prevention: 2021 update. Retrieved from: https://ginasthma.org/wp-content/uploads/2021/05/GINA-Main-Report-2021-V2-WMS.pdf

- Raghu, G., Remy-Jardin, M., Myers, J. L., et al. (2018). Diagnosis of idiopathic pulmonary fibrosis: An official ATS/ERS/JRS/ALAT clinical practice guideline. American Journal of Respiratory and Critical Care Medicine, 198(5), e44-e68.
- Statement on sarcoidosis. (1999). Joint Statement of the American Thoracic Society (ATS), the European Respiratory Society (ERS) and the World Association of Sarcoidosis and Other Granulomatous Disorders (WASOG) adopted by the ATS Board of Directors and by the ERS Executive Committee, February 1999. American Journal of Respiratory and Critical Care Medicine, 160(2), 736-755.
- Vasakova, M., Morell, F., Walsh, S., et al. (2017). Hypersensitivity pneumonitis: Perspectives in diagnosis and management. American Journal of Respiratory and Critical Care Medicine, 196(6), 680-689.
- Epstein, L. J., Kristo, D., Strollo Jr, P. J., et al. (2009). Clinical guideline for the evaluation, management and long-term care of obstructive sleep apnea in adults. Journal of Clinical Sleep Medicine, 5(3), 263-276.
- Bell, S. C., Mall, M. A., Gutierrez, H., et al. (2020). The future of cystic fibrosis care: A global perspective. The Lancet Respiratory Medicine, 8(1), 65-124.
- Light, R. W. (2002). Clinical practice: Pleural effusion. New England Journal of Medicine, 346(25), 1971-1977.
- Galie, N., Humbert, M., Vachiery, J. L., et al. (2015). 2015 ESC/ERS guidelines for the diagnosis and treatment of pulmonary hypertension. European Respiratory Journal, 46(4), 903-975.

Chapter 6. Gastrointestinal Disorders

Reviewed by
Henry Hoang Nguyen, MD, PhD, RPH, FACHE

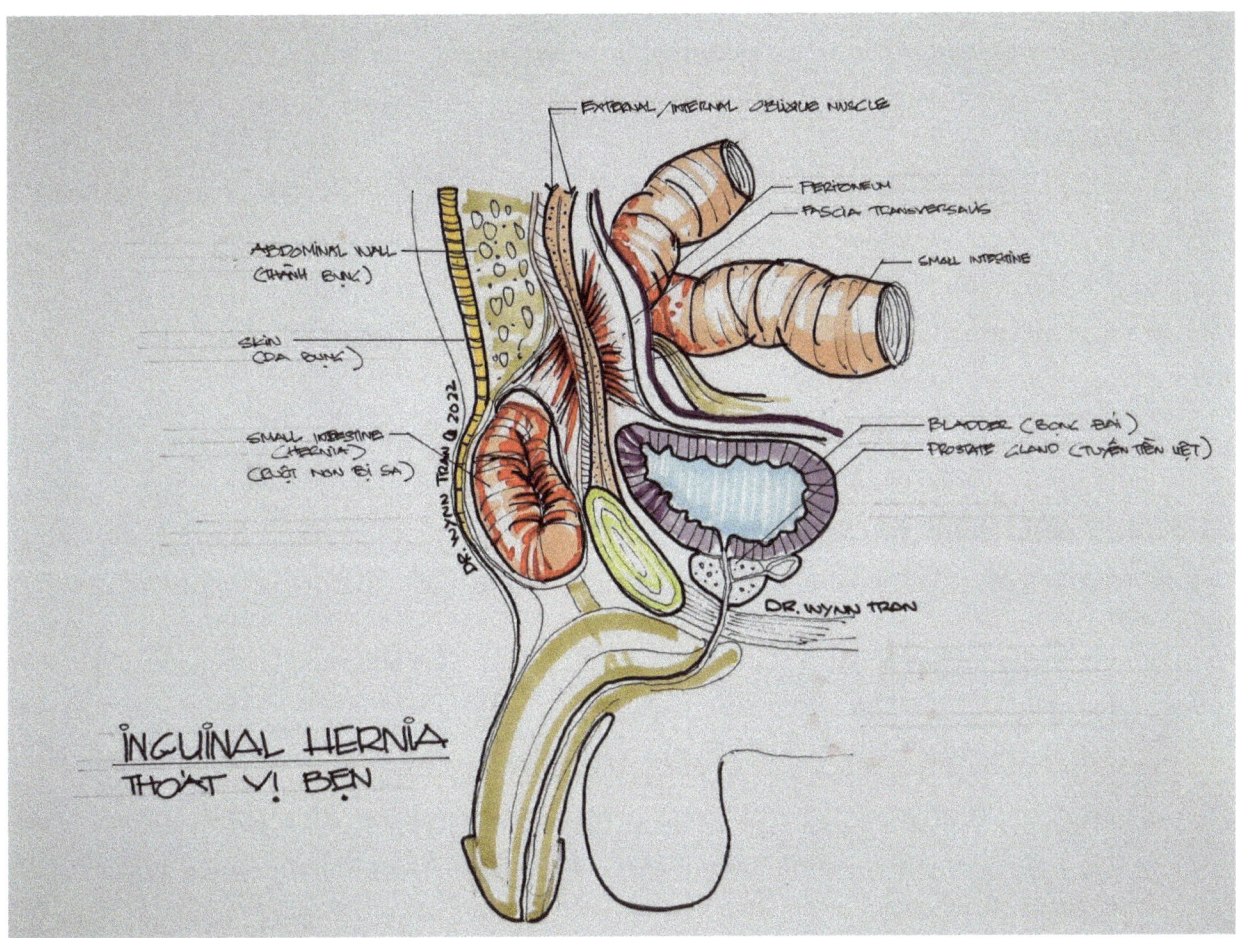

The APh should be familiar with the presentation, diagnosis, and management of these common GI disorders to provide appropriate care and referral to the gastroenterologist when necessary.

6.1. Abdominal Pain

> ➤ *Abdominal pain is a common symptom with various potential causes, ranging from indigestion to serious medical conditions.*
>
> ➤ *It can manifest as cramping, sharp, dull, or burning sensations, often accompanied by other symptoms such as nausea, vomiting, or diarrhea.*
>
> ➤ *Accurate diagnosis often requires medical evaluation to determine the underlying cause and appropriate treatment.*

Symptoms:

Abdominal pain can range from mild to severe and may be characterized by:

- Sharp, dull, or cramping pain.
- Localized in quadrants (RUQ, RLQ, LLQ, LUQ) or diffuse.
- Acute or chronic.
- Accompanied by other symptoms such as nausea, vomiting, diarrhea, fever, bloating, or loss of appetite.

Causes and Risk Factors:

Risk factors for abdominal pain depend on the specific condition but can include:

- Dietary choices (e.g., high consumption of fatty, spicy, or greasy foods).
- Lifestyle factors (e.g., stress, sedentary lifestyle).
- Medical history (e.g., history of gastrointestinal diseases, infections).
- Use of certain medications (e.g., NSAIDs) that can irritate the stomach lining.
- Alcohol and tobacco use.

Epidemiology:

The prevalence of abdominal pain varies greatly depending on geographical region, age, gender, and underlying health conditions. It is a common reason for visits to primary care physicians and emergency departments worldwide.

Diagnosis:

Given the wide range of potential causes, accurately diagnosing abdominal pain often requires careful consideration of patient history, physical findings, and diagnostic testing. It's crucial to evaluate life-threatening conditions early.

- Detailed medical history and physical examination focusing on the pain's characteristics, location, and timing.
- Laboratory tests (blood, urine, stool tests) to detect infections, inflammation, or metabolic conditions.
- Imaging studies (ultrasound, X-ray, CT scan, MRI) to visualize organs and structures within the abdomen.
- Endoscopic procedures (e.g., gastroscopy, colonoscopy) for a closer examination of the gastrointestinal tract.

Gastrointestinal Causes

- Appendicitis: Inflammation of the appendix, typically causing acute sharp pain in the lower right abdomen.
- Gastroenteritis: Infection or irritation of the stomach and intestines, often leading to cramping, diarrhea, and vomiting.
- Peptic Ulcers: Sores on the stomach or small intestine lining causing burning or gnawing pain.
- Inflammatory Bowel Disease (IBD): Including Crohn's disease and ulcerative colitis, causing chronic inflammation of the GI tract.
- Gastroesophageal Reflux Disease (GERD): Acid reflux causing burning pain or discomfort in the upper abdomen or below the sternum.
- Bowel Obstruction: Blockage in the intestines causing cramping and bloating.

Hepatobiliary Causes

- Gallstones: Hardened deposits in the gallbladder that can cause severe pain in the upper right abdomen.
- Hepatitis: Inflammation of the liver, causing upper abdominal pain, often with jaundice.

Renal and Urological Causes

- Kidney Stones: Hard deposits formed in the kidneys, causing severe flank pain.
- Urinary Tract Infection (UTI): Infection in the urinary system, sometimes causing lower abdominal pain and dysuria.

Gynecological Causes

- Ectopic Pregnancy: A pregnancy outside the uterus, causing sharp, one-sided abdominal pain.
- Ovarian Cyst: A fluid-filled sac within the ovary, potentially causing intermittent or sharp pain.
- Pelvic Inflammatory Disease (PID): Infection of the female reproductive organs, often causing lower abdominal pain.

Vascular Causes
- Aortic Aneurysm: Enlargement of the aorta that can lead to sudden, severe abdominal pain if ruptured.

Musculoskeletal Causes
- Muscle Strain: Overuse or injury to abdominal muscles, causing localized pain.

Neurological Causes
- Herpes Zoster: Reactivation of the chickenpox virus, causing pain before a rash appears in a band-like pattern.

Metabolic/Endocrine Causes
- Diabetic Ketoacidosis: A serious complication of diabetes causing abdominal pain, nausea, and vomiting.

Treatment:

- Dietary and lifestyle modifications: a diet low in inflammatory foods (like dairy and gluten for sensitive individuals), high in fiber, and maintain hydration, alongside stress management and regular physical activity.
- Over-the-counter or prescription medications: to relieve pain, reduce inflammation, or treat infections
- Surgical intervention: for conditions such as appendicitis, hernias, or obstructive diseases
- Management of chronic conditions: (e.g., Crohn's disease, ulcerative colitis, irritable bowel syndrome) with a combination of diet, medication, and sometimes surgery

6.2. Gastroesophageal Reflux Disease

> ➢ *Gastroesophageal reflux disease (GERD) is a chronic condition where stomach acid frequently flows back into the esophagus, causing irritation and inflammation.*
> ➢ *Symptoms include heartburn, regurgitation, chest pain, and difficulty swallowing, often worsening after eating or lying down.*
> ➢ *Treatment involves lifestyle changes, medications to reduce acid production or neutralize acid, and in severe cases, surgery to reinforce the lower esophageal sphincter.*

Symptoms:
- Heartburn: A burning sensation in the chest, often after eating, which may worsen when lying down or bending over.
- Regurgitation: Sour or bitter-tasting acid backing up into the throat or mouth.
- Chest pain: Chest discomfort or pain that can mimic heart-related conditions.
- Difficulty swallowing: A sensation of food sticking in the throat or the sensation of a lump in the throat.
- Chronic cough: A persistent cough, especially at night, often due to irritation from stomach acid.

Causes and Risk Factors:
- Hiatal hernia: A condition where a portion of the stomach protrudes into the chest cavity, increasing the risk of reflux.
- Obesity: Excess body weight can put pressure on the abdomen and increase the likelihood of GERD.
- Pregnancy: Hormonal changes and increased pressure on the abdomen during pregnancy can contribute to GERD.
- Smoking: Smoking weakens the lower esophageal sphincter (LES), allowing stomach acid to reflux into the esophagus.
- Certain foods and beverages: Spicy, acidic, fatty, or fried foods, as well as caffeine, alcohol, and carbonated drinks, can trigger or worsen GERD symptoms.

Diagnosis:
- <u>Symptom evaluation:</u> Diagnosis is often based on symptoms such as heartburn and regurgitation.
- <u>Endoscopy:</u>

A procedure where a flexible tube with a camera is inserted into the esophagus to visualize the lining and look for signs of inflammation, erosions, or complications like Barrett's esophagus.

- Esophageal pH monitoring: A test to measure the amount of acid reflux into the esophagus over a period of time, usually 24 hours.
- Upper gastrointestinal (GI) series:

    A series of X-rays taken after swallowing a contrast material to evaluate the anatomy of the esophagus, stomach, and upper intestine.

Treatment:
- Lifestyle modifications:
    - Avoid triggering foods and beverages.
    - Eat smaller, more frequent meals.
    - Avoid lying down or bending over after eating.
    - Elevate the head of the bed.
    - Quit smoking.
- Medications:
    - Antacids: Neutralize stomach acid.
    - H2-receptor antagonists (e.g., ranitidine, famotidine): Reduce acid production.
    - Proton pump inhibitors (PPIs) (e.g., omeprazole, esomeprazole): Block stomach acid production and promote healing of the esophagus.
- Surgery (in severe cases or when medications are ineffective):
    - Fundoplication: A procedure to reinforce the LES and prevent reflux.
    - LINX device: A small ring of magnetic beads placed around the LES to prevent acid reflux while allowing food to pass through.

6.3. Peptic Ulcer Disease

> ➢ *Peptic Ulcer Disease (PUD) is a condition characterized by the formation of open sores (ulcers) in the lining of the stomach, small intestine, or esophagus.*
>
> ➢ *The most common cause is infection with Helicobacter pylori bacteria or long-term use of nonsteroidal anti-inflammatory drugs (NSAIDs). Diagnosis typically involves endoscopy, biopsy, or imaging tests.*
>
> ➢ *Treatment aims to alleviate symptoms, heal the ulcer, and prevent recurrence. It often involves antibiotics to eradicate H. pylori, proton pump inhibitors to reduce stomach acid, and lifestyle modifications.*

Symptoms:
- Abdominal pain: Typically described as burning or gnawing pain in the upper abdomen, often occurring between meals or during the night.
- Heartburn: A burning sensation in the chest, similar to symptoms of gastroesophageal reflux disease (GERD).
- Nausea and vomiting: Some patients with PUD may experience nausea and vomiting, especially if the ulcer is causing obstruction or inflammation.
- Loss of appetite: Due to discomfort and pain associated with eating.
- Weight loss: In severe cases where eating exacerbates symptoms or leads to decreased food intake.

Causes and Risk Factors:
- Helicobacter pylori infection: This bacterium is a major risk factor for PUD, as it can weaken the protective lining of the stomach and duodenum, making them more susceptible to damage from stomach acid.
- Nonsteroidal anti-inflammatory drugs (NSAIDs): Long-term use of NSAIDs, such as aspirin, ibuprofen, and naproxen, can irritate the stomach lining and increase the risk of developing ulcers.
- Smoking: Smoking cigarettes increases the risk of developing peptic ulcers and can delay healing.
- Excessive alcohol consumption: Alcohol can irritate the stomach lining and increase acid production, contributing to the development of ulcers.
- Stress: While stress itself does not cause ulcers, it can exacerbate symptoms and delay healing in patients with PUD.

Diagnosis:
- Upper gastrointestinal endoscopy:

    A procedure where a flexible tube with a camera is inserted into the esophagus, stomach, and duodenum to visualize any ulcers or inflammation.

- Blood tests: Testing for the presence of Helicobacter pylori antibodies or antigens can help diagnose an active infection.
- Stool tests: Testing for the presence of Helicobacter pylori antigens in the stool can also be used to diagnose an active infection.
- Upper GI series:

    A series of X-rays taken after swallowing a contrast material to visualize any ulcers or abnormalities in the esophagus, stomach, or duodenum.

Treatment:
- Medications:
    - Proton pump inhibitors (PPIs): Reduce stomach acid production and promote healing of the ulcer.
    - Antibiotics: Used to eradicate Helicobacter pylori infection in patients with PUD caused by this bacterium.
    - H2-receptor antagonists: Reduce acid production in the stomach.
    - Antacids: Provide temporary relief by neutralizing stomach acid.
- Lifestyle modifications:
    - Avoiding NSAIDs and other irritants.
    - Quitting smoking.
    - Limiting alcohol consumption.
    - Managing stress through relaxation techniques.
- Surgery:

    In rare cases where ulcers do not respond to medications or if complications such as bleeding or perforation occur, surgery may be necessary to remove the affected portion of the stomach or duodenum.

6.4. Cirrhosis

> ➢ *Cirrhosis is the late stage of liver scarring due to various liver diseases, notably chronic alcoholism and hepatitis.*
> ➢ *Symptoms often remain silent until significant damage occurs, manifesting as jaundice, fluid accumulation, and weakness.*
> ➢ *Treatment focuses on managing the cause, symptoms, and complications, with liver transplantation being an option for advanced cases.*

Symptoms:
- Fatigue and weakness
- Loss of appetite, weight loss
- Nausea or vomiting
- Easy bruising or bleeding
- Jaundice
- Itchy skin
- Ascites
- Swelling in the legs
- Spider angioma

Causes and Risk Factors:
- Chronic alcohol abuse
- Chronic viral hepatitis (hepatitis B, C, and D)
- Fat accumulating in the liver (non-alcoholic fatty liver disease)
- Other causes include autoimmune hepatitis, bile duct disorders, and inherited diseases such as Wilson's disease and hemochromatosis.
- Excessive alcohol consumption
- Obesity
- Type 2 diabetes
- Having viral hepatitis

Epidemiology:

Globally, cirrhosis is a leading cause of mortality and morbidity. The prevalence varies widely depending on the geographic region and the predominant causes in the population, such as hepatitis B and C infections or alcohol consumption. It's more common in men than in women and usually affects middle-aged or older individuals.

Cirrhosis Score:

1. Child-Pugh Score
    - This score assesses the prognosis of chronic liver disease, mainly cirrhosis. It uses five clinical measures: bilirubin, albumin, prothrombin time/INR, ascites, and hepatic encephalopathy.
    - Patients are classified into Child-Pugh Class A (well-compensated disease), Class B (significant functional compromise), or Class C (decompensated disease). Higher scores correlate with increased severity and worse prognosis.
2. Model for End-Stage Liver Disease (MELD) Score
    - The MELD score is used to prioritize patients for liver transplantation, based on the patient's risk of dying from liver disease within the next three months. It includes values for bilirubin, INR (a measure of blood clotting), creatinine (a measure of kidney function), and sometimes sodium levels.
    - The MELD score ranges from 6 to 40, with higher scores indicating more severe disease and a higher urgency for liver transplantation.

Diagnosis:

- Blood Tests: To assess liver function (liver enzymes, bilirubin, albumin) and screen for viral hepatitis.
- Imaging Tests: Ultrasound, CT scans, and MRI can detect liver abnormalities.
- Liver Biopsy: Though not always necessary, it is the definitive test for cirrhosis, allowing direct examination of the liver tissue.

Treatment:

- Addressing the Underlying Cause: Such as antiviral drugs for hepatitis or weight loss for non-alcoholic fatty liver disease.
- Alcohol Abstinence: Essential for those with alcohol-related liver disease.
- Medications: To manage symptoms and complications, such as diuretics for fluid accumulation and beta-blockers for portal hypertension.
- Liver Transplant: For advanced cirrhosis with liver failure, a transplant may be the only option.

6.5. Inflammatory Bowel Disease - Crohn's disease

> ➢ *Crohn's disease is a type of inflammatory bowel disease (IBD) characterized by chronic inflammation of the digestive tract, typically affecting the small intestine and colon.*
>
> ➢ *Symptoms include abdominal pain, diarrhea, weight loss, and fatigue, with complications such as bowel obstruction or fistulas.*
>
> ➢ *Treatment aims to reduce inflammation with medications like corticosteroids or immunosuppressants, and in severe cases, surgery may be necessary to remove damaged portions of the intestine.*

Symptoms:

- Abdominal pain and cramping: Often occurs in the lower right abdomen but can occur anywhere in the abdomen.
- Diarrhea: May be persistent and watery, sometimes containing blood.
- Weight loss: Due to loss of appetite, malabsorption, and inflammation.
- Fatigue: Can be severe and debilitating.
- Fever: Often accompanies active disease flare-ups.
- Other symptoms: Nausea, vomiting, reduced appetite, and anal fissures or fistulas may also occur.

Causes and Risk Factors:

- Genetics: Family history of Crohn's disease increases the risk.
- Immune system: Abnormal immune responses may contribute to the development of Crohn's disease.
- Environmental factors: Smoking, diet, and certain infections may increase the risk.
- Age and ethnicity: Crohn's disease can occur at any age but is more common in young adults. It affects patients of all ethnic backgrounds but is more common in Caucasians.

Epidemiology:

- Crohn's disease is more prevalent in developed countries, particularly North America and Europe.
- The incidence and prevalence of Crohn's disease have been increasing worldwide.
- It affects approximately 3 in every 1,000 patients in North America and Europe.

Diagnosis:

Diagnosis is based on a combination of clinical symptoms, imaging studies, endoscopy, and biopsy.

- Imaging tests:

    X-rays, CT scans, MRI, and capsule endoscopy may be used to visualize the gastrointestinal tract and identify areas of inflammation or complications.

- Endoscopy:

    Colonoscopy or upper endoscopy allows direct visualization of the intestines and collection of tissue samples (biopsy) for examination under a microscope.

- Blood tests: Elevated inflammatory markers such as C-reactive protein (CRP) and erythrocyte sedimentation rate (ESR) may be present.

Treatment:

- Medications:

    The goals of treatment are to induce and maintain remission, control inflammation, and alleviate symptoms. Medications include aminosalicylates, corticosteroids, immunomodulators, biologic therapies (such as anti-TNF agents), and antibiotics.

- Nutrition therapy: In some cases, nutritional supplementation or exclusive enteral nutrition may be used to manage symptoms and promote healing.

- Surgery:

    Surgery may be necessary to remove diseased portions of the intestine, treat complications such as strictures or fistulas, or manage severe symptoms that do not respond to medication.

- Lifestyle modifications: Dietary changes, stress management, smoking cessation, and regular exercise may help improve symptoms and overall well-being.

6.6. Inflammatory Bowel Disease - Ulcerative colitis

> ➤ *Ulcerative colitis is a form of inflammatory bowel disease (IBD) characterized by chronic inflammation and ulcers in the colon and rectum lining.*
>
> ➤ *Symptoms include abdominal pain, diarrhea with blood or pus, rectal bleeding, and urgency to defecate.*
>
> ➤ *Treatment aims to reduce inflammation with medications like corticosteroids, immunosuppressants, or biologics, and in severe cases, surgery to remove the colon may be necessary.*

Symptoms:
- Bloody diarrhea: One of the hallmark symptoms of UC, often accompanied by abdominal pain and urgency to have a bowel movement.
- Rectal bleeding: Blood may be present in the stool or on toilet paper.
- Abdominal pain and cramping: Can range from mild to severe.
- Urgency: Feeling the need to have a bowel movement urgently, even when the bowel is empty.
- Tenesmus: The feeling of incomplete bowel emptying, despite having a bowel movement.
- Fatigue: Due to anemia, inflammation, and the chronic nature of the disease.
- Weight loss: Often due to loss of appetite and malabsorption.

Causes and Risk Factors:
- Genetics: Family history of UC or other autoimmune diseases increases the risk.
- Environmental factors: Smoking, diet, and certain infections may play a role.
- Age and ethnicity: UC can occur at any age but is more common in young adults. It affects patients of all ethnic backgrounds but is more common in Caucasians.

Epidemiology:
- UC is less common than Crohn's disease but still affects a significant number of patients worldwide.
- It is more prevalent in developed countries, particularly North America and Europe.
- The incidence and prevalence of UC have been increasing globally.

Diagnosis:

Diagnosis is based on a combination of clinical symptoms, endoscopy, and biopsy.

- Colonoscopy:

    Direct visualization of the colon and rectum allows the healthcare provider to assess the extent and severity of inflammation and collect tissue samples (biopsy) for examination under a microscope.

- Blood tests: Elevated inflammatory markers such as C-reactive protein (CRP) and erythrocyte sedimentation rate (ESR) may be present.

- Stool tests: To rule out infectious causes of diarrhea and assess for markers of inflammation.

Treatment:

- Medications:

    The goals of treatment are to induce and maintain remission, control inflammation, and alleviate symptoms. Medications include aminosalicylates, corticosteroids, immunomodulators, biologic therapies (such as anti-TNF agents), and antibiotics.

- Nutrition therapy: In some cases, nutritional supplementation or exclusive enteral nutrition may be used to manage symptoms and promote healing.

- Surgery:

    Surgery may be necessary for severe or refractory cases of UC, particularly if complications such as toxic megacolon or colorectal cancer develop. Surgical options include colectomy with or without ileal pouch-anal anastomosis (IPAA) or ileostomy.

- Lifestyle modifications: Dietary changes, stress management, smoking cessation, and regular exercise may help improve symptoms and overall well-being.

6.7. Gastroenteritis

> ➤ *Gastroenteritis, commonly known as stomach flu, is inflammation of the stomach and intestines caused by viral, bacterial, or parasitic infections.*
> ➤ *Symptoms include diarrhea, vomiting, abdominal cramps, nausea, and sometimes fever.*
> ➤ *It is typically self-limiting, with treatment focusing on hydration, rest, and symptomatic relief. Severe cases may require medical intervention to prevent dehydration.*

Symptoms:
- Diarrhea: Watery or loose stools are common, often accompanied by urgency and frequent bowel movements.
- Nausea and vomiting: Patients may experience nausea, vomiting, or both, which can contribute to dehydration.
- Abdominal pain and cramps: Discomfort or cramping in the abdominal region may occur.
- Fever: In some cases, patients may develop a fever, particularly with bacterial or parasitic infections.
- Dehydration: Symptoms such as dry mouth, decreased urination, thirst, fatigue, and dizziness may indicate dehydration, especially in severe cases.

Causes and Risk Factors:
- Contaminated food or water: Consumption of contaminated food or water is a common risk factor for gastroenteritis.
- Poor sanitation: Inadequate handwashing, unsanitary food handling practices, and exposure to contaminated environments increase the risk of infection.
- Immunosuppression: patients with weakened immune systems, such as the elderly, young children, pregnant women, and those with underlying health conditions, are at increased risk of developing gastroenteritis and experiencing severe complications.
- Travel to high-risk areas: Traveling to regions with poor sanitation or endemic gastrointestinal infections increases the risk of acquiring gastroenteritis.

Epidemiology:
- Gastroenteritis is a common condition worldwide, with millions of cases reported annually.

- The incidence of gastroenteritis varies by geographic region, season, and circulating pathogens.
- Viral gastroenteritis is the most common form and is often seen in outbreaks, particularly in settings such as healthcare facilities, schools, and cruise ships.
- Bacterial and parasitic gastroenteritis may occur sporadically or as outbreaks associated with contaminated food or water sources.

Diagnosis:

- Clinical evaluation: Diagnosis is primarily based on the patient's history, symptoms, and physical examination findings.
- Stool studies:

    Laboratory tests, including stool culture, stool antigen testing, and stool microscopy, may be performed to identify the causative pathogen, particularly in cases of suspected bacterial or parasitic gastroenteritis.

- Imaging studies:

    In severe cases or when complications are suspected, imaging tests such as abdominal ultrasound or CT scan may be indicated to evaluate the gastrointestinal tract.

Treatment:

- Supportive care:

    Treatment focuses on managing symptoms and preventing dehydration. This may include oral rehydration solutions, intravenous fluids, and antiemetic medications to control nausea and vomiting.

- Antimicrobial therapy:

    Antibiotics may be prescribed for bacterial gastroenteritis, particularly in severe or high-risk cases. However, they are not routinely recommended for viral gastroenteritis, as they do not shorten the duration of illness and may contribute to antimicrobial resistance.

- Antiparasitic medication:

    In cases of parasitic gastroenteritis, such as those caused by Giardia or Cryptosporidium, specific antiparasitic medications may be prescribed.

6.8. Appendicitis

> ➤ *Appendicitis is an inflammation of the appendix, marked by pain in the lower right abdomen, nausea, and fever.*
>
> ➤ *It's primarily caused by a blockage that leads to infection, affecting mainly individuals between 10 and 30 years old.*
>
> ➤ *Treatment typically involves surgical removal of the appendix, appropriate antibiotic, and to prevent complications like rupture and peritonitis.*

Symptoms:

- A sudden pain that begins right lower quadrant, or periumbilical and often shifts to lower right abdomen
- Pain that worsens with activities such as cough, walk, or make other jarring movements
- Nausea and vomiting
- Loss of appetite
- Low-grade fever that may worsen as the illness progresses
- Constipation or diarrhea
- Abdominal bloating

Cause and Risk Factors

The exact cause of appendicitis is often unclear, but it is believed to occur when the appendix becomes blocked, often by stool, a foreign body, or cancer. Blockage may also occur from infection, since the appendix can swell in response to any infection in the body.

Risk factors include:

- Age: Appendicitis most commonly affects people between the ages of 10 and 30.
- Sex: Males are slightly more likely to develop appendicitis than females.
- Family history: People with a family history of appendicitis may be at higher risk.
- Other gastrointestinal infections

Epidemiology:

Appendicitis is a common condition. It is one of the most common causes of emergency abdominal surgery in the United States, with around 250,000 appendectomies performed each year.

Workup and Diagnosis:

- Physical examination to assess pain in the RLQ
- Blood test to look for infection and rule out other abdominal causes
- Urine test to rule out urinary tract infection or kidney stones
- Imaging tests, such as an abdominal ultrasound, CT scan, or MRI, to confirm appendicitis or find other causes of pain

Appendicitis Score

The Alvarado Score assesses the probability of appendicitis using eight criteria.

Symptoms:
- Migratory right lower quadrant (RLQ) pain (1 point)
- Anorexia (1 point)
- Nausea or vomiting (1 point)

Signs:
- Tenderness in RLQ (2 points)
- Rebound pain (1 point)
- Elevated temperature (1 point)

Laboratory:
- Leukocytosis (white blood cell count > 10,000/mm³) (2 points)
- Left shift (elevated neutrophils) (1 point)

Interpretation

- Score of 1-4: Low probability of appendicitis. Further observation, diagnostic imaging, or discharge with follow-up may be considered based on clinical judgment.
- Score of 5-6: Intermediate probability of appendicitis. Additional diagnostic testing, such as imaging (ultrasound or CT scan), is often recommended.
- Score of 7-10: High probability of appendicitis. The patient may be considered for surgical intervention or further diagnostic imaging if not already performed.

Treatment:
The standard treatment for acute appendicitis is appendectomy. The surgery can be performed through open surgery or laparoscopically. In some cases, if an abscess is present, the infection may be drained, and surgery may be delayed.

For uncomplicated appendicitis, a course of antibiotics can be an effective first-line treatment, potentially avoiding the need for immediate surgery. Antibiotic therapy usually includes a combination of anaerobic and aerobic coverage.

For adults, this might involve regimens such as ticarcillin-clavulanate, piperacillin-tazobactam, or a combination of metronidazole with a fluoroquinolone like ciprofloxacin or a third-generation cephalosporin like ceftriaxone.

6.9. Diverticulitis

> ➤ *Diverticulitis occurs when small pouches (diverticula) in the colon become inflamed or infected, leading to abdominal pain, fever, and changes in bowel habits.*
> ➤ *Risk factors include age, a low-fiber diet, obesity, and lack of exercise.*
> ➤ *Treatment typically involves antibiotics, dietary modifications, and in severe cases, surgery may be necessary to remove the affected portion of the colon.*

Symptoms:
- Abdominal pain: Typically localized in the lower left side of the abdomen, though it can occur on the right side or be diffuse.
- Fever: Often accompanies diverticulitis, indicating inflammation or infection.
- Change in bowel habits: Symptoms may include diarrhea, constipation, or alternating between the two.
- Nausea and vomiting: Some patients may experience these symptoms, particularly if there is associated bowel obstruction.
- Rectal bleeding: Blood in the stool may occur if diverticulitis leads to bleeding from inflamed or ruptured diverticula.

- Bloating and gas: Some patients may experience bloating and increased gas production.

Causes and Risk Factors:
- Aging: Diverticulitis becomes more common with age, particularly after the age of 40.
- Diet: A low-fiber diet, high in refined foods and low in fruits, vegetables, and whole grains, increases the risk of diverticulitis.
- Obesity: Being overweight or obese is associated with an increased risk of developing diverticulitis.
- Lack of physical activity: Sedentary lifestyle and lack of regular exercise may contribute to the development of diverticulitis.
- Genetics: There may be a genetic predisposition to diverticulitis, as it tends to run in families.
- Previous history of diverticulosis: patients with diverticulosis are at risk of developing diverticulitis.

Epidemiology:
- Diverticulitis is a common condition, particularly in Western countries such as the United States and Europe.
- The prevalence of diverticulitis increases with age, affecting approximately 10-25% of patients over the age of 50.
- Diverticulitis is less common in populations with high-fiber diets and lifestyles that promote regular bowel movements.

Diagnosis:
- <u>Clinical evaluation:</u> Diagnosis is based on a combination of clinical symptoms, physical examination findings, and diagnostic tests.
- <u>Imaging studies:</u>
    - CT scan of the abdomen and pelvis is the preferred imaging modality for diagnosing diverticulitis. It can identify inflamed or infected diverticula, as well as complications such as abscesses or perforation.
- <u>Blood tests:</u> Laboratory tests such as complete blood count (CBC) may show elevated white blood cell count, indicating inflammation or infection.

Treatment:
- <u>Mild diverticulitis:</u> Treatment may include bowel rest, a clear liquid diet, and oral antibiotics such as ciprofloxacin and metronidazole.
- <u>Severe or complicated diverticulitis:</u>

Hospitalization may be necessary for intravenous antibiotics, bowel rest, and possible drainage of abscesses or surgical intervention in cases of perforation, fistula formation, or severe complications.
- Prevention: Adopting a high-fiber diet, drinking plenty of fluids, regular exercise, and maintaining a healthy weight can help prevent diverticulitis and manage symptoms.

6.10. Cholelithiasis

> ➤ *Gallstones are hardened deposits that form in the gallbladder, often composed of cholesterol or bilirubin.*
> ➤ *Symptoms include abdominal pain, nausea, vomiting, and jaundice, with complications such as pancreatitis or cholecystitis.*
> ➤ *Treatment ranges from medications to surgical removal of the gallbladder (cholecystectomy) depending on severity and symptoms.*

Symptoms:

Many patients with gallstones may not experience any symptoms and may only discover them incidentally during medical tests for unrelated conditions. When symptoms do occur, they often include:

- Sudden and intense pain in the upper right abdomen, which may radiate to the back or right shoulder blade.
- Nausea and vomiting.
- Jaundice
- Clay-colored stools.
- Fever and chills

Causes and Risk Factors:

- Gender: Women are more likely to develop gallstones than men, particularly during pregnancy or while taking hormone replacement therapy or birth control pills.
- Age: Gallstones are more common in older adults.
- Obesity: Excess body weight, especially central obesity, increases the risk of gallstones.
- Diet: High-fat and low-fiber diets may contribute to gallstone formation.
- Rapid weight loss: Losing weight quickly, whether through dieting or bariatric surgery, can increase the risk of gallstones.

- Family history: Having a family history of gallstones increases the likelihood of developing them.
- Certain medical conditions: Conditions such as diabetes, liver disease, and certain blood disorders can increase the risk of gallstones.

Epidemiology:

- Gallstones are common, affecting approximately 10-15% of adults in the United States.
- The prevalence of gallstones varies depending on factors such as age, gender, ethnicity, and geographic location.

Diagnosis:

Gallstones are often diagnosed based on a combination of clinical symptoms, physical examination, and imaging studies.

- Imaging tests: such as ultrasound, computed tomography (CT) scan, or magnetic resonance cholangiopancreatography (MRCP) can visualize gallstones and assess the severity of gallbladder inflammation or obstruction.
- Blood tests: may be performed to evaluate liver function and check for signs of infection or inflammation.

Treatment:

- Observation: Asymptomatic gallstones may not require treatment, particularly if they're not causing any symptoms.
- Medications: Oral medications such as ursodeoxycholic acid may be prescribed to dissolve cholesterol gallstones in some cases.
- Surgery:

    The most definitive treatment for symptomatic gallstones is cholecystectomy. This can be performed via laparoscopic or open surgery.

- Non-surgical procedures:

    In some cases, non-surgical techniques such as endoscopic retrograde cholangiopancreatography (ERCP) with sphincterotomy or shock wave lithotripsy may be used to break up or remove gallstones.

6.11. Constipation

> ➤ *Constipation is a common digestive issue characterized by infrequent bowel movements or difficulty passing stools.*
> ➤ *Symptoms include straining during bowel movements, hard or lumpy stools, and a feeling of incomplete evacuation.*
> ➤ *Treatment involves dietary changes, increased fluid intake, exercise, and occasionally medications to soften stools or stimulate bowel movements.*

Symptoms:
- Infrequent bowel movements (typically fewer than three bowel movements per week).
- Difficulty passing stools, which may be hard, dry, or lumpy.
- Straining during bowel movements.
- Feeling of incomplete evacuation after bowel movements.
- Abdominal discomfort or bloating.
- Rectal bleeding or hemorrhoids due to straining.

Causes and Risk Factors:
- Inadequate fiber intake: Diets low in fiber can contribute to constipation by slowing down bowel movements.
- Inadequate fluid intake: Dehydration can lead to harder stools and difficulty passing them.
- Sedentary lifestyle: Lack of physical activity can contribute to sluggish bowel movements.
- Certain medications: Some medications, including opioids, antacids containing aluminum or calcium, certain antidepressants, and anticholinergic drugs, can cause constipation.
- Aging: Constipation becomes more common with age due to changes in bowel habits and decreased mobility.
- Chronic medical conditions: Conditions such as irritable bowel syndrome (IBS), hypothyroidism, diabetes, and neurological disorders can increase the risk of constipation.
- Pregnancy: Hormonal changes during pregnancy can slow down bowel movements and lead to constipation.

Epidemiology:

Constipation is a common gastrointestinal complaint, affecting patients of all ages, although it tends to be more prevalent in older adults. According to some estimates, up to 20% of the general population experiences constipation at any given time.

Diagnosis:

Diagnosis of constipation is usually based on clinical evaluation, including a thorough medical history and physical examination.

- Laboratory tests or imaging studies: may be ordered if there are concerns about underlying medical conditions contributing to constipation.
- Additional tests: such as colonoscopy may be recommended for patients with alarm symptoms such as rectal bleeding, unexplained weight loss, or a family history of colon cancer.

Treatment:

- Dietary and lifestyle modifications:

    Increasing fiber intake through fruits, vegetables, whole grains, and legumes can help soften stools and promote regular bowel movements. Drinking plenty of fluids and engaging in regular physical activity can also help prevent constipation.

- Over-the-counter laxatives:

    Various types of laxatives, including bulk-forming agents, osmotic laxatives, stimulant laxatives, and stool softeners, may be used to relieve constipation. However, long-term use of laxatives should be avoided without medical supervision.

- Prescription medications:

    In some cases, prescription medications such as prokinetic agents or lubiprostone may be prescribed to stimulate bowel movements or improve intestinal motility.

- Biofeedback therapy:

    Biofeedback techniques can help patients with chronic constipation learn to better control their pelvic muscles and improve bowel function.

- Surgery:

    In rare cases of severe constipation that do not respond to other treatments, surgical procedures such as colectomy may be considered.

6.12. Hemorrhoids

> ➢ *Hemorrhoids are swollen veins in the lower rectum or anus, leading to discomfort, itching, and bleeding during bowel movements.*
> ➢ *Common causes include straining during bowel movements, chronic constipation, or pregnancy.*
> ➢ *Treatment involves lifestyle modifications, topical creams, and in severe cases, procedures like rubber band ligation or surgery may be necessary.*

Symptoms:
- Rectal bleeding: Bright red blood may be seen on toilet paper or in the toilet bowl after bowel movements.
- Itching or irritation: Anus may become itchy or irritated, particularly during or after bowel movements.
- Pain or discomfort: Hemorrhoids can cause pain, discomfort, or a feeling of fullness in the rectum or anus, especially during bowel movements or when sitting for prolonged periods.
- Swelling or lump: External hemorrhoids may appear as a tender lump or swelling near the anal opening.
- Protrusion: Internal hemorrhoids may protrude through the anal opening during bowel movements, known as prolapse, and may require manual reduction.
- Mucous discharge: Excessive mucous discharge from the anus may occur in some cases, particularly with internal hemorrhoids.

Causes and Risk Factors:
- Straining during bowel movements: Constipation, diarrhea, or prolonged straining during bowel movements can increase pressure on the veins in the rectum and anus, leading to hemorrhoid formation.
- Pregnancy: Increased abdominal pressure and hormonal changes during pregnancy can contribute to the development of hemorrhoids.
- Chronic constipation or diarrhea: Conditions that cause frequent or prolonged episodes of constipation or diarrhea can predispose patients to hemorrhoids.
- Obesity: Excess body weight can increase pressure on the pelvic veins and exacerbate hemorrhoid symptoms.

- Sedentary lifestyle: Lack of physical activity or prolonged sitting or standing can impair venous circulation and contribute to hemorrhoid formation.
- Heavy lifting: Straining during heavy lifting or strenuous physical activity can increase intra-abdominal pressure and exacerbate hemorrhoid symptoms.
- Age: Hemorrhoids become more common with age, as the connective tissues and vascular structures in the rectal area may weaken over time.
- Family history: patients with a family history of hemorrhoids may be at increased risk of developing the condition due to genetic predisposition.

Epidemiology:

Hemorrhoids are a common condition, affecting millions of patients worldwide. While precise prevalence rates vary depending on the population studied and diagnostic criteria used, hemorrhoids are estimated to affect approximately 4-5% of the general population. The condition is more prevalent in adults aged 45-65 years, but it can occur at any age.

Diagnosis:

- Medical history and physical examination:

    A healthcare provider will perform a thorough medical history and physical examination, including a digital rectal examination, to assess for signs and symptoms of hemorrhoids.

- Visualization:

    Anoscopy, proctoscopy, or sigmoidoscopy may be performed to visualize the anal canal and rectum and assess for hemorrhoid presence, size, and location.

- Stool examination:

    Stool may be examined for occult blood to rule out other causes of rectal bleeding, such as colorectal cancer or inflammatory bowel disease.

Treatment:

- Lifestyle modifications:

    Dietary changes, including increasing fiber intake, staying hydrated, and adopting regular bowel habits, can help prevent constipation and reduce strain during bowel movements.

- Topical treatments:

    Over-the-counter creams, ointments, or suppositories containing corticosteroids, witch hazel, or lidocaine may provide symptomatic relief from itching, pain, or swelling associated with hemorrhoids.

- Warm baths:

    Soaking in a warm bath (sitz bath) for 10-15 minutes several times a day can help alleviate discomfort and promote healing of hemorrhoids.

- Stool softeners:

    Oral stool softeners or fiber supplements may be recommended to soften stools and reduce straining during bowel movements.

- Minimally invasive procedures:

    Rubber band ligation, sclerotherapy, or infrared coagulation may be performed in-office to shrink internal hemorrhoids by cutting off their blood supply.

- Surgical intervention:

    For severe or persistent hemorrhoids that do not respond to conservative measures, surgical procedures such as hemorrhoidectomy or stapled hemorrhoidopexy may be considered to remove or reduce the size of hemorrhoidal tissue.

6.13. Celiac Disease

> *Celiac disease is an autoimmune disorder triggered by gluten consumption, causing damage to the small intestine lining.*
>
> *Symptoms include gastrointestinal issues like diarrhea, bloating, and abdominal pain, along with fatigue and nutrient deficiencies.*
>
> *Treatment involves adhering to a strict gluten-free diet to manage symptoms and prevent complications.*

Symptoms:

- Digestive symptoms: These may include diarrhea, constipation, abdominal pain, bloating, gas, and nausea.
- Fatigue and weakness.
- Weight loss or failure to thrive (in children).
- Anemia: Due to deficiencies in iron, folate, and vitamin B12.

- Dermatitis herpetiformis: An itchy, blistering skin rash.
- Joint pain.
- Osteoporosis or osteopenia: Weakening of the bones.
- Infertility or recurrent miscarriages.
- Neurological symptoms: Including headaches, peripheral neuropathy, and seizures.
- Mouth ulcers.
- Delayed puberty (in adolescents).

Causes and Risk Factors:
- Family history: Having a first-degree relative with celiac disease increases the risk.
- Certain genetic factors: The presence of specific genetic markers such as HLA-DQ2 and HLA-DQ8.
- Autoimmune diseases: patients with other autoimmune disorders such as type 1 diabetes, autoimmune thyroid disease, or autoimmune liver disease have a higher risk.
- Environmental factors: Early exposure to gluten, such as during infancy, and certain infections may contribute to the development of celiac disease.

Epidemiology:
- Celiac disease is relatively common, affecting approximately 1% of the population worldwide.
- It can occur in patients of any age, including children and adults.
- The prevalence varies among different ethnic and racial groups.

Diagnosis:
- <u>Blood tests:</u>

    Initial screening involves blood tests to detect specific antibodies associated with celiac disease, such as anti-tissue transglutaminase (anti-tTG) antibodies and anti-endomysial antibodies (EMA).

- <u>Intestinal biopsy:</u>

    A definitive diagnosis is usually made by obtaining a biopsy of the small intestine through an upper endoscopy. The biopsy shows characteristic changes in the intestinal lining, including villous atrophy and inflammation.

- Genetic testing:

    HLA typing may be performed to identify genetic markers associated with celiac disease, although it is not used for diagnostic purposes alone.

Treatment:

- Gluten-free diet:

    The cornerstone of treatment for celiac disease is strict adherence to a gluten-free diet, which involves avoiding all sources of gluten, including wheat, barley, rye, and their derivatives.

- Nutritional support: Patients may require nutritional supplementation, especially if they have deficiencies in vitamins or minerals due to malabsorption.

- Monitoring:

    Regular follow-up with a healthcare provider, including monitoring of symptoms, blood tests, and sometimes repeat intestinal biopsies, is important to assess response to treatment and detect any complications.

6.14. Non-Alcoholic Fatty Liver Disease

> - *Non-alcoholic fatty liver disease (NAFLD) is a condition characterized by excessive fat buildup in the liver, not caused by alcohol consumption.*
> - *It ranges from simple fatty liver to non-alcoholic steatohepatitis (NASH), potentially leading to liver inflammation, fibrosis, and cirrhosis.*
> - *Management involves lifestyle changes such as weight loss, dietary modifications, and exercise, along with monitoring for complications and addressing underlying risk factors.*

Symptoms:

- NAFLD is often asymptomatic, especially in the early stages.
- When symptoms do occur, they may include fatigue, weakness, discomfort in the upper right abdomen, and mild jaundice.
- In more advanced stages or if complications develop, symptoms may include ascites, edema, and hepatic encephalopathy.

Causes and Risk Factors:
- Obesity: Excess body weight, particularly central obesity, is strongly associated with NAFLD.
- Insulin resistance and type 2 diabetes: Insulin resistance, often accompanied by type 2 diabetes, is a significant risk factor for NAFLD.
- Dyslipidemia: High levels of triglycerides and low levels of high-density lipoprotein (HDL) cholesterol are common in patients with NAFLD.
- Metabolic syndrome: NAFLD is closely linked to metabolic syndrome, a cluster of conditions including obesity, insulin resistance, dyslipidemia, and hypertension.
- Sedentary lifestyle: Lack of physical activity contributes to the development and progression of NAFLD.
- Genetics: Certain genetic factors may predispose patients to NAFLD, although the exact mechanisms are not fully understood.

Epidemiology:
- NAFLD is the most common liver disorder worldwide, with prevalence rates varying by region and population.
- It is estimated to affect approximately 25% of the global population.
- Prevalence rates are increasing in parallel with the rising rates of obesity, type 2 diabetes, and metabolic syndrome.

Diagnosis:
Diagnosis of NAFLD typically begins with a thorough medical history, physical examination, and assessment of risk factors.
- <u>Blood tests:</u> Liver function tests (LFTs) may show elevated levels of liver enzymes, although they are not specific to NAFLD.
- <u>Imaging studies:</u> Ultrasonography, computed tomography (CT), or magnetic resonance imaging (MRI) may reveal the presence of fatty liver.
- <u>Liver biopsy:</u>
  > A liver biopsy may be performed to confirm the diagnosis and assess the degree of liver inflammation and fibrosis. However, it is usually reserved for cases where the diagnosis is uncertain or when advanced liver disease is suspected.

Treatment:
- <u>Lifestyle modifications:</u>

Weight loss through a combination of dietary changes and increased physical activity is the cornerstone of NAFLD treatment. Gradual weight loss of 5-10% can improve liver health and reduce the risk of disease progression.

- Diet:

    A balanced, calorie-controlled diet that emphasizes fruits, vegetables, whole grains, and lean proteins is recommended. Limiting intake of refined carbohydrates, saturated fats, and added sugars is important.

- Exercise: Regular aerobic exercise, such as brisk walking or cycling, can help improve insulin sensitivity, reduce liver fat, and promote overall health.

- Medications:

    In some cases, medications may be prescribed to manage underlying conditions such as diabetes, dyslipidemia, or hypertension. However, there are currently no specific medications approved for the treatment of NAFLD.

6.15. Acute Pancreatitis

> ➤ *Acute pancreatitis is a sudden inflammation of the pancreas, often triggered by gallstones or excessive alcohol consumption.*
> ➤ *Symptoms include severe abdominal pain, nausea, vomiting, and elevated pancreatic enzymes.*
> ➤ *Treatment involves hospitalization for pain management, intravenous fluids, and addressing underlying causes such as gallstone removal or alcohol cessation.*

Symptoms:

- Sudden and severe abdominal pain, often radiating to the back or shoulder blades.
- Nausea and vomiting.
- Abdominal tenderness and distension.
- Fever and rapid pulse.
- In severe cases, signs of shock, such as low blood pressure and rapid heartbeat, may occur.

Causes and Risk Factors:
- Gallstones: One of the most common causes of acute pancreatitis, especially in women.
- Alcohol consumption: Heavy and chronic alcohol use can lead to pancreatitis.
- Trauma or injury to the abdomen.
- Certain medications, such as corticosteroids, diuretics, and some antibiotics.
- High levels of triglycerides in the blood.
- Infections, such as mumps or viral hepatitis.
- Family history of pancreatitis or pancreatic disorders.
- Smoking.
- Certain medical conditions, including cystic fibrosis and autoimmune disorders.

Epidemiology:
- Acute pancreatitis is relatively common, with an annual incidence of approximately 10-20 cases per 100,000 patients.
- It can occur at any age but is more common in adults, particularly those aged 40-60 years.
- The incidence of acute pancreatitis has been increasing in recent years, possibly due to changes in lifestyle factors such as alcohol consumption and obesity.

Diagnosis:
- <u>History and physical examination:</u> The APP will inquire about symptoms and conduct a physical examination to assess for signs of acute pancreatitis, such as abdominal tenderness.
- <u>Blood tests:</u>

    Elevated levels of pancreatic enzymes, such as amylase and lipase, in the blood are suggestive of pancreatitis. Other blood tests may be performed to assess complications and underlying causes.

- <u>Imaging studies:</u>

    Abdominal ultrasound, computed tomography (CT) scan, or magnetic resonance imaging (MRI) may be used to visualize the pancreas and surrounding structures, assess for inflammation or fluid collections, and identify potential causes such as gallstones or tumors.

- Endoscopic retrograde cholangiopancreatography (ERCP): This procedure may be performed to evaluate the pancreatic duct and bile ducts for obstruction or other abnormalities.

Treatment:
- Supportive care:

    Treatment initially focuses on relieving symptoms and providing supportive care, such as intravenous fluids to prevent dehydration and pain management with analgesic medications.

- NPO status:

    Patients may be advised to refrain from eating or drinking to allow the pancreas to rest and reduce stimulation of pancreatic enzyme secretion.

- Management of underlying causes:

    Treatment may involve addressing the underlying cause of pancreatitis, such as removing gallstones or discontinuing medications that may be contributing to the condition.

- Nutritional support:

    In severe cases or when oral intake is not possible, enteral or parenteral nutrition may be administered to meet nutritional needs and support healing.

- Surgery: In some cases, surgery may be necessary to drain fluid collections, remove obstructions, or treat complications such as infected necrosis.

6.16. Chronic Pancreatitis

> ➤ *Chronic pancreatitis is a long-term inflammation of the pancreas, often caused by repeated episodes of acute pancreatitis, alcohol abuse, or underlying genetic conditions.*
>
> ➤ *Symptoms include persistent abdominal pain, weight loss, digestive issues, and diabetes.*
>
> ➤ *Treatment focuses on pain management, enzyme replacement therapy, dietary modifications, and addressing underlying causes to prevent complications like pancreatic insufficiency or pancreatic cancer.*

Symptoms:
- Persistent or recurrent abdominal pain, typically located in the upper abdomen and radiating to the back.

- Nausea and vomiting.
- Unintentional weight loss.
- Steatorrhea due to malabsorption of fats.
- Jaundice in cases with obstruction of the bile duct.
- Diabetes mellitus may develop in advanced stages due to pancreatic damage affecting insulin production.

Causes and Risk Factors:
- Chronic alcohol consumption: Heavy and prolonged alcohol use is the leading cause of chronic pancreatitis in developed countries.
- Smoking: Tobacco use is a significant risk factor for the development and progression of chronic pancreatitis.
- Genetic factors: Mutations in genes such as PRSS1, CFTR, SPINK1, and CTRC have been implicated in the development of chronic pancreatitis.
- Autoimmune conditions: Autoimmune pancreatitis is a rare form of chronic pancreatitis associated with autoimmune diseases such as autoimmune pancreatitis.
- Obstructive causes: Conditions such as pancreatic duct strictures, pancreatic tumors, or choledocholithiasis can lead to chronic pancreatitis.

Epidemiology:
- Chronic pancreatitis is less common than acute pancreatitis but can lead to significant morbidity and complications.
- It typically affects adults, with the peak incidence occurring between the ages of 30 and 40 years.
- Men are more commonly affected than women.
- The prevalence of chronic pancreatitis varies widely across populations and regions, with higher rates reported in countries with high alcohol consumption.

Diagnosis:
- History and physical examination:

    The APP will inquire about symptoms and conduct a physical examination to assess for signs of chronic pancreatitis, such as abdominal tenderness or palpable masses.

- Imaging studies:

    Imaging tests such as abdominal ultrasound, computed tomography (CT) scan, magnetic resonance imaging (MRI), or endoscopic ultrasound (EUS) may be used to visualize the pancreas and assess for structural abnormalities, calcifications, or pancreatic duct dilation.

- Laboratory tests:

    Blood tests may be performed to evaluate pancreatic function, assess for signs of inflammation, and screen for complications such as diabetes mellitus.

- Endoscopic retrograde cholangiopancreatography (ERCP) or magnetic resonance cholangiopancreatography (MRCP): may be performed to evaluate the pancreatic duct and bile ducts for strictures, stones, or other abnormalities.

Treatment:

- Pain management:

    Treatment aims to alleviate abdominal pain and improve quality of life. This may involve lifestyle modifications, such as avoiding alcohol and smoking, and medications to control pain.

- Enzyme replacement therapy: Pancreatic enzyme supplements may be prescribed to aid in the digestion and absorption of nutrients.

- Nutritional support: Dietary counseling and supplementation may be necessary to address malabsorption and prevent nutritional deficiencies.

- Treatment of complications:

    Interventions may be required to manage complications such as pancreatic pseudocysts, bile duct obstruction, or diabetes mellitus.

- Surgical intervention:

    In severe cases or when conservative measures fail, surgical procedures such as pancreatic duct drainage, pancreatic resection, or total pancreatectomy may be considered.

6.17. Gallstones

> ➤ *Gallstones (Cholelithiasis) are hard deposits formed in the gallbladder, often causing no symptoms unless they block a bile duct, leading to pain, nausea, and potential complications.*
> ➤ *Risk factors include being female, overweight, and dietary habits.*
> ➤ *Treatment typically involves surgery to remove the gallbladder, especially in symptomatic cases or when complications arise.*

Symptoms:

- Sudden and rapidly intensifying pain in the upper right portion of your abdomen
- Sudden and rapidly intensifying pain in the center of your abdomen, just below your breastbone
- Back pain between your shoulder blades
- Pain in your right shoulder
- Nausea or vomiting
- Gallstone pain may last several minutes to a few hours

Risk Factors and Causes

- Diet, with high cholesterol and high-fat diets, as well as low-fiber diets, being linked to gallstone formation.
- Being female
- Being age 40 or older
- Being overweight or obese
- Eating a high-fat or high-cholesterol diet
- Having a family history of gallstones
- Experiencing rapid weight loss
- Having diabetes
- Taking medications that contain estrogen

Epidemiology:

Gallstones are a common digestive problem. They are particularly prevalent among certain populations and regions, affecting millions worldwide. The prevalence varies but is higher in some Native American tribes and among people of European descent. Women are more likely to develop gallstones than men, especially those who are pregnant, overweight, or over the age of 40.

Workup and Diagnosis:

- Ultrasound: to evaluate gallstones.
- CT scan: Which can show gallstones or complications such as infection.
- Blood tests: To check for signs of infection or blockage, and liver function tests.

Treatment

- Cholecystectomy: The most common treatment for symptomatic gallstones is surgical removal of the gallbladder.
- Medications: In some cases, medications can be used to dissolve gallstones, but this treatment is less common and may take years.
- ERCP (Endoscopic Retrograde Cholangiopancreatography): An endoscopic procedure used to remove gallstones from the bile duct.

When is surgery needed?

- Symptomatic Gallstones: If the patient experiences recurrent gallstone attack, surgery is often recommended to prevent future episodes and complications.
- Complications: Surgery is advised if gallstones lead to complications such as:
    - Cholecystitis
    - Pancreatitis
    - Cholangitis
    - Gallstone ileus
    - Jaundice or severe liver dysfunction caused by blocked bile ducts
- Non-functioning Gallbladder: A gallbladder that is not functioning properly (e.g., due to chronic cholecystitis) even if symptomatic gallstones are not present.
- Asymptomatic Gallstones with High Risk of Cancer: Although rare, in certain high-risk cases, such as porcelain gallbladder, surgery might be recommended to prevent gallbladder cancer.
- Asymptomatic Gallstones in Certain Situations: Surgery may be considered for people with asymptomatic gallstones who have a high risk of complications due to other medical conditions or are undergoing other abdominal surgeries **for different reasons.**

6.18. Functional Dyspepsia

> ➤ *Functional dyspepsia is a chronic disorder characterized by persistent upper abdominal discomfort or pain, often accompanied by symptoms like early satiety, bloating, nausea, and belching.*
>
> ➤ *It lacks an identifiable organic cause, and diagnosis is made based on symptom criteria after excluding other gastrointestinal conditions.*
>
> ➤ *Treatment involves lifestyle modifications, dietary changes, symptom management, and occasionally medications targeting gastric motility or acid secretion.*

Symptoms:

- Functional dyspepsia is characterized by chronic or recurrent upper abdominal discomfort or pain without evidence of an organic cause.
- Common symptoms include:
- Epigastric pain or burning sensation
- Feeling uncomfortably full or bloated after eating
- Early satiety
- Nausea
- Belching
- Regurgitation

Causes and Risk Factors:

- The exact cause of functional dyspepsia is not well understood, but several factors may contribute to its development:
- Helicobacter pylori infection: patients with H. pylori infection may have an increased risk of developing functional dyspepsia.
- Psychological factors: Stress, anxiety, and depression may exacerbate symptoms of functional dyspepsia.
- Diet and lifestyle: Certain dietary factors (e.g., spicy or fatty foods) and lifestyle habits (e.g., smoking, excessive alcohol consumption) may trigger or worsen symptoms.
- Female gender: Functional dyspepsia is more common in women than men.

Epidemiology:

- Functional dyspepsia is a common gastrointestinal disorder, affecting millions of patients worldwide.

- The prevalence of functional dyspepsia varies across populations and is estimated to range from 10% to 30%.
- It can occur at any age but is more commonly diagnosed in adults between the ages of 30 and 50.
- Functional dyspepsia may have a significant impact on quality of life, leading to decreased productivity and social functioning.

Diagnosis:
- Diagnosis of functional dyspepsia:

    Diagnosis is based on clinical criteria and the exclusion of other gastrointestinal disorders with similar symptoms. The APP may perform a thorough medical history and physical examination to assess symptoms and rule out potential organic causes.

- Diagnostic tests:

    Tests such as upper endoscopy, abdominal ultrasound, or laboratory tests (e.g., H. pylori testing) may be performed to rule out structural abnormalities or other conditions.

Treatment:

Treatment of functional dyspepsia focuses on symptom management and may include:

- Lifestyle modifications: Avoiding trigger foods, eating smaller, more frequent meals, reducing stress, and avoiding smoking and excessive alcohol consumption.
- Pharmacological therapy:

    Medications such as proton pump inhibitors (PPIs), histamine H2-receptor antagonists, prokinetic agents, and antacids may be prescribed to alleviate symptoms.

- Psychological interventions:

    Cognitive-behavioral therapy (CBT), relaxation techniques, and stress management strategies may help reduce symptoms in patients with functional dyspepsia.

- Dietary modifications: Some patients may benefit from dietary changes, such as avoiding spicy or fatty foods, caffeine, and carbonated beverages.

6.19. Anal Fissure

> ➤ Anal fissure is a tear or split in the lining of the anal canal, typically causing sharp pain and bleeding during bowel movements.
>
> ➤ Common symptoms include pain during or after defecation, bright red blood on toilet paper or in stools, and spasms of the anal sphincter.
>
> ➤ Treatment often involves dietary modifications, stool softeners, topical medications (such as nitroglycerin or calcium channel blockers), and in severe cases, surgical intervention.

Symptoms:

Anal fissures are small tears or cracks in the lining of the anal canal, which can cause pain and discomfort during bowel movements. Common symptoms include:

- Pain during or after bowel movements, often described as sharp or stabbing
- Bright red blood on toilet paper or in the toilet bowl after wiping
- Itching or burning around the anal area
- Fissures may cause spasms of the anal sphincter muscles, leading to further pain and difficulty with bowel movements.

Causes and Risk Factors:

- Constipation: Passing hard stools or straining during bowel movements can increase the risk of developing anal fissures.
- Diarrhea: Chronic diarrhea or frequent bowel movements can irritate the anal canal and contribute to fissure formation.
- Anal trauma: Trauma to the anal region from childbirth, anal intercourse, or insertion of foreign objects can predispose patients to anal fissures.
- Inflammatory bowel disease (IBD): Conditions such as Crohn's disease or ulcerative colitis can increase the risk of anal fissures.
- Aging: Older adults may be more prone to developing anal fissures due to changes in bowel habits and decreased elasticity of the anal tissues.

Epidemiology:

- Anal fissures are a common problem, affecting patients of all ages, but they are more prevalent in younger adults.

- While the exact prevalence of anal fissures is not well established, they are considered one of the most common causes of anorectal pain and bleeding.
- Anal fissures can occur in both men and women, although they may be more common in women due to factors such as childbirth.

Diagnosis:

Diagnosis of anal fissures is typically based on clinical examination and medical history.

- Digital rectal exam: may be performed by APP to assess for signs of fissures, such as tenderness, swelling, or the presence of a skin tag (sentinel pile) near the anal opening.
- Anoscopy or proctoscopy: may be performed to visualize the inside of the anal canal and confirm the diagnosis.

Treatment:

Initial treatment for anal fissures often involves conservative measures aimed at relieving symptoms and promoting healing.

- Dietary modifications:
    Increasing fiber intake to soften stools and prevent constipation, drinking plenty of fluids, and avoiding straining during bowel movements.
- Topical treatments:
    Over-the-counter or prescription creams containing local anesthetics, corticosteroids, or calcium channel blockers may help reduce pain and promote healing.
- Sitz baths: Warm water baths taken several times a day can help soothe the anal area and promote relaxation of the anal sphincter muscles.
- Medications: In some cases, medications such as stool softeners or laxatives may be prescribed to help alleviate constipation and reduce strain during bowel movements.
- Surgical intervention:
    If conservative measures fail to provide relief, surgical procedures such as lateral internal sphincterotomy or botulinum toxin injection may be considered to relax the anal sphincter muscles and promote healing.

6.20. Anal Abscess

> ➢ An anal abscess is a painful collection of pus near the anus or rectum, typically caused by a bacterial infection in an anal gland.
>
> ➢ Symptoms include swelling, redness, pain, and sometimes fever or drainage of pus.
>
> ➢ Treatment involves drainage of the abscess, antibiotics, and measures to prevent recurrence, such as maintaining good hygiene and addressing underlying conditions like inflammatory bowel disease.

Symptoms:
- Pain and swelling around the anus or rectum are the hallmark symptoms of an anal abscess.
- Other common symptoms include:
- Redness and warmth in the affected area
- Fever and chills
- Painful bowel movements
- Discharge of pus or blood from the anus
- Feeling of fullness or pressure in the rectal area

Causes and Risk Factors:
- Conditions that lead to the blockage of anal glands, such as constipation or inflammatory bowel disease, can increase the risk of developing an anal abscess.
- Sexually transmitted infections (STIs) such as gonorrhea or chlamydia can also predispose patients to anal abscesses.
- Immunosuppression, diabetes, or other medical conditions that weaken the immune system may increase susceptibility to infections.
- Anal trauma or injury, including anal intercourse or insertion of foreign objects, can introduce bacteria into the anal region and lead to abscess formation.

Epidemiology:
- Anal abscesses are relatively common and can affect patients of any age, although they are more prevalent in adults.
- Men are more likely to develop anal abscesses than women.
- The incidence of anal abscesses may vary depending on factors such as access to healthcare, hygiene practices, and prevalence of risk factors in a given population.

Diagnosis:
- Physical examination of the anal area: to assess for signs of swelling, redness, or tenderness.
- Imaging studies: in some cases, ultrasound or MRI may be ordered to evaluate the extent of the abscess and rule out complications such as fistulas.

Treatment:
- Incision and drainage:

    The primary treatment for an anal abscess involves surgical drainage to evacuate pus and relieve pressure. This is usually performed under local anesthesia in outpatient clinics.

- Antibiotic therapy:

    In cases where the abscess is associated with cellulitis or systemic symptoms, antibiotic therapy may be prescribed to control infection and prevent further complications.

- Pain management:

    Analgesic medications such as nonsteroidal anti-inflammatory drugs (NSAIDs) or opioids may be prescribed to manage pain and discomfort.

- Warm compresses: Applying warm compresses to the affected area may help reduce pain and promote drainage of the abscess.
- Follow-up care: Patients may require follow-up visits with the APP or other healthcare providers to monitor healing and assess for recurrence or complications.

6.21. Eosinophilic Esophagitis

> - Eosinophilic esophagitis (EoE) is a chronic inflammatory condition of the esophagus, characterized by an excessive number of eosinophils in the esophageal tissue.
> - Symptoms include difficulty swallowing, chest pain, and food impaction, often triggered by allergies or immune-mediated responses.
> - Management involves dietary modifications, medication, and in some cases, endoscopic dilation or steroid therapy to alleviate symptoms and prevent complications.

Symptoms:
- Difficulty swallowing is the most common symptom of EoE, especially for solid foods.
- Other symptoms may include:
- Food impaction
- Chest pain or discomfort, often mistaken for heartburn
- Heartburn or acid reflux symptoms
- Regurgitation
- Nausea and vomiting
- Failure to thrive or poor weight gain in children
- Food refusal or aversion in children

Causes and Risk Factors:
- EoE is believed to be an allergic or immune-mediated disorder, so patients with a history of allergic conditions such as asthma, allergic rhinitis, eczema, or food allergies may be at higher risk.
- Family history of EoE or other allergic conditions may increase susceptibility.
- Environmental factors, such as exposure to allergens or pollutants, may also play a role.

Epidemiology:
- EoE is increasingly recognized as a chronic condition, particularly in Western countries.
- It can affect patients of any age but is more common in children and young adults.
- The prevalence of EoE appears to be rising, although this may be due in part to increased awareness and improved diagnostic techniques.

Diagnosis:

Diagnosis of EoE typically involves a combination of clinical evaluation, endoscopy, and histological assessment.

- Endoscopy:

    During an upper endoscopy (esophagogastroduodenoscopy or EGD), the esophagus may appear inflamed, with features such as rings, furrows, or white plaques.

- Biopsy:

    Tissue samples (biopsies) are taken from the esophagus during endoscopy to assess for the presence of eosinophils, a type of white blood cell indicative of inflammation. A high number of eosinophils (>15-20 per high-power field) in the esophageal tissue is consistent with EoE.

- Other tests:

    Additional tests may be performed to rule out other causes of esophageal inflammation or symptoms, such as pH monitoring to assess for acid reflux.

Treatment:

- Dietary management:

    The first-line treatment for EoE often involves dietary modifications, such as elimination diets to identify and avoid trigger foods that may be causing inflammation. Common trigger foods include dairy, wheat, soy, eggs, and seafood.

- Topical steroids:

    Inhaled corticosteroids or swallowed steroid preparations may be prescribed to reduce esophageal inflammation and eosinophilic infiltration.

- Proton pump inhibitors (PPIs):

    These medications may be used to suppress acid reflux symptoms in some patients with EoE, although they may not address the underlying inflammation.

- Esophageal dilation:

    In cases of severe narrowing or dysphagia that does not respond to other treatments, esophageal dilation may be performed to widen the esophagus and improve swallowing.

- Immunomodulators or biologic agents: These medications may be considered for patients with refractory EoE or those who cannot tolerate other treatments.

6.22. Gastrointestinal Bleeding

> ➤ *Gastrointestinal bleeding refers to bleeding within the digestive tract, often presenting as blood in vomit or stool.*
>
> ➤ *Causes range from peptic ulcers and gastritis to more severe conditions like colorectal cancer or diverticulosis.*
>
> ➤ *Diagnosis involves endoscopy, imaging, and treatment may include medications, endoscopic procedures, or surgery depending on the cause and severity.*

Symptoms:
- Bright red or maroon-colored blood in vomit
- Dark, tarry, or black stools
- Blood in the stool, which may appear red or maroon
- Fatigue
- Weakness
- Dizziness or lightheadedness
- Fainting (syncope) in severe cases

Causes and Risk Factors:
- Peptic ulcer disease
- Gastritis
- Esophagitis
- Gastrointestinal cancers
- Mallory-Weiss tears
- Esophageal varices
- Diverticulosis
- Inflammatory bowel disease (Crohn's disease, ulcerative colitis)
- Medication use, such as nonsteroidal anti-inflammatory drugs (NSAIDs), aspirin, or anticoagulants
- Alcohol abuse
- Liver cirrhosis
- Helicobacter pylori infection

Epidemiology:
- GI bleeding is a common medical emergency and can occur at any age, although it is more common in older adults.
- Upper GI bleeding (involving the esophagus, stomach, or duodenum) accounts for the majority of cases.
- Lower GI bleeding (involving the colon, rectum, or anus) is less common but can also be serious.

Diagnosis:
- Endoscopy/Colonoscopy:

    Upper endoscopy (esophagogastroduodenoscopy or EGD) or colonoscopy may be performed to visualize the gastrointestinal tract and identify the source of bleeding.

- Imaging studies:

    Radiographic imaging, such as abdominal computed tomography (CT) scans or angiography, may be used to locate the bleeding site if endoscopy is inconclusive.
- Laboratory tests: Blood tests may be performed to assess hemoglobin levels, coagulation status, and other parameters.

Treatment:
- Supportive care:

    Initial management may involve stabilization of the patient, intravenous fluids, blood transfusions (if significant blood loss), and correction of coagulopathy if present.
- Endoscopic therapy:

    Various endoscopic techniques, such as injection therapy, thermal coagulation, or hemostatic clipping, may be used to stop bleeding lesions identified during endoscopy.
- Medications:

    Proton pump inhibitors (PPIs) may be prescribed to reduce gastric acid secretion and promote healing of peptic ulcers or erosive gastritis.
- Surgery:

    Surgical intervention may be necessary in cases of severe or refractory bleeding, such as arterial embolization or surgical resection of bleeding lesions.

6.23. Barrett's Esophagus

> ➤ *Barrett's esophagus is a condition where the tissue lining the esophagus is replaced by tissue similar to the lining of the intestine, often due to chronic acid reflux. It increases the risk of esophageal adenocarcinoma.*
>
> ➤ *Monitoring and treatment aim to prevent cancer development, typically through surveillance endoscopy and medications to manage reflux.*

Symptoms:
- Barrett's Esophagus itself typically does not cause symptoms. However, it is often associated with gastroesophageal reflux disease (GERD), which may present with symptoms such as:

- Heartburn
- Regurgitation of stomach acid or food
- Difficulty swallowing
- Chest pain
- Persistent cough
- Hoarseness or voice changes

Causes and Risk Factors:
- Chronic gastroesophageal reflux disease (GERD): Frequent exposure of the esophagus to stomach acid increases the risk of developing Barrett's Esophagus.
- Male gender: Men are more likely than women to develop Barrett's Esophagus.
- Age: Barrett's Esophagus is more common in older adults.
- Hiatal hernia: Having a hiatal hernia, where part of the stomach protrudes into the chest cavity through the diaphragm, is a risk factor.
- Obesity: Being overweight or obese increases the risk of developing Barrett's Esophagus.
- Tobacco smoking: Smoking cigarettes or using other tobacco products is associated with an increased risk.
- Family history: Having a family history of Barrett's Esophagus or esophageal cancer may increase the risk.

Epidemiology:
- Barrett's Esophagus is relatively common, particularly in patients with long-standing GERD.
- It is estimated that 1% to 2% of adults in Western countries have Barrett's Esophagus.
- The prevalence of Barrett's Esophagus increases with age, and it is more common in men than in women.

Workup and Diagnosis:
- <u>Endoscopy:</u>

    Barrett's Esophagus is typically diagnosed through upper endoscopy (esophagogastroduodenoscopy or EGD) with biopsy. During endoscopy, the gastroenterologist examines the lining of the esophagus and may take biopsies from any suspicious areas.

- Biopsy: Samples are examined under a microscope to confirm the presence of specialized intestinal metaplasia, which is characteristic of Barrett's Esophagus.

Treatment:
- Management of Barrett's Esophagus: focuses on controlling GERD symptoms and surveillance to monitor for dysplasia (pre-cancerous changes) or progression to esophageal cancer.
- Treatment options for GERD:

    Treatment may include lifestyle modifications (e.g., weight loss, dietary changes), medications (e.g., proton pump inhibitors), and, in some cases, surgical procedures to strengthen the lower esophageal sphincter or repair a hiatal hernia.

- Surveillance endoscopy with biopsy:

    This may be recommended periodically to monitor for dysplasia or cancerous changes. If high-grade dysplasia or early-stage cancer is detected, treatment options may include endoscopic mucosal resection (EMR), radiofrequency ablation (RFA), or surgical resection.

6.24. Intestinal Obstruction

> ➤ *Intestinal obstruction occurs when there's a partial or complete blockage in the intestines, preventing the passage of food, fluids, and gas.*
>
> ➤ *Symptoms include severe abdominal pain, vomiting, bloating, and inability to pass stool or gas.*
>
> ➤ *Treatment involves identifying and addressing the cause, often requiring hospitalization for bowel rest, hydration, and, in severe cases, surgery to remove the obstruction.*

Symptoms:
- Abdominal pain: Typically, the pain starts as crampy abdominal discomfort and progresses to severe, colicky pain.
- Abdominal distension: The abdomen may become visibly swollen and bloated.
- Nausea and vomiting: Due to the obstruction, food and fluid cannot pass through the intestine, leading to nausea and vomiting.

- Inability to pass gas or stool: Patients may experience a lack of bowel movements and the inability to pass gas.
- Constipation or diarrhea: Depending on the location and severity of the obstruction, patients may experience either constipation or diarrhea.
- Abdominal tenderness: Palpation of the abdomen may reveal areas of tenderness or discomfort.

Causes and Risk Factors:
- Prior abdominal surgery: Previous abdominal surgeries, especially those involving the intestines, increase the risk of developing adhesions or scar tissue that can cause obstruction.
- Hernias: Inguinal, femoral, or umbilical hernias can lead to intestinal obstruction if the bowel becomes trapped within the hernia sac.
- Intestinal tumors: Benign or malignant tumors within the intestine can obstruct the passage of stool or fluid.
- Inflammatory bowel disease (IBD): Conditions such as Crohn's disease or ulcerative colitis can cause inflammation and narrowing of the intestinal lumen, leading to obstruction.
- Intestinal adhesions: Adhesions can form as a result of abdominal surgery, radiation therapy, or intra-abdominal infections.
- Volvulus: Twisting of the intestine upon itself can cause obstruction, especially in conditions such as sigmoid volvulus or cecal volvulus.

Epidemiology:
- Intestinal obstruction can occur at any age but is more common in older adults due to increased prevalence of conditions such as adhesions, hernias, and tumors.
- The incidence of intestinal obstruction varies depending on the underlying cause and population studied.

Workup and Diagnosis:
- <u>Physical examination:</u> Abdominal examination may reveal distension, tenderness, and abnormal bowel sounds (e.g., high-pitched tinkling sounds).
- <u>Imaging studies:</u> Abdominal X-rays, CT scans, or ultrasound may be performed to visualize the location and cause of the obstruction.
- <u>Blood tests:</u> Laboratory tests such as complete blood count (CBC) and electrolyte panel may be ordered to assess for signs of dehydration or infection.

Treatment:
- Fluid resuscitation: Intravenous fluids are administered to correct dehydration and electrolyte imbalances.
- Nasogastric decompression: A nasogastric tube may be inserted to decompress the stomach and relieve vomiting and distension.
- Bowel rest: Patients are typically kept nil per os (NPO) to allow the bowel to rest and reduce the risk of further complications.
- Surgical intervention:
    In cases of mechanical obstruction or ischemic bowel, surgical intervention may be necessary to relieve the obstruction, resect damaged bowel, and repair any underlying pathology.

6.25. Small Intestinal Bacterial Overgrowth

> ➤ *Small intestinal bacterial overgrowth (SIBO) is a condition characterized by an abnormal increase in bacteria in the small intestine, often leading to gastrointestinal symptoms.*
> ➤ *Symptoms include bloating, diarrhea, abdominal pain, and malabsorption of nutrients.*
> ➤ *Treatment involves antibiotics to reduce bacterial overgrowth, along with dietary modifications to manage symptoms and prevent recurrence.*

Symptoms:
- Abdominal bloating and distension
- Abdominal pain or discomfort, often relieved by bowel movements
- Excessive gas
- Diarrhea, often watery or loose stools
- Constipation or alternating diarrhea and constipation
- Fatigue and weakness
- Weight loss or malnutrition, especially in severe cases
- Symptoms may worsen after eating certain foods, especially those high in fermentable carbohydrates (FODMAPs).

Causes and Risk Factors:
- Conditions that affect gastrointestinal motility, such as gastroparesis or intestinal dysmotility

- Anatomical abnormalities or surgical interventions that alter the normal anatomy or function of the gastrointestinal tract
- Use of medications that affect gastrointestinal motility or suppress gastric acid production, such as proton pump inhibitors (PPIs)
- Chronic conditions that predispose to SIBO, such as inflammatory bowel disease (IBD) or celiac disease
- Aging, as gastrointestinal motility tends to decrease with age
- Previous intestinal surgery or radiation therapy to the abdomen

Epidemiology:
- The prevalence of SIBO varies depending on the population studied and the diagnostic criteria used.
- It is more common in patients with conditions that affect gastrointestinal motility or disrupt the normal balance of gut microbiota.

Workup and Diagnosis:
- Breath tests:

    Hydrogen breath tests are commonly used to diagnose SIBO. Patients ingest a substrate (usually lactulose or glucose), and breath samples are collected over several hours to measure the production of hydrogen and methane gases by bacteria in the small intestine.

- Small bowel aspirate:

    Direct sampling of fluid from the small intestine via endoscopy can provide a definitive diagnosis of SIBO by quantifying bacterial overgrowth.

- Blood tests:

    Elevated levels of markers such as C-reactive protein (CRP) or fecal calprotectin may indicate inflammation or infection in the gastrointestinal tract.

Treatment:
- Antibiotics:

    The primary treatment for SIBO involves antibiotics to eradicate the overgrowth of bacteria in the small intestine. Commonly used antibiotics include rifaximin, metronidazole, and tetracycline.

- Probiotics: Certain probiotic strains may help restore a healthy balance of gut microbiota and prevent recurrences of SIBO.

- Dietary modifications: Following a low-FODMAP diet or other dietary interventions may help alleviate symptoms and prevent bacterial overgrowth.
- Addressing underlying conditions: Treating underlying conditions such as gastroparesis, IBD, or celiac disease may help reduce the risk of SIBO recurrence.
- Symptomatic management: Medications to alleviate symptoms such as abdominal pain, bloating, or diarrhea may be prescribed as needed.

6.26. Malabsorption Syndromes

> ➤ *Malabsorption syndromes refer to a group of disorders where the intestines are unable to properly absorb nutrients from food.*
> ➤ *Symptoms include diarrhea, weight loss, bloating, and nutrient deficiencies.*
> ➤ *Treatment involves dietary changes, supplementation, managing underlying conditions, and sometimes medications to alleviate symptoms and improve nutrient absorption.*

Symptoms:
- Diarrhea
- Steatorrhea
- Abdominal bloating and cramps
- Gas (flatulence)
- Weight loss
- Weakness and fatigue due to malnutrition
- Anemia (due to malabsorption of nutrients like iron, folate, and vitamin B12)
- Bone pain or fractures (due to calcium and vitamin D deficiency)

Causes and Risk Factors:
- Genetics: Some malabsorption syndromes, such as lactose intolerance, can have a genetic component.
- Age: Certain conditions, such as lactose intolerance, may become more common with age due to a decrease in lactase enzyme production.

- Gastrointestinal surgeries or diseases: Conditions such as celiac disease, Crohn's disease, and surgical resection of parts of the intestine can lead to malabsorption.
- Medications: Some medications, such as proton pump inhibitors (PPIs), can interfere with nutrient absorption.
- Infections: Gastrointestinal infections or overgrowth of bacteria in the small intestine can disrupt normal nutrient absorption.

Epidemiology:

- The prevalence of malabsorption syndromes varies depending on the specific condition and population studied.
- Lactose intolerance, for example, is estimated to affect approximately 65% of the global population to some degree.

Workup and Diagnosis:

Lactose intolerance:

- Lactose tolerance test: Measures blood glucose levels after ingesting a lactose solution.
- Hydrogen breath test: Measures breath hydrogen levels after ingesting a lactose solution.
- Stool acidity test: Measures acidity in the stool after lactose ingestion.

Other malabsorption syndromes:

- Blood tests: Assess levels of specific nutrients (e.g., vitamin B12, iron) or markers of malabsorption (e.g., fecal fat).
- Endoscopy with biopsy: Used to diagnose conditions like celiac disease by examining the small intestine's lining.
- Stool tests: Check for fat malabsorption or evidence of bacterial overgrowth.

Treatment:

Lactose intolerance:

- Dietary modification: Avoiding or reducing lactose-containing foods and beverages.
- Lactase enzyme supplements: Taken before consuming dairy products to aid lactose digestion.

Other malabsorption syndromes:

- Dietary modifications: Adjusting the diet to minimize symptoms and ensure adequate nutrient intake.

- **Nutritional supplements:** Taking supplements to address specific nutrient deficiencies.
- **Treatment of underlying conditions:** Managing conditions like celiac disease or Crohn's disease to improve nutrient absorption.
- **Medications:** Some medications may help alleviate symptoms or improve nutrient absorption in certain cases.

6.27. Gastrointestinal Motility Disorders

> ➤ *Gastrointestinal motility disorders involve abnormal movements or function of the digestive tract, affecting the passage of food and waste.*
> ➤ *Symptoms include abdominal pain, bloating, constipation, diarrhea, and difficulty swallowing.*
> ➤ *Treatment focuses on managing symptoms through dietary changes, medications, and sometimes surgical interventions to improve motility and alleviate discomfort.*

Symptoms:
- Abdominal pain or discomfort
- Bloating
- Nausea or vomiting
- Difficulty swallowing
- Regurgitation
- Heartburn or gastroesophageal reflux
- Changes in bowel habits (diarrhea, constipation, or alternating between the two)
- Feeling of fullness after eating small amounts
- Unintended weight loss or malnutrition

Causes and Risk Factors:
- Aging: GI motility disorders may become more common with age due to changes in the muscles and nerves of the digestive system.
- Neurological conditions: Disorders affecting the nervous system, such as Parkinson's disease or multiple sclerosis, can disrupt normal GI motility.
- Diabetes: Diabetic neuropathy can affect the nerves controlling GI function.

- Medications: Certain medications, such as opioids, anticholinergics, and some antidepressants, can slow down GI motility.
- Surgery: Previous abdominal surgeries, especially those involving the stomach or intestines, can lead to motility issues.

Epidemiology:
- The prevalence of GI motility disorders varies depending on the specific condition.
- Conditions like gastroesophageal reflux disease (GERD) and irritable bowel syndrome (IBS) are relatively common, affecting millions of patients worldwide.

Workup and Diagnosis:
- <u>Medical history and physical examination:</u> Including a detailed history of symptoms and risk factors.
- <u>Imaging tests:</u> Such as upper GI series, barium swallow, or esophagogastroduodenoscopy (EGD) to evaluate the structure and function of the GI tract.
- <u>Manometry:</u> Measures pressure and movement in the GI tract to assess motility.
- <u>Breath tests:</u> Used to diagnose conditions like bacterial overgrowth or lactose intolerance.
- <u>Blood tests:</u> To check for signs of inflammation or nutritional deficiencies.
- <u>Stool tests:</u> To evaluate for infection, inflammation, or malabsorption.

Treatment:
- <u>Dietary modifications:</u> Including changes in fiber intake, avoiding trigger foods, and consuming smaller, more frequent meals.
- <u>Medications:</u> Such as prokinetic agents to enhance GI motility or acid-suppressing drugs for GERD.
- <u>Behavioral therapies:</u> Such as biofeedback or relaxation techniques to manage symptoms.
- <u>Surgical interventions:</u> In severe cases, surgical procedures may be necessary to correct structural abnormalities or improve motility.
- <u>Lifestyle changes:</u> Including regular exercise, stress management, and adequate hydration.
- <u>Symptom management:</u> Addressing specific symptoms like heartburn, bloating, or constipation with appropriate medications or interventions.

6.28. Inguinal Hernia and Ventral Hernia

> ➢ Inguinal hernia involves protrusion of tissue through a weak spot in the groin area, causing a bulge and discomfort, commonly due to strain or muscle weakness.
>
> ➢ Ventral hernia occurs when tissue pushes through weakened abdominal muscles, often at a surgical scar site, causing a visible bulge and discomfort, with surgery typically required for repair in both cases.

6.28.1. Inguinal Hernia:

Symptoms:
- Bulge or swelling in the groin area, which may become more prominent when coughing, straining, or standing upright.
- Pain or discomfort in the groin, particularly when lifting heavy objects, coughing, or bending over.
- A sensation of heaviness or pressure in the groin.
- Burning or aching sensation at the site of the hernia.
- Sometimes, an inguinal hernia may be asymptomatic and only discovered during a physical examination.

Causes and Risk Factors:
- Male gender (inguinal hernias are more common in men than women).
- Older age.
- Family history of hernias.
- Chronic coughing or straining during bowel movements.
- Obesity.
- Smoking.
- Previous abdominal surgery.
- Congenital factors, such as weak abdominal muscles or defects in the abdominal wall.

Epidemiology:
- Inguinal hernias are the most common type of hernia, accounting for approximately 75% of all hernias.
- They are more common in men, with a lifetime risk of around 25%, compared to approximately 2% in women.

Workup and Diagnosis:

- Physical examination: The APP can typically diagnose an inguinal hernia by feeling for a bulge in the groin area during a physical examination.
- Imaging tests: Ultrasound or MRI may be used to confirm the diagnosis and evaluate the size and extent of the hernia.

Treatment:

- Observation:

    Asymptomatic inguinal hernias may be monitored without immediate treatment, particularly if they are small and not causing symptoms.

- Hernia truss:

    A supportive garment called a hernia truss may be worn to help hold the hernia in place and reduce discomfort, although this is not typically recommended as a long-term solution.

- Surgery:

    Surgical repair is the definitive treatment for inguinal hernias and may involve open or laparoscopic techniques to push the hernia back into place and reinforce the abdominal wall with mesh.

6.28.2. Ventral Hernia:

Symptoms:

- Visible bulge or swelling in the abdominal wall.
- Pain or discomfort at the site of the hernia, particularly when lifting heavy objects or straining.
- Changes in the appearance of the abdomen, such as a noticeable bulge or protrusion.

Causes and Risk Factors:

- Previous abdominal surgery.
- Obesity.
- Pregnancy.
- Chronic coughing or straining.
- Aging.
- Connective tissue disorders.
- Conditions that increase intra-abdominal pressure, such as ascites or chronic constipation.

Epidemiology:
- Ventral hernias are less common than inguinal hernias but can occur in both men and women.
- The incidence of ventral hernias increases with age and is more common in patients who have undergone abdominal surgery.

Workup and Diagnosis:
- Physical examination:

    A healthcare provider can often diagnose a ventral hernia by feeling for a bulge or mass in the abdominal wall during a physical examination.
- Imaging tests: Ultrasound, CT scan, or MRI may be used to confirm the diagnosis and evaluate the size and extent of the hernia.

Treatment:
- Observation:

    Asymptomatic ventral hernias may be monitored without immediate treatment, particularly if they are small and not causing symptoms.
- Hernia truss:

    Similar to inguinal hernias, a hernia truss may be worn to provide support and reduce discomfort, although this is not typically recommended as a long-term solution.
- Surgery:

    Surgical repair is the main treatment for ventral hernias and may involve open or laparoscopic techniques to push the hernia contents back into place and reinforce the abdominal wall with mesh.

References
- Katz, P. O., Gerson, L. B., & Vela, M. F. (2013). Guidelines for the diagnosis and management of gastroesophageal reflux disease. American Journal of Gastroenterology, 108(3), 308-328.
- Chey, W. D., Leontiadis, G. I., Howden, C. W., & Moss, S. F. (2017). ACG clinical guideline: Treatment of Helicobacter pylori infection. American Journal of Gastroenterology, 112(2), 212-239.
- Ford, A. C., Lacy, B. E., Talley, N. J., & et al. (2017). Effect of antidepressants and psychological therapies, including hypnotherapy, in irritable bowel syndrome: Systematic review and meta-analysis. American Journal of Gastroenterology, 109(9), 1350-1365.

- Lichtenstein, G. R., Loftus Jr, E. V., Isaacs, K. L., et al. (2018). ACG clinical guideline: Management of Crohn's disease in adults. American Journal of Gastroenterology, 113(4), 481-517.
- Rubin, D. T., Ananthakrishnan, A. N., Siegel, C. A., et al. (2019). ACG clinical guideline: Ulcerative colitis in adults. American Journal of Gastroenterology, 114(3), 384-413.
- Riddle, M. S., DuPont, H. L., & Connor, B. A. (2016). ACG clinical guideline: Diagnosis and treatment of acute diarrhea. American Journal of Gastroenterology, 111(5), 602-622.
- Stollman, N., & Raskin, J. B. (2004). Diverticular disease of the colon. The Lancet, 363(9409), 631-639.
- Friedman, L. S. (2010). Gallstones. New England Journal of Medicine, 363(19), 1911-1923.
- Bharucha, A. E., Pemberton, J. H., & Locke III, G. R. (2013). American Gastroenterological Association technical review on constipation. Gastroenterology, 144(1), 218-238.
- Davis, B. R., Lee-Kong, S. A., & Migaly, J. (2016). The American Society of Colon and Rectal Surgeons clinical practice guidelines for the management of hemorrhoids. Diseases of the Colon & Rectum, 59(12), 479-492.
- Rubio-Tapia, A., Hill, I. D., Kelly, C. P., Calderwood, A. H., & Murray, J. A. (2013). ACG clinical guidelines: Diagnosis and management of celiac disease. American Journal of Gastroenterology, 108(5), 656-676.
- Chalasani, N., Younossi, Z., Lavine, J. E., et al. (2018). The diagnosis and management of nonalcoholic fatty liver disease: Practice guidance from the American Association for the Study of Liver Diseases. Hepatology, 67(1), 328-357.
- Tenner, S., Baillie, J., DeWitt, J., et al. (2013). American College of Gastroenterology guideline: Management of acute pancreatitis. American Journal of Gastroenterology, 108(9), 1400-1415.
- American Gastroenterological Association. (2019). AGA clinical practice guidelines on the role of endoscopy in the diagnosis and management of chronic pancreatitis. Gastroenterology, 156(1), 199-214.
- Gurusamy, K., Junnarkar, S., Farouk, M., Davidson, B. R. (2013). Cholecystectomy for suspected gallbladder dyskinesia. Cochrane Database of Systematic Reviews, (4), CD006233.
- Talley, N. J., Ford, A. C., & et al. (2017). Guidelines on the management of dyspepsia. American Journal of Gastroenterology, 112(7), 988-1013.
- Lohsiriwat, V. (2016). Treatment of chronic anal fissure: A systematic review and meta-analysis. World Journal of Surgery, 40(1), 179-187.
- DeBord, J. R., & Luchtefeld, M. A. (2016). Perianal abscess and fistula-in-ano: Diagnosis and management. American Family Physician, 93(10), 830-836.

- Strate, L. L., Gralnek, I. M., & et al. (2016). ACG clinical guideline: Management of patients with acute lower gastrointestinal bleeding. American Journal of Gastroenterology, 111(4), 459-474.
- Shaheen, N. J., Falk, G. W., Iyer, P. G., Gerson, L. B. (2016). ACG clinical guideline: Diagnosis and management of Barrett's esophagus. American Journal of Gastroenterology, 111(1), 30-50.
- Di Saverio, S., Catena, F., & et al. (2017). Bologna guidelines for diagnosis and management of adhesive small bowel obstruction (ASBO): 2017 evidence-based guidelines of the World Society of Emergency Surgery. World Journal of Emergency Surgery, 12(1), 38.
- Rezaie, A., Buresi, M., & et al. (2020). Hydrogen and methane-based breath testing in gastrointestinal disorders: The North American Consensus. American Journal of Gastroenterology, 115(5), 775-789.
- Heizer, W. D., Southern, S., & McGovern, S. (2009). The role of diet in symptoms of irritable bowel syndrome in adults: A narrative review. Journal of the American Dietetic Association, 109(7), 1204-1214.
- Camilleri, M., Parkman, H. P., Shafi, M. A., Abell, T. L., Gerson, L. (2013). Clinical guideline: Management of gastroparesis. American Journal of Gastroenterology, 108(1), 18-37.
- Itani, K. M. F., Hur, K., & Kim, L. T. (2016). Comparison of laparoscopic and open repair with mesh for the treatment of ventral incisional hernia: A randomized trial. Archives of Surgery, 146(4), 362-367.

Chapter 7. Endocrine and Metabolism Disorders

Reviewed by
Thanh Hoang, DO, FACP, FACE

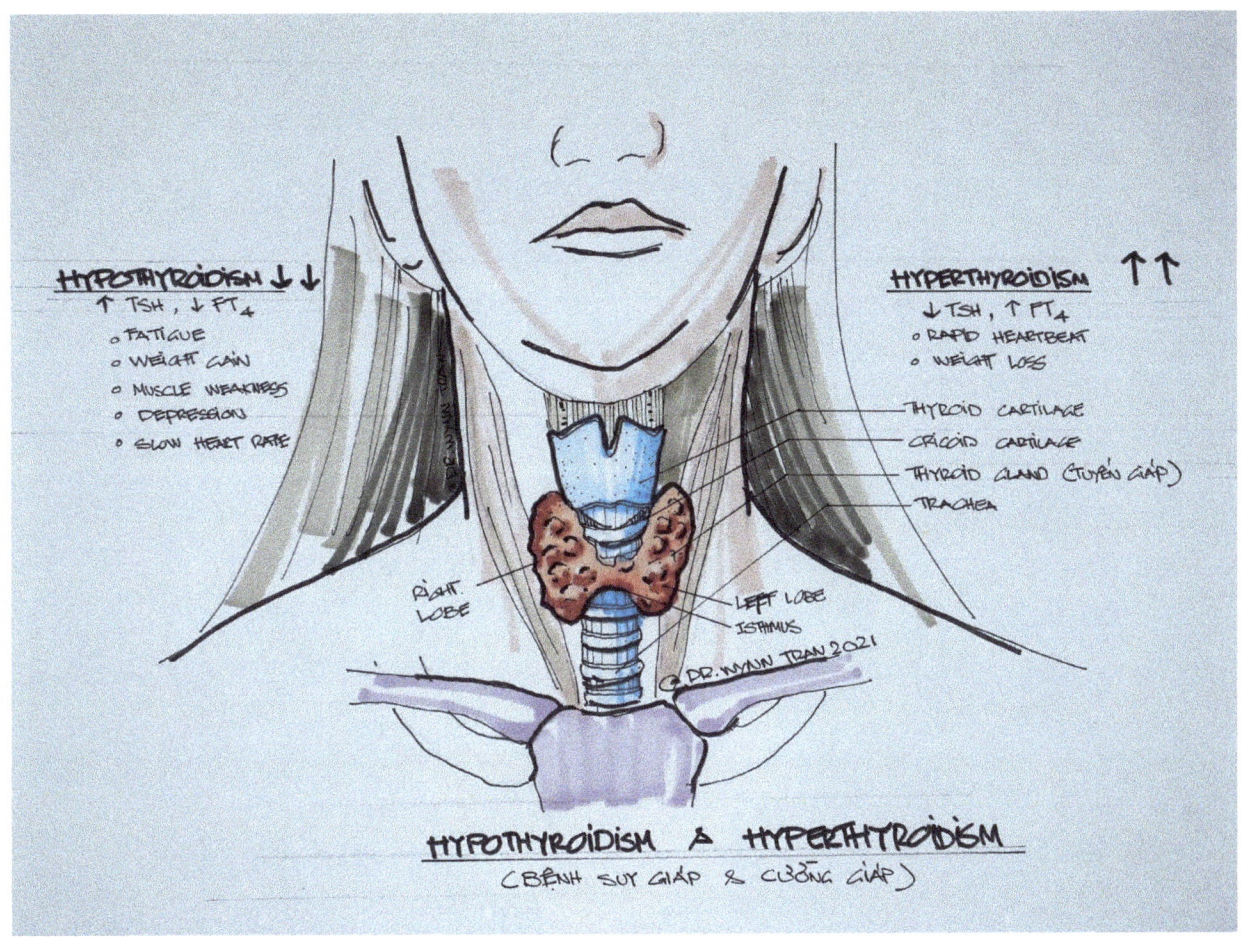

The APh should be familiar with the presentation, diagnosis, and management of these common endocrine disorders to provide appropriate care and referral to the endocrinologist when necessary.

7.1. Diabetes Mellitus Type 2

> ➤ *Type 2 diabetes is a chronic condition characterized by insulin resistance and high blood sugar levels due to inadequate insulin production or utilization.*
>
> ➤ *Risk factors include obesity, sedentary lifestyle, and genetic predisposition, with symptoms including increased thirst, frequent urination, fatigue, and blurred vision.*
>
> ➤ *Management involves lifestyle modifications, oral medications, insulin therapy, and regular monitoring to prevent complications like cardiovascular disease and neuropathy.*

Symptoms:

- Polyuria: Excessive urination volume, often leading to increased frequency of urination.
- Polydipsia: Excessive thirst, often accompanied by drinking large volumes of fluid.
- Polyphagia: Increased hunger and appetite, despite adequate food intake.
- Feeling tired or fatigued, often due to the body's inability to properly utilize glucose for energy.
- Unintentional weight loss, particularly when diabetes is poorly controlled.
- Blurred vision: Fluctuations in blood sugar levels can affect the shape of the lens in the eye, leading to temporary visual changes.
- Slow wound healing: High blood sugar levels can impair the body's ability to heal wounds and infections.

Causes and Risk Factors:

- Obesity: particularly abdominal obesity, is a major risk factor for type 2 diabetes.
- Sedentary lifestyle: Lack of physical activity and exercise increases the risk of developing insulin resistance and type 2 diabetes.
- Family history of type 2 diabetes: increases risk of developing the condition.
- Age, particularly after age 45.
- Certain racial and ethnic groups, including African Americans, Hispanics, Native Americans, and Asian Americans are at higher risk of developing type 2 diabetes.

- Gestational diabetes: increases risk of developing type 2 diabetes later in life.
- Polycystic ovary syndrome (PCOS): Women with PCOS have an increased risk of insulin resistance and type 2 diabetes.
- Hypertension: increases risk of type 2 diabetes.

Workup and Diagnosis:
- Fasting plasma glucose (FPG) test: A blood test to measure glucose levels after an overnight fast.
- Oral glucose tolerance test (OGTT): A blood test to measure glucose levels before and after consuming a sugary drink.
- Hemoglobin A1c (HbA1c) test: A blood test that measures average blood sugar levels over the past two to three months.
- Random plasma glucose test: A blood test to measure glucose levels at any time of the day, regardless of when the patient last ate.
- Symptom evaluation: Symptoms of diabetes, along with abnormal blood glucose levels, are used to diagnose diabetes.

Treatment:
- Lifestyle modifications:
    - Healthy diet: Emphasizing fruits, vegetables, whole grains, lean proteins, and healthy fats, and limiting refined carbohydrates and sugars.
    - Regular exercise: Engaging in at least 150 minutes of moderate-intensity aerobic activity per week.
    - Weight management: Achieving and maintaining a healthy weight through diet and exercise.
- Medications:
    - Oral antidiabetic medications: Such as metformin, sulfonylureas, meglitinides, dipeptidyl peptidase-4 (DPP-4) inhibitors, sodium-glucose cotransporter-2 (SGLT2) inhibitors, and glucagon-like peptide-1 (GLP-1) receptor agonists.
    - Insulin therapy: For patients who are unable to achieve glycemic control with oral medications alone.
- Blood sugar monitoring: Regular monitoring of blood glucose levels to assess glycemic control and adjust treatment as needed.
- Education and support: Diabetes self-management education and support programs to help patients learn how to manage their condition effectively and prevent complications.

7.2. Diabetes Mellitus Type 1

> ➤ Type 1 diabetes is an autoimmune condition where the pancreas produces little to no insulin, leading to high blood sugar levels.
>
> ➤ It often develops in childhood or adolescence and requires lifelong insulin therapy to manage blood sugar levels.
>
> ➤ Symptoms include increased thirst, frequent urination, weight loss, and fatigue, with management involving insulin injections, blood sugar monitoring, and lifestyle adjustments.

Symptoms:

- Polyphagia: Increased hunger and appetite, despite adequate food intake.
- Unintentional weight loss despite increased appetite and food intake.
- Feeling tired or fatigued, often due to the body's inability to properly utilize glucose for energy.
- Blurred vision: Fluctuations in blood sugar levels can affect the shape of the lens in the eye, leading to temporary changes in vision.
- Nausea and vomiting: Especially in cases of diabetic ketoacidosis (DKA), a serious complication of uncontrolled type 1 diabetes.

Causes and Risk Factors:

- Autoimmune factors: Type 1 diabetes is primarily an autoimmune condition where the body's immune system attacks and destroys insulin-producing beta cells in the pancreas.
- Patients with a family history of type 1 diabetes are at increased risk.
- Genetics: Certain genes are associated with an increased susceptibility to developing type 1 diabetes.
- Environmental factors: Exposure to certain environmental triggers, such as viral infections or toxins, may play a role in triggering the autoimmune response.
- Age: Type 1 diabetes can occur at any age but is more commonly diagnosed in children, adolescents, and young adults.
- Race and ethnicity: Certain racial and ethnic groups, including Caucasian patients, are at higher risk of developing type 1 diabetes.

Workup and Diagnosis:
- Blood tests:
    - Measurement of blood glucose levels using fasting plasma glucose (FPG) test, oral glucose tolerance test (OGTT), or hemoglobin A1c (HbA1c) test.
- Urine tests: Detection of ketones in the urine, especially in cases of suspected diabetic ketoacidosis (DKA).
- Autoantibody tests:
    - Detection of antibodies that target pancreatic beta cells, such as glutamic acid decarboxylase (GAD) antibodies, islet cell antibodies (ICA), insulin autoantibodies (IAA), and zinc transporter 8 antibodies (ZnT8), to confirm autoimmune destruction of beta cells.
- Clinical evaluation: Assessment of symptoms and medical history, including family history of diabetes.

Treatment:
- Insulin therapy:
    - Lifelong insulin replacement therapy is the mainstay of treatment for type 1 diabetes. Multiple daily injections of insulin or continuous subcutaneous insulin infusion (insulin pump) are used to mimic physiological insulin secretion.
- Blood sugar monitoring: Regular monitoring of blood glucose levels using blood glucose meters to adjust insulin doses and maintain glycemic control.
- Carbohydrate counting: Patients with type 1 diabetes often learn to count carbohydrates in their meals and adjust insulin doses accordingly.
- Healthy lifestyle: Emphasis on healthy eating, regular physical activity, and weight management to optimize overall health and glycemic control.
- Continuous glucose monitoring (CGM): Use of CGM devices to continuously monitor interstitial glucose levels and provide real-time feedback on blood sugar trends.
- Education and support:
    - Diabetes self-management education and support programs to help patients with type 1 diabetes learn how to manage their condition effectively, prevent complications, and cope with the psychosocial aspects of living with diabetes.

7.3. Hypothyroidism

> ➢ *Hypothyroidism is a condition where the thyroid gland does not produce enough thyroid hormone, leading to a slowdown in bodily functions.*
>
> ➢ *Symptoms include fatigue, weight gain, constipation, dry skin, and sensitivity to cold, with treatment typically involving thyroid hormone replacement therapy to restore hormone levels and alleviate symptoms.*
>
> ➢ *Regular monitoring and adjustments to medication dosage are often necessary for optimal management.*

Symptoms:

- Fatigue: Feeling tired, sluggish, and lacking energy despite adequate rest.
- Weight gain: Unexplained weight gain or difficulty losing weight, even with reduced caloric intake.
- Cold intolerance: Feeling unusually cold, especially in the extremities, and having a low tolerance for cold temperatures.
- Dry skin and hair: Dry, flaky skin and brittle hair that may become coarse and thin.
- Constipation: Difficulty passing stools and decreased frequency of bowel movements.
- Muscle weakness: Weakness, aching, or stiffness in the muscles, especially in the arms and legs.
- Depression: Feelings of sadness, low mood, and decreased interest in activities.
- Memory problems: Difficulty concentrating, forgetfulness, and impaired memory.
- Menstrual irregularities: Irregular menstrual periods, including heavier or lighter bleeding than usual, or missed periods.
- Hoarseness: Changes in the voice, including hoarseness or a deepening of the voice.
- Bradycardia: Slow heart rate, often accompanied by palpitations or irregular heartbeats.

Causes and Risk Factors:

- Gender: Hypothyroidism is more common in women than men.

- Age: Risk of hypothyroidism increases with age, particularly after age 60.
- Autoimmune thyroiditis: Conditions such as Hashimoto's thyroiditis, an autoimmune disorder where the body's immune system attacks the thyroid gland, increase the risk of hypothyroidism.
- Family history: patients with a family history of thyroid disorders are at increased risk.
- Previous thyroid surgery or radiation therapy: Previous thyroid surgery or radiation therapy to the neck area can damage the thyroid gland and increase the risk of hypothyroidism.
- Certain medications: Some medications, such as lithium, amiodarone, and certain anti-thyroid medications, can interfere with thyroid function and increase the risk of hypothyroidism.

Workup and Diagnosis:
- Thyroid function tests:

    Measurement of thyroid hormone levels, including thyroid-stimulating hormone (TSH), free thyroxine (T4), and triiodothyronine (T3) levels.
- Antibody tests:

    Detection of antibodies associated with autoimmune thyroiditis, such as thyroid peroxidase antibodies (TPOAb) and thyroglobulin antibodies (TgAb).
- Clinical evaluation: Assessment of symptoms and physical examination, including examination of the thyroid gland for enlargement or nodules.
- Imaging tests:

    Ultrasound imaging of the thyroid gland may be performed to evaluate the size, shape, and structure of the thyroid gland, as well as to detect any nodules or abnormalities.

Treatment:
- Thyroid hormone replacement therapy:

    Oral administration of synthetic thyroid hormone (levothyroxine) to replace deficient thyroid hormone levels and restore normal thyroid function.
- Regular monitoring:

    Periodic monitoring of thyroid hormone levels and TSH levels to adjust levothyroxine dosage as needed and ensure optimal thyroid function.

- Lifestyle modifications:

    Healthy lifestyle habits, including regular exercise, balanced nutrition, stress management, and adequate sleep, to support overall health and well-being.

- Education and support:

    Education about hypothyroidism, its management, and the importance of adherence to medication therapy, as well as support from The APh and support groups.

7.4. Hyperthyroidism

> ➤ *Hyperthyroidism, commonly caused by Graves' disease, is a condition where the thyroid gland overproduces thyroid hormones, leading to increased metabolism.*
>
> ➤ *Symptoms include weight loss, rapid heartbeat, anxiety, tremors, and heat intolerance.*
>
> ➤ *Treatment options include medications, radioactive iodine therapy, or surgery to control hormone levels and alleviate symptoms.*

Symptoms:

- Rapid heartbeat: A noticeably fast heartbeat, even at rest.
- Palpitations: Sensations of irregular or forceful heartbeats.
- Tremors: Fine trembling or shaking of the hands or fingers.
- Weight loss: Unexplained weight loss, despite increased appetite and food intake.
- Heat intolerance: Feeling excessively hot or sweaty, even in cooler temperatures.
- Increased sweating: Profuse sweating, particularly at night.
- Fatigue: Feeling tired or exhausted, despite adequate rest.
- Anxiety and nervousness: Feelings of anxiety, nervousness, or irritability.
- Restlessness: Feeling jittery or unable to sit still.
- Difficulty sleeping: Difficulty falling asleep or staying asleep.
- Frequent bowel movements: Increased frequency of bowel movements or diarrhea.
- Muscle weakness: Weakness or fatigue in the muscles, especially in the arms and legs.

- Changes in menstrual patterns: Irregular menstrual periods, including lighter or missed periods.
- Enlargement of the thyroid gland: Visible swelling or enlargement of the thyroid gland in the neck.

Causes and Risk Factors:
- Autoimmune factors: Graves' disease is an autoimmune disorder where the body's immune system mistakenly attacks the thyroid gland, leading to overproduction of thyroid hormones.
- Family history: patients with a family history of Graves' disease or other autoimmune disorders are at increased risk.
- Gender: Graves' disease is more common in women than men.
- Age: Although Graves' disease can occur at any age, it most commonly affects patients between the ages of 20 and 40.
- Stress: Stressful life events or chronic stress may trigger the onset or exacerbation of Graves' disease.
- Smoking: Cigarette smoking has been associated with an increased risk of Graves' disease and worsening of symptoms.

Workup and Diagnosis:
- Thyroid function tests:

    Measurement of thyroid hormone levels, including thyroxine (T4), triiodothyronine (T3), and thyroid-stimulating hormone (TSH) levels.

- Thyroid antibody tests:

    Detection of antibodies associated with Graves' disease, such as thyroid-stimulating immunoglobulins (TSI), thyroid peroxidase antibodies (TPOAb), and thyroglobulin antibodies (TgAb).

- Radioactive iodine uptake (RAIU) test:

    A nuclear medicine scan to measure the amount of radioactive iodine absorbed by the thyroid gland, which can help differentiate Graves' disease from other causes of hyperthyroidism.

- Thyroid ultrasound:

    Imaging of the thyroid gland using ultrasound to evaluate the size, shape, and structure of the thyroid gland, as well as to detect any nodules or abnormalities.

Treatment:

- <u>Antithyroid medications:</u>

    Medications such as methimazole or propylthiouracil (PTU) to block the production of thyroid hormones and reduce thyroid gland activity.

- <u>Radioactive iodine therapy (RAI):</u> Oral administration of radioactive iodine to destroy thyroid cells and reduce thyroid hormone production.

- <u>Beta-blockers:</u> Medications such as propranolol or atenolol to control symptoms such as rapid heartbeat, palpitations, and tremors.

- <u>Thyroidectomy:</u>

    Surgical removal of part or all of the thyroid gland (thyroidectomy) to reduce thyroid hormone levels in cases where other treatments are ineffective or contraindicated.

7.5. Thyroid Nodules

> ➤ *Thyroid nodules are abnormal growths or lumps that form within the thyroid gland, often discovered incidentally during imaging studies.*
>
> ➤ *Most nodules are benign, but some can be cancerous, warranting further evaluation with ultrasound, fine-needle aspiration biopsy, or molecular testing.*
>
> ➤ *Treatment depends on the size, characteristics, and risk of malignancy, ranging from observation to surgery or radioactive iodine therapy.*

Symptoms:

Most thyroid nodules do not cause symptoms and are discovered incidentally during a physical examination or imaging tests for other reasons.

In some cases, thyroid nodules may cause symptoms such as:

- Visible swelling or enlargement of the thyroid gland in the neck.
- Difficulty swallowing or a feeling of fullness in the throat.
- Hoarseness or voice changes due to compression of the nearby structures.
- Neck pain or discomfort, especially if the nodule is large or growing rapidly.

- Rarely, hyperthyroidism if the nodule produces excess thyroid hormones.

Causes and Risk Factors:
- Age: Thyroid nodules are more common with increasing age, particularly after age 40.
- Gender: Women are more likely to develop thyroid nodules than men.
- History of radiation exposure: Previous exposure to radiation, especially during childhood, increases the risk of developing thyroid nodules.
- Family history: patients with a family history of thyroid nodules or thyroid cancer are at increased risk.
- Iodine deficiency: Insufficient intake of iodine, an essential nutrient for thyroid hormone production, may increase the risk of thyroid nodules, particularly in regions with iodine deficiency.
- Hashimoto's thyroiditis: Chronic inflammation of the thyroid gland, as seen in Hashimoto's thyroiditis, may increase the risk of developing thyroid nodules.
- Age: Thyroid nodules are more common with increasing age, particularly after age 40.
- Gender: Women are more likely to develop thyroid nodules than men.
- History of radiation exposure: Previous exposure to radiation, especially during childhood, increases the risk of developing thyroid nodules.
- Family history: patients with a family history of thyroid nodules or thyroid cancer are at increased risk.
- Iodine deficiency: Insufficient intake of iodine, an essential nutrient for thyroid hormone production, may increase the risk of thyroid nodules, particularly in regions with iodine deficiency.
- Hashimoto's thyroiditis: Chronic inflammation of the thyroid gland, as seen in Hashimoto's thyroiditis, may increase the risk of developing thyroid nodules.

Workup and Diagnosis:
- Physical examination: A healthcare provider may palpate the thyroid gland in the neck to detect any enlargement or nodules.

- Imaging tests:
    - Ultrasound: Imaging of the thyroid gland using ultrasound to visualize the size, shape, and characteristics of thyroid nodules.
    - Thyroid scan: A nuclear medicine scan to evaluate the function and activity of thyroid nodules, particularly if they are overactive or suspicious for cancer.
- Fine-needle aspiration biopsy (FNAB):

    A procedure to obtain a small sample of cells from thyroid nodules for microscopic examination and analysis. FNAB helps determine whether a nodule is benign, malignant, or indeterminate.
- Blood tests:

    Measurement of thyroid function tests, including thyroid-stimulating hormone (TSH), free thyroxine (T4), and thyroglobulin levels, to assess thyroid function and rule out hyperthyroidism or hypothyroidism.

Treatment:
- Observation:

    Many thyroid nodules, especially small and non-suspicious nodules, may not require immediate treatment and can be monitored over time with follow-up examinations and imaging tests.
- Medications:

    Thyroid hormone replacement therapy with levothyroxine may be prescribed to suppress the growth of benign thyroid nodules and reduce the risk of recurrence.
- Radioactive iodine therapy (RAI):

    Oral administration of radioactive iodine to shrink or destroy overactive thyroid nodules, particularly those causing hyperthyroidism.
- Fine-needle aspiration biopsy (FNAB):

    A procedure to obtain a small sample of cells from thyroid nodules for microscopic examination and analysis. FNAB helps determine whether a nodule is benign , malignant, or indeterminate.

- Surgery:

    Surgical removal of thyroid nodules may be recommended for nodules that are suspicious for cancer, causing compressive symptoms, or causing hyperthyroidism.

7.6. Hashimoto's Thyroiditis

> ➢ *Hashimoto's thyroiditis is an autoimmune condition where the immune system attacks the thyroid gland, leading to inflammation and reduced thyroid hormone production.*
> ➢ *Symptoms include fatigue, weight gain, sensitivity to cold, dry skin, and swelling in the neck.*
> ➢ *Treatment involves thyroid hormone replacement therapy to manage hypothyroidism and regular monitoring of thyroid function and antibody levels.*

Symptoms:
- Fatigue: Feeling tired or exhausted, despite adequate rest.
- Weight gain: Unexplained weight gain, despite normal eating habits.
- Cold intolerance: Feeling unusually cold, especially in the extremities, and having a low tolerance for cold temperatures.
- Dry skin and hair: Dry, flaky skin and brittle hair that may become coarse and thin.
- Constipation: Difficulty passing stools and decreased frequency of bowel movements.
- Muscle weakness: Weakness or fatigue in the muscles, especially in the arms and legs.
- Joint pain and stiffness: Aching or stiffness in the joints, especially in the hands and feet.
- Depression: Feelings of sadness, low mood, and decreased interest in activities.
- Menstrual irregularities: Irregular menstrual periods, including heavier or lighter bleeding than usual, or missed periods.
- Bradycardia: Slow heart rate, often accompanied by palpitations or irregular heartbeats.

Causes and Risk Factors:
- Autoimmune factors: Hashimoto's thyroiditis is an autoimmune disorder where the body's immune system mistakenly attacks the

thyroid gland, leading to inflammation and destruction of thyroid tissue.

- Family history: patients with a family history of Hashimoto's thyroiditis or other autoimmune disorders are at increased risk.
- Gender: Hashimoto's thyroiditis is more common in women than men.
- Age: Hashimoto's thyroiditis can occur at any age but is more commonly diagnosed in middle-aged patients.
- Other autoimmune disorders: patients with other autoimmune disorders, such as type 1 diabetes, rheumatoid arthritis, or lupus, are at increased risk of developing Hashimoto's thyroiditis.

Workup and Diagnosis:

- Thyroid function tests:

    Measurement of thyroid hormone levels, including thyroid-stimulating hormone (TSH), free thyroxine (T4), and triiodothyronine (T3) levels.

- Thyroid antibody tests:

    Detection of antibodies associated with Hashimoto's thyroiditis, such as thyroid peroxidase antibodies (TPOAb) and thyroglobulin antibodies (TgAb).

- Thyroid ultrasound:

    Imaging of the thyroid gland using ultrasound to evaluate the size, shape, and structure of the thyroid gland, as well as to detect any nodules or abnormalities.

Treatment:

- Thyroid hormone replacement therapy:

    Oral administration of synthetic thyroid hormone (levothyroxine) to replace deficient thyroid hormone levels and restore normal thyroid function.

- Regular monitoring:

    Periodic monitoring of thyroid hormone levels and TSH levels to adjust levothyroxine dosage as needed and ensure optimal thyroid function.

- Lifestyle modifications:

    Healthy lifestyle habits, including regular exercise, balanced nutrition, stress management, and adequate sleep, to support overall health and well-being.

- Education and support:

    Education about Hashimoto's thyroiditis, its management, and the importance of adherence to medication therapy, as well as support from The APh and support groups.

7.7. Addison's Disease

> ➢ *Addison's disease is a rare condition where the adrenal glands do not produce enough cortisol and sometimes aldosterone.*
> ➢ *Symptoms include fatigue, weight loss, low blood pressure, darkening of the skin, and salt cravings.*
> ➢ *Treatment involves lifelong hormone replacement therapy with glucocorticoids and mineralocorticoids to manage symptoms and prevent adrenal crisis.*

Symptoms:

- Fatigue and weakness: Persistent tiredness and weakness, even with adequate rest.
- Weight loss: Unexplained weight loss, despite normal eating habits.
- Hyperpigmentation: Darkening of the skin, particularly in areas exposed to sun or pressure, such as elbows, knees, and scars.
- Hypotension: Low blood pressure, which may cause dizziness, lightheadedness, or fainting.
- Salt cravings: Intense cravings for salty foods or beverages due to electrolyte imbalances.
- Nausea, vomiting, and abdominal pain: Digestive symptoms such as nausea, vomiting, and abdominal discomfort.
- Hypoglycemia: Low blood sugar levels, leading to symptoms such as weakness, confusion, and sweating.
- Muscle or joint pain: Aching muscles or joints, often accompanied by stiffness or discomfort.
- Depression or mood changes: Feelings of sadness, irritability, or anxiety.
- Loss of appetite: Decreased appetite and interest in food.
- Menstrual irregularities: Irregular menstrual periods or loss of menstrual periods in women.

- Orthostatic hypotension: A drop in blood pressure upon standing up from a seated or lying position, leading to dizziness or lightheadedness.

Causes and Risk Factors:
- Autoimmune disorders: Addison's disease is most commonly caused by autoimmune destruction of the adrenal glands, where the body's immune system mistakenly attacks and destroys the adrenal cortex.
- Tuberculosis: Infections such as tuberculosis can damage the adrenal glands and increase the risk of adrenal insufficiency.
- Cancer: Metastatic cancer or primary cancer of the adrenal glands can impair adrenal function and lead to adrenal insufficiency.
- Previous adrenal surgery: Surgical removal of the adrenal glands or certain adrenal tumors can result in adrenal insufficiency.
- Medications: Long-term use of certain medications, such as corticosteroids, can suppress adrenal function and increase the risk of adrenal insufficiency.

Workup and Diagnosis:
- Blood tests:
  - Measurement of cortisol levels: Low cortisol levels in the blood, particularly in the morning, may indicate adrenal insufficiency.
  - Adrenocorticotropic hormone (ACTH) stimulation test: Administration of synthetic ACTH and measurement of cortisol levels before and after stimulation to assess adrenal gland function.
- Imaging tests:
  - Imaging of the adrenal glands using computed tomography (CT) or magnetic resonance imaging (MRI) to evaluate the size, shape, and structure of the adrenal glands, as well as to detect any abnormalities.
- Other tests:
  - Electrolyte levels: Measurement of electrolyte levels, such as sodium and potassium, to assess for electrolyte imbalances associated with adrenal insufficiency.
  - Blood glucose levels: Measurement of blood glucose levels to assess for hypoglycemia, which may occur in adrenal crisis.

Treatment:

- Hormone replacement therapy:

    Oral administration of synthetic glucocorticoids (such as hydrocortisone, prednisone, or dexamethasone) and mineralocorticoids (such as fludrocortisone) to replace deficient adrenal hormones and restore normal adrenal function.

- Medication adjustments:

    Individualized dosing and adjustments of hormone replacement therapy based on symptoms, blood tests, and response to treatment.

- Education and support:

    Education about Addison's disease, its management, and the importance of medication adherence, as well as support from healthcare providers and support groups.

- Emergency treatment:

    In cases of adrenal crisis (severe adrenal insufficiency), prompt treatment with intravenous fluids, glucocorticoids, and electrolyte replacement to stabilize blood pressure and correct electrolyte imbalances.

7.8. Cushing's Syndrome

> ➤ *Cushing's syndrome is a rare condition caused by prolonged exposure to high levels of cortisol, often due to tumors in the adrenal glands or pituitary gland.*
>
> ➤ *Symptoms include weight gain, particularly in the face and abdomen, thinning skin, easy bruising, muscle weakness, and high blood pressure.*
>
> ➤ *Treatment involves addressing the underlying cause, such as surgery or medication, to normalize cortisol levels and alleviate symptoms.*

Symptoms:

- Weight gain: Particularly in the face (moon face), upper back (buffalo hump), and abdomen (central obesity), while the limbs remain relatively thin.

- Fatigue and weakness: Persistent tiredness and weakness, despite adequate rest.

- Muscle weakness: Weakness or loss of muscle mass, especially in the proximal muscles of the arms and legs.

- Skin changes: Thin, fragile skin that bruises easily, purple or pink stretch marks on the abdomen, thighs, and breasts, and slow wound healing.
- Hyperpigmentation: Darkening of the skin, particularly in skin folds, scars, and creases.
- Hirsutism: Excessive hair growth on the face, chest, back, or abdomen in women.
- Menstrual irregularities: Irregular menstrual periods or loss of menstrual periods in women.
- Acne and oily skin: Increased oil production in the skin, leading to acne and oily skin.
- Hypertension: High blood pressure, which may cause headaches, dizziness, or visual disturbances.
- Mood changes: Irritability, anxiety, depression, or mood swings.
- Cognitive changes: Difficulty concentrating, memory problems, and cognitive impairment.
- Hyperglycemia: Elevated blood sugar levels, leading to increased thirst, frequent urination, and fatigue.
- Osteoporosis: Decreased bone density and increased risk of fractures due to long-term exposure to excess cortisol.

Causes and Risk Factors:
- Exogenous glucocorticoid use: Prolonged use of corticosteroid medications, such as prednisone or dexamethasone, for the treatment of conditions such as asthma, autoimmune disorders, or organ transplantation, can cause Cushing's syndrome.
- Pituitary adenoma: Benign tumors of the pituitary gland (pituitary adenomas) that secrete excess adrenocorticotropic hormone (ACTH) can stimulate the adrenal glands to produce excess cortisol, leading to Cushing's syndrome (Cushing's disease).
- Adrenal adenoma or carcinoma: Benign or malignant tumors of the adrenal glands that produce excess cortisol independently of ACTH stimulation can cause Cushing's syndrome.
- Ectopic ACTH syndrome: Non-pituitary tumors, such as small cell lung cancer or carcinoid tumors, that produce ACTH can stimulate the adrenal glands to produce excess cortisol, leading to Cushing's syndrome.

Workup and Diagnosis:
- Laboratory tests:
  - Measurement of cortisol levels: Elevated cortisol levels in the blood, urine, or saliva samples, particularly in the morning or after overnight dexamethasone suppression test, may indicate Cushing's syndrome.
  - Measurement of adrenocorticotropic hormone (ACTH) levels: Differentiating between ACTH-dependent and ACTH-independent causes of Cushing's syndrome.
- Imaging tests:
  - Imaging of the pituitary gland using magnetic resonance imaging (MRI) to evaluate for pituitary adenomas (Cushing's disease).
  - Imaging of the adrenal glands using computed tomography (CT) or MRI to evaluate for adrenal tumors (adrenal adenomas or carcinomas).
- Dexamethasone suppression test: Administration of synthetic glucocorticoid (dexamethasone) and measurement of cortisol levels before and after suppression to assess adrenal gland function and differentiate between Cushing's syndrome and other causes of hypercortisolism.

Treatment:
- Surgery:

    Surgical removal of pituitary tumors (transsphenoidal surgery) or adrenal tumors (adrenalectomy) to remove the source of excess cortisol production.

- Radiation therapy:

    External beam radiation therapy (EBRT) or stereotactic radiosurgery (Gamma Knife) to shrink or destroy pituitary tumors (Cushing's disease) that cannot be surgically removed or recur after surgery.

- Medications:

    Medications such as ketoconazole, metyrapone, or mitotane to inhibit cortisol production or block adrenal steroidogenesis in cases where surgery or radiation therapy is not feasible or effective.

- **Supportive therapy:**

    Symptomatic treatment of complications associated with Cushing's syndrome, such as hypertension, hyperglycemia, osteoporosis, and mood disorders.

- **Long-term monitoring:**

    Regular monitoring of cortisol levels and clinical symptoms to assess treatment response, monitor for recurrence, and manage potential complications.

7.9. Hyperparathyroidism

> ➤ *Hyperparathyroidism is a condition where the parathyroid glands produce too much parathyroid hormone (PTH), leading to elevated calcium levels in the blood.*
>
> ➤ *Symptoms include fatigue, weakness, bone pain, kidney stones, and digestive issues.*
>
> ➤ *Treatment involves surgical removal of the overactive parathyroid gland or medication to regulate calcium levels and manage symptoms.*

Symptoms:

- Fatigue: Persistent tiredness and lack of energy.
- Weakness: Generalized weakness, especially in the muscles.
- Bone pain: Aching or tenderness in the bones, particularly in the ribs, spine, and long bones.
- Kidney stones: Formation of kidney stones due to elevated calcium levels in the blood.
- Abdominal pain: Discomfort or pain in the abdomen, often associated with pancreatitis or peptic ulcers.
- Polyuria and polydipsia: Increased urination and thirst due to hypercalcemia-induced dehydration.
- Constipation: Difficulty passing stools and decreased frequency of bowel movements.
- Depression or cognitive changes: Mood swings, irritability, depression, memory problems, or difficulty concentrating.
- Osteoporosis: Decreased bone density and increased risk of fractures due to calcium loss from bones.
- Nausea, vomiting, and loss of appetite: Digestive symptoms associated with hypercalcemia.

- Hypertension: High blood pressure, which may cause headaches or visual disturbances.
- Heart palpitations: Irregular heartbeats or sensations of fluttering in the chest.
- Shortness of breath: Difficulty breathing, especially with exertion.
- Weight loss: Unintentional weight loss, particularly in severe cases of hyperparathyroidism.

Causes and Risk Factors:
- Age: Hyperparathyroidism is more common in older adults, particularly postmenopausal women.
- Gender: Women are more likely to develop hyperparathyroidism than men.
- Family history: patients with a family history of hyperparathyroidism or multiple endocrine neoplasia type 1 (MEN1) syndrome are at increased risk.
- Radiation exposure: Previous exposure to head and neck radiation therapy, particularly during childhood, may increase the risk of developing hyperparathyroidism.
- Certain medical conditions: Chronic kidney disease, vitamin D deficiency, gastrointestinal disorders, and certain autoimmune disorders may increase the risk of hyperparathyroidism.
- Medications: Long-term use of medications such as lithium, thiazide diuretics, or proton pump inhibitors (PPIs) may increase the risk of hyperparathyroidism.

Epidemiology:
- Primary hyperparathyroidism is the most common cause of hypercalcemia in outpatient settings.
- The prevalence of primary hyperparathyroidism increases with age, with the highest incidence observed in postmenopausal women.
- Secondary hyperparathyroidism is more common in patients with chronic kidney disease or vitamin D deficiency.
- Tertiary hyperparathyroidism may occur in patients with long-standing secondary hyperparathyroidism, particularly after renal transplantation.

Workup and Diagnosis:
- <u>Laboratory tests:</u>
  - Measurement of serum calcium levels: Elevated serum calcium levels (>10.4 mg/dL) are suggestive of hyperparathyroidism.

- Measurement of parathyroid hormone (PTH) levels: Elevated or inappropriately normal PTH levels (>65 pg/mL) in the setting of hypercalcemia support the diagnosis of primary hyperparathyroidism.
- Measurement of 25-hydroxyvitamin D levels: Assessment of vitamin D status to evaluate for vitamin D deficiency, which can contribute to secondary hyperparathyroidism.

- Imaging studies:
    - Neck ultrasound: Imaging of the neck using ultrasound to visualize the parathyroid glands and detect any abnormalities, such as adenomas or hyperplasia.
    - Sestamibi scan: Nuclear medicine imaging using technetium-99m sestamibi to localize abnormal parathyroid glands, particularly adenomas.

- Bone mineral density (BMD) testing:

    Dual-energy X-ray absorptiometry (DEXA) scanning to assess bone density and evaluate for osteoporosis or osteopenia associated with hyperparathyroidism.

- Renal imaging: Imaging of the kidneys using ultrasound or CT scan to assess for kidney stones or nephrocalcinosis.

Treatment:

- Observation:

    Observation with periodic monitoring may be appropriate for asymptomatic or mild cases of primary hyperparathyroidism with stable calcium levels and preserved kidney function.

- Surgical intervention:

    Parathyroidectomy, surgical removal of the abnormal parathyroid gland(s), is the definitive treatment for primary hyperparathyroidism, particularly in symptomatic cases or those with complications such as severe hypercalcemia, kidney stones, osteoporosis, or renal impairment.

- Medications:
    - Bisphosphonates: Medications such as alendronate or zoledronic acid may be prescribed to treat osteoporosis associated with hyperparathyroidism and reduce the risk of fractures.
    - Cinacalcet: Calcimimetic medication that reduces PTH secretion and can be used to manage hypercalcemia in

patients who are not candidates for surgery or have persistent hypercalcemia after surgery.

- Fluids and diuretics:

    Intravenous hydration with normal saline and loop diuretics (e.g., furosemide) may be used to promote urinary calcium excretion and manage hypercalcemia in acute settings.

7.10. Hypoparathyroidism

> ➢ *Hypoparathyroidism is a rare condition characterized by insufficient production of parathyroid hormone (PTH), leading to low calcium levels in the blood.*
> ➢ *Symptoms include muscle cramps, tingling sensations, seizures, and weakened bones (osteoporosis).*
> ➢ *Treatment involves calcium and vitamin D supplementation to maintain normal blood calcium levels and prevent complications like tetany and seizures.*

Symptoms:

- Tetany: Muscle cramps, spasms, or twitching, particularly in the hands, feet, or face, due to hypocalcemia.
- Paresthesias: Tingling or numbness, often in the fingertips, toes, or lips, caused by low calcium levels.
- Muscle weakness: Weakness or fatigue, especially with exertion, due to impaired muscle function.
- Chvostek's sign: Facial twitching or spasm elicited by tapping over the facial nerve at the angle of the jaw.
- Trousseau's sign: Carpal spasm induced by inflating a blood pressure cuff above systolic pressure for several minutes.
- Seizures: Convulsions or seizures, particularly in severe cases of hypocalcemia.
- Dyspnea: Shortness of breath or difficulty breathing, especially with exertion.
- Dry skin and hair: Dry, rough skin and brittle hair due to impaired calcium-dependent cellular processes.
- Cognitive symptoms: Confusion, memory problems, or mood changes, including irritability or depression.

- Dental abnormalities: Enamel defects, tooth decay, or delayed tooth eruption in children due to impaired calcium metabolism.
- Cardiac arrhythmias: Abnormal heart rhythms, such as prolonged QT interval or ventricular arrhythmias, associated with severe hypocalcemia.
- Ophthalmic manifestations: Cataracts, retinal abnormalities, or optic neuropathy in chronic cases of hypoparathyroidism.

Causes and Risk Factors:
- Surgery: Surgical removal or damage to the parathyroid glands during neck surgery, particularly thyroidectomy or parathyroidectomy, is the most common cause of hypoparathyroidism.
- Autoimmune disorders: Autoimmune destruction of the parathyroid glands, such as autoimmune polyendocrine syndrome type 1 (APS-1) or autoimmune polyglandular syndrome type 2 (APS-2), may lead to hypoparathyroidism.
- Genetic factors: Inherited genetic mutations associated with syndromes such as DiGeorge syndrome (22q11.2 deletion syndrome) or familial isolated hypoparathyroidism can cause hypoparathyroidism.
- Radiation therapy: Previous exposure to head and neck radiation therapy for the treatment of cancer or other conditions may damage the parathyroid glands and lead to hypoparathyroidism.
- Idiopathic: Idiopathic or sporadic hypoparathyroidism, with no identifiable cause, may occur in some cases.
- Medications: Certain medications, such as antiepileptic drugs (phenytoin, phenobarbital), can interfere with calcium metabolism and increase the risk of hypoparathyroidism.

Epidemiology:
- Hypoparathyroidism is a rare disorder, with an estimated prevalence of approximately 25-37 cases per 100,000 patients.
- The incidence of hypoparathyroidism varies depending on the underlying cause, with surgical causes (e.g., thyroidectomy) being the most common.
- Hypoparathyroidism can occur at any age but is more common in adults than in children.
- Autoimmune hypoparathyroidism may be associated with other autoimmune disorders, such as autoimmune thyroid disease or type 1 diabetes mellitus.

Workup and Diagnosis:

- Laboratory tests:
  - Measurement of serum calcium levels: Low serum calcium levels (<8.5 mg/dL) are indicative of hypocalcemia.
  - Measurement of parathyroid hormone (PTH) levels: Inappropriately low or undetectable PTH levels (<15 pg/mL) in the setting of hypocalcemia support the diagnosis of hypoparathyroidism.
  - Measurement of magnesium levels: Assessment of magnesium levels, as hypomagnesemia can impair PTH secretion and exacerbate hypocalcemia.

- Electrocardiogram (ECG):

  ECG may reveal characteristic changes associated with hypocalcemia, such as prolonged QT interval or ST-segment abnormalities.

- Imaging studies:

  Imaging of the neck using ultrasound or nuclear medicine scans may be performed to evaluate the size and morphology of the parathyroid glands and assess for any abnormalities or damage.

- Other tests:

  Assessment of renal function, vitamin D levels, and urinary calcium excretion may be performed to evaluate for secondary causes of hypocalcemia.

Treatment:

- Calcium supplementation:

  Oral calcium supplements, such as calcium carbonate or calcium citrate, are administered to correct hypocalcemia and maintain serum calcium levels within the normal range.

- Active vitamin D analogs:

  Calcitriol (1,25-dihydroxyvitamin D) or other active vitamin D analogs are prescribed to enhance intestinal calcium absorption and facilitate calcium reabsorption in the kidneys.

- Magnesium replacement:

  Magnesium supplementation may be required in patients with concurrent hypomagnesemia to optimize PTH secretion and calcium metabolism.

- Symptomatic management:

    Treatment of acute symptoms of hypocalcemia, such as tetany or seizures, with intravenous calcium gluconate or calcium chloride.

- Long-term monitoring:

    Regular monitoring of serum calcium, phosphate, and PTH levels, as well as renal function and bone health, to assess treatment response, adjust medication dosages, and prevent complications such as renal calcifications or nephrolithiasis.

7.11. Pituitary Adenoma

> ➤ A pituitary adenoma is a benign tumor that develops in the pituitary gland, often causing hormonal imbalances.
>
> ➤ Symptoms vary depending on the size and location of the tumor but may include headaches, vision changes, hormonal disturbances, and symptoms related to excess hormone production.
>
> ➤ Treatment options include medication, surgery, or radiation therapy to manage hormone levels and alleviate symptoms.

Symptoms:

- Vision changes: Visual disturbances, such as blurry vision, double vision, or loss of peripheral vision, due to compression of the optic chiasm by the growing tumor.

- Headaches: Persistent or recurrent headaches, often located in the frontal or temporal regions, which may worsen over time and be associated with nausea or vomiting.

- Hormonal disturbances: Pituitary adenomas can disrupt normal hormone secretion, leading to various endocrine symptoms, including:

    - Hyperprolactinemia: Galactorrhea, amenorrhea or oligomenorrhea, infertility, or decreased libido in women, and erectile dysfunction or gynecomastia in men.

    - Acromegaly: Enlargement of the hands, feet, and facial features, joint pain, excessive sweating, snoring or sleep apnea, and visual changes due to tumor compression.

    - Cushing's disease: Weight gain, central obesity, moon face, buffalo hump, thinning of the skin, easy bruising, hypertension,

diabetes mellitus, mood changes, and menstrual irregularities in women.
    - Hypopituitarism: Fatigue, weakness, cold intolerance, weight loss or weight gain, loss of libido, menstrual irregularities, and symptoms of adrenal insufficiency (weakness, dizziness, hypotension) or thyroid dysfunction (dry skin, constipation, hair loss).
- Neurological deficits: Depending on the size and location of the tumor, pituitary adenomas may cause neurological deficits, such as cranial nerve palsies (e.g., visual disturbances, facial numbness), hypopituitarism, or hydrocephalus due to obstructive hydrocephalus.
- Behavioral changes: Mood swings, irritability, depression, or cognitive impairment, particularly in cases of hormone-secreting pituitary adenomas.

Causes and Risk Factors:
- Age: Pituitary adenomas can occur at any age but are more common in adults, with peak incidence in the fourth to sixth decades of life.
- Gender: Pituitary adenomas affect both men and women, although certain subtypes may have a slight predilection for one gender over the other (e.g., prolactinomas are more common in women).
- Genetic predisposition: Rare genetic syndromes, such as multiple endocrine neoplasia type 1 (MEN1), familial isolated pituitary adenoma (FIPA), or Carney complex, may increase the risk of developing pituitary adenomas.
- Radiation exposure: Previous exposure to head and neck radiation therapy, particularly during childhood, may increase the risk of developing pituitary adenomas later in life.
- Hormonal factors: Hormonal changes or imbalances, such as estrogen excess in women or androgen deficiency in men, may contribute to the development or growth of pituitary adenomas.

Epidemiology:
- Pituitary adenomas are the most common type of intracranial neoplasm, accounting for approximately 10-15% of all primary brain tumors.
- The estimated annual incidence of pituitary adenomas is approximately 3-4 cases per 100,000 patients.
- Pituitary adenomas are typically benign, slow-growing tumors, although they can cause significant morbidity and mortality if left untreated or inadequately managed.

- The prevalence of pituitary adenomas may vary depending on geographic region, population characteristics, and diagnostic criteria used.

Workup and Diagnosis:
- Clinical evaluation: Comprehensive history and physical examination to assess for symptoms suggestive of pituitary adenomas, including visual disturbances, headaches, hormonal imbalances, and neurological deficits.
- Laboratory tests:
    - Hormonal assays: Measurement of serum levels of pituitary hormones (e.g., prolactin, growth hormone, adrenocorticotropic hormone, thyroid-stimulating hormone, luteinizing hormone, follicle-stimulating hormone) and peripheral hormones (e.g., cortisol, insulin-like growth factor 1) to assess for hormone hypersecretion or hyposecretion.
    - Biochemical tests: Assessment of metabolic parameters, such as glucose tolerance, lipid profile, and calcium levels, to evaluate for associated metabolic abnormalities.
- Imaging studies:
    - Magnetic resonance imaging (MRI) of the brain with contrast: Preferred imaging modality for visualizing pituitary adenomas and assessing tumor size, location, extent of invasion, and involvement of surrounding structures.
    - Computed tomography (CT) scan: May be used in cases where MRI is contraindicated or unavailable, although MRI is more sensitive for detecting pituitary adenomas.
- Visual field testing: Formal assessment of visual fields using perimeter to detect visual field defects associated with optic chiasm compression by pituitary adenomas.

Treatment:
- Observation:

    In cases of asymptomatic or incidental pituitary adenomas with no evidence of hormonal hypersecretion or visual compromise, close observation with periodic monitoring may be appropriate.

- Medical therapy:
    - Dopamine agonists: Medications such as cabergoline or bromocriptine may be used to treat prolactin-secreting pituitary adenomas (prolactinomas) and reduce prolactin levels,

normalize menstrual cycles, restore fertility, and shrink tumor size.
- Somatostatin analogs: Medications such as octreotide or lanreotide may be prescribed to control growth hormone hypersecretion and mitigate symptoms of acromegaly, including soft tissue swelling, arthralgia, and glucose intolerance.
- Growth hormone receptor antagonists: Medications such as pegvisomant may be used to block the effects of growth hormone in cases of acromegaly refractory to other treatments or in patients who cannot tolerate somatostatin analogs.
- Stereotactic radiosurgery: Precise delivery of focused radiation to the pituitary adenoma using techniques such as gamma knife radiosurgery or CyberKnife may be considered for small, residual, or recurrent tumors that are not amenable to surgical resection.

- Surgical intervention:
  - Transsphenoidal surgery: Endoscopic or microscopic surgical removal of pituitary adenomas through the nasal cavity and sphenoid sinus, with preservation of normal pituitary gland function and adjacent structures, is the primary treatment for most pituitary adenomas.
  - Transcranial surgery: Open surgical resection of pituitary adenomas via a craniotomy approach may be necessary for large, invasive, or complex tumors that cannot be adequately addressed through a transsphenoidal approach.

- Hormone replacement therapy:

  Hormone replacement with glucocorticoids, thyroid hormone, sex steroids, or other pituitary hormones may be required in patients with hypopituitarism following surgical resection of pituitary adenomas to restore normal endocrine function.

7.12. Hypopituitarism

> ➤ *Hypopituitarism is a rare condition where the pituitary gland fails to produce one or more hormones, affecting various bodily functions.*
>
> ➤ *Symptoms depend on the deficient hormone(s) but may include fatigue, weight loss, low blood pressure, infertility, and growth abnormalities.*
>
> ➤ *Treatment involves hormone replacement therapy to restore hormone levels and manage symptoms, with regular monitoring to adjust therapy as needed.*

Symptoms:

- Fatigue: Persistent tiredness or lack of energy, often accompanied by decreased physical stamina and exercise intolerance.
- Weight changes: Unexplained weight gain or weight loss, which may occur despite changes in dietary habits or physical activity levels.
- Cold intolerance: Sensitivity to cold temperatures, with a tendency to feel cold or chilled even in warm environments.
- Hypoglycemia: Episodes of low blood sugar, characterized by symptoms such as shakiness, sweating, palpitations, confusion, or loss of consciousness.
- Amenorrhea or oligomenorrhea: Absent or irregular menstrual periods in women, often accompanied by infertility or difficulty conceiving.
- Erectile dysfunction: Difficulty achieving or maintaining erections in men, often accompanied by decreased libido or loss of sexual desire.
- Galactorrhea: Spontaneous milk production from the breasts in women, unrelated to breastfeeding or pregnancy.
- Infertility: Difficulty conceiving or achieving pregnancy, often associated with hormonal imbalances affecting reproductive function.
- Decreased libido: Reduced interest in sexual activity or diminished sexual desire, affecting both men and women.
- Growth failure: Slow growth or short stature in children, resulting from impaired secretion of growth hormone or other pituitary hormones.
- Hypothyroidism: Symptoms of thyroid hormone deficiency, including fatigue, weight gain, cold intolerance, dry skin, constipation, and hair loss.

- Adrenal insufficiency: Symptoms of adrenal hormone deficiency, such as weakness, fatigue, hypotension, dizziness, salt cravings, and hyperpigmentation of the skin.
- Hypogonadism: Symptoms of sex hormone deficiency, including decreased muscle mass, loss of body hair, breast enlargement in men, and menstrual irregularities or vaginal dryness in women.
- Polyuria and polydipsia: Increased urination and thirst due to impaired secretion of antidiuretic hormone (ADH), leading to diabetes insipidus.
- Visual changes: Visual disturbances, such as blurred vision, double vision, or loss of peripheral vision, due to compression of the optic chiasm by pituitary adenomas.

Causes and Risk Factors:
- Pituitary adenomas: Benign tumors of the pituitary gland are the most common cause of hypopituitarism, often resulting from pituitary adenomas or other space-occupying lesions within the sellar or parasellar region.
- Pituitary surgery: Surgical removal of pituitary adenomas or other pituitary lesions, such as craniopharyngiomas or Rathke's cleft cysts, may lead to hypopituitarism due to damage to the pituitary gland or disruption of normal hormone secretion.
- Radiation therapy: Previous exposure to head and neck radiation therapy for the treatment of brain tumors, nasopharyngeal cancers, or other conditions may damage the pituitary gland and result in hypopituitarism.
- Traumatic brain injury: Severe head trauma or traumatic brain injury (TBI) may cause damage to the pituitary gland or hypothalamus, leading to hypopituitarism or dysfunction of other hormonal axes.
- Autoimmune disorders: Autoimmune diseases affecting the pituitary gland or hypothalamus, such as lymphocytic hypophysitis or autoimmune hypopituitarism, may result in progressive destruction of pituitary tissue and hormonal deficiencies.
- Genetic syndromes: Rare genetic syndromes, such as septo-optic dysplasia (de Morsier syndrome), Kallmann syndrome, or familial isolated pituitary adenoma (FIPA), may be associated with hypopituitarism or pituitary hormone deficiencies.
- Infiltrative disorders: Infiltrative diseases affecting the pituitary gland, such as sarcoidosis, hemochromatosis, or histiocytosis, may lead to hypopituitarism due to infiltration of pituitary tissue by abnormal cells or deposits.

Epidemiology:
- The exact prevalence of hypopituitarism is difficult to determine due to variability in diagnostic criteria, population characteristics, and underlying etiologies.
- Hypopituitarism is considered a rare disorder, with an estimated prevalence ranging from 45 to 125 cases per 100,000 patients in population-based studies.
- The incidence of hypopituitarism may vary depending on geographic region, age distribution, and underlying causes, with higher rates reported in older adults and certain high-risk populations.
- Pituitary adenomas are the most common cause of hypopituitarism in adults, accounting for approximately 70-80% of cases, while other etiologies, such as pituitary surgery, radiation therapy, or traumatic brain injury, may contribute to a smaller proportion of cases.

Workup and Diagnosis:
- Clinical evaluation:
    Comprehensive history and physical examination to assess for symptoms suggestive of hypopituitarism, including hormonal deficiencies, growth failure, visual changes, or neurological deficits.
- Hormonal testing:
    - Basal hormone levels: Measurement of basal serum levels of pituitary hormones (e.g., growth hormone, adrenocorticotropic hormone, thyroid-stimulating hormone, luteinizing hormone, follicle-stimulating hormone) and peripheral hormones (e.g., cortisol, thyroid hormones, sex steroids) to screen for hormonal deficiencies.
    - Stimulation tests: Dynamic testing with provocative stimuli (e.g., insulin-induced hypoglycemia, synthetic corticotropin-releasing hormone, thyrotropin-releasing hormone, gonadotropin-releasing hormone) to assess the responsiveness of the pituitary gland to physiological stimuli and confirm hormonal deficiencies.
- Imaging studies:
    - Magnetic resonance imaging (MRI) of the brain with contrast: Preferred imaging modality for visualizing the pituitary gland and hypothalamus, detecting structural abnormalities (e.g., pituitary adenomas, cysts, or tumors), and evaluating for mass effects or compression of adjacent structures.

- Computed tomography (CT) scan: May be used in cases where MRI is contraindicated or unavailable, although MRI is more sensitive for detecting pituitary lesions and assessing soft tissue structures.
- <u>Visual field testing:</u> Formal assessment of visual fields using perimetry to detect visual field defects associated with optic chiasm compression by pituitary adenomas or other lesions.
- <u>Laboratory investigations:</u>

    Additional laboratory tests, such as complete blood count (CBC), comprehensive metabolic panel (CMP), serum electrolytes, and urinary osmolality, may be performed to evaluate for associated metabolic abnormalities, renal function, or diabetes insipidus.

Treatment:
- <u>Hormone replacement therapy:</u>

    Hormone replacement with synthetic or recombinant forms of deficient pituitary hormones (e.g., hydrocortisone, levothyroxine, sex steroids, growth hormone) to restore normal endocrine function and alleviate symptoms of hormonal deficiency.
- <u>Individualized management:</u>

    Treatment should be individualized based on the specific hormonal deficiencies, severity of symptoms, underlying etiology, patient preferences, and response to therapy.
- <u>Regular monitoring:</u>

    Close monitoring of hormonal levels, clinical symptoms, growth parameters, metabolic parameters, and other relevant parameters to assess treatment response, adjust medication dosages, and prevent complications.
- <u>Multidisciplinary care:</u>

    Collaboration among endocrinologists, neurosurgeons, ophthalmologists, radiologists, and other healthcare providers to optimize patient care, coordinate treatment modalities, and address associated comorbidities or complications.

7.13. Growth Hormone Deficiency

> ➤ *Growth hormone deficiency (GHD) is a condition where the pituitary gland does not produce enough growth hormone, affecting growth and development in children and metabolism in adults.*
>
> ➤ *Symptoms in children include short stature and delayed growth, while adults may experience fatigue, weight gain, and reduced bone density.*
>
> ➤ *Treatment involves growth hormone replacement therapy to promote growth and metabolic balance.*

Symptoms:

- Growth retardation: Slow growth or short stature in children, with height below the third percentile for age and sex, often apparent by early childhood.

- Delayed milestones: Delayed development of motor skills, such as sitting, crawling, or walking, in infancy or early childhood.

- Reduced growth velocity: Slowed rate of linear growth over time, with height measurements consistently below expected growth curves for age and sex.

- Short stature: Adult height significantly below the mid-parental height or the height of unaffected siblings or family members.

- Immature appearance: Childlike or juvenile facial features, with delayed skeletal maturation and delayed eruption of permanent teeth.

- Increased body fat: Excessive adiposity or central adiposity, particularly around the trunk and abdomen, despite normal or decreased muscle mass.

- Delayed puberty: Delayed onset of puberty or incomplete pubertal development, characterized by delayed menarche in girls or delayed onset of secondary sexual characteristics in boys.

- Hypoglycemia: Episodes of low blood sugar, particularly during fasting or prolonged periods without food, due to impaired gluconeogenesis and glycogenolysis.

- Fatigue and weakness: Persistent tiredness or lack of energy, with reduced physical stamina, exercise intolerance, and decreased muscle strength.

- Psychological symptoms: Decreased self-esteem, social withdrawal, or psychological distress related to short stature or delayed growth compared to peers.

- Dyslipidemia: Abnormal lipid profile, including elevated levels of total cholesterol, low-density lipoprotein (LDL) cholesterol, and triglycerides, despite normal body weight or body mass index (BMI).
- Osteopenia or osteoporosis: Decreased bone mineral density and increased risk of fractures or bone deformities due to inadequate bone formation and delayed skeletal maturation.

Causes and Risk Factors:
- Congenital causes: Genetic mutations or congenital malformations affecting the pituitary gland, hypothalamus, or other components of the hypothalamic-pituitary axis, leading to impaired synthesis or secretion of growth hormone (GH).
- Acquired causes: Acquired or secondary GHD resulting from factors such as pituitary or hypothalamic tumors, brain trauma or injury, radiation therapy, surgery, infections, infiltrative disorders, or vascular lesions affecting the pituitary gland.
- Idiopathic GHD: Idiopathic or isolated GHD of unknown cause, often diagnosed in children with short stature and delayed growth without identifiable genetic or structural abnormalities.
- Genetic syndromes: Genetic syndromes associated with GHD, such as septo-optic dysplasia (de Morsier syndrome), Prader-Willi syndrome, Turner syndrome, or Noonan syndrome, may present with characteristic clinical features and growth patterns.
- Prematurity: Preterm birth or low birth weight may increase the risk of GHD due to immaturity of the hypothalamic-pituitary axis or complications of neonatal illness or treatment.
- Brain tumors or lesions: Tumors or lesions affecting the hypothalamus, pituitary gland, or adjacent structures may disrupt normal GH secretion or impair hypothalamic-pituitary function, leading to GHD.
- Radiation therapy: Previous exposure to cranial or craniospinal radiation therapy for the treatment of brain tumors, leukemia, or other malignancies may damage the hypothalamus or pituitary gland and result in GHD.

Epidemiology:
- The prevalence of GHD varies depending on the population studied, diagnostic criteria used, and underlying etiologies.
- GHD is relatively rare, with estimated prevalence rates ranging from 1 in 3,500 to 1 in 10,000 children, and higher rates reported in certain high-risk populations or clinical settings.

- The incidence of GHD may be higher in children with short stature, delayed growth, or other features suggestive of pituitary dysfunction, as well as in patients with known risk factors or predisposing conditions for GHD.
- GHD can occur at any age but is most commonly diagnosed in childhood or adolescence, when growth failure or delayed growth becomes apparent, although adult-onset GHD may also occur in later life due to acquired or secondary causes.

Workup and Diagnosis:
- Clinical evaluation: Comprehensive history and physical examination to assess for symptoms suggestive of GHD, including short stature, delayed growth, delayed milestones, or other features of pituitary dysfunction.
- Growth assessment: Measurement of height, weight, and growth velocity over time, with plotting on growth charts or growth curves to assess growth patterns and detect deviations from normal.
- Laboratory tests:
  - Measurement of serum insulin-like growth factor 1 (IGF-1) levels: Low or subnormal levels of IGF-1, a surrogate marker of GH action, may suggest GHD but should be interpreted in conjunction with age and pubertal status.
  - GH stimulation tests: Dynamic testing with provocative stimuli (e.g., arginine, clonidine, glucagon, insulin, or growth hormone-releasing hormone [GHRH]) to assess the pituitary gland's ability to produce GH in response to physiological stimuli.
- Imaging studies:
  - Magnetic resonance imaging (MRI) of the brain: Preferred imaging modality for visualizing the hypothalamus and pituitary gland, detecting structural abnormalities (e.g., tumors, cysts, or lesions), and assessing the integrity of the hypothalamic-pituitary axis.
  - Computed tomography (CT) scan: May be used in cases where MRI is contraindicated or unavailable, although MRI is more sensitive for detecting pituitary lesions and soft tissue structures.
- Bone age assessment: Radiographic evaluation of skeletal maturation using hand-wrist radiographs to assess bone age relative to chronological age and evaluate growth potential.

Treatment:

- <u>Growth hormone replacement therapy:</u>

    Recombinant human growth hormone (rhGH) therapy administered via subcutaneous injections to replace deficient GH and stimulate linear growth, bone maturation, and somatic development.

- <u>Individualized dosing:</u>

    GH replacement therapy should be individualized based on factors such as age, weight, growth response, pubertal status, bone age, and treatment goals, with regular monitoring of growth parameters and hormone levels to optimize treatment efficacy and safety.

- <u>Monitoring and follow-up:</u>

    Close monitoring of growth velocity, height measurements, bone age, IGF-1 levels, and other relevant parameters to assess treatment response, adjust medication dosages, and identify potential adverse effects or complications.

- <u>Multidisciplinary care:</u>

    Collaboration among pediatric endocrinologists, pediatricians, nurses, dietitians, and other healthcare providers to coordinate care, provide education and support, address psychosocial needs, and optimize outcomes for patients with GHD.

- <u>Long-term management:</u>

    Continuation of GH replacement therapy into adulthood for patients with persistent or lifelong GHD, with regular monitoring of bone health, metabolic parameters, cardiovascular risk factors, and quality of life to optimize long-term outcomes and prevent complications associated with untreated GHD.

7.14. Hyperaldosteronism

> ➤ *Hyperaldosteronism is a condition characterized by excessive production of aldosterone hormone by the adrenal glands, leading to high blood pressure and low potassium levels.*
>
> ➤ *Symptoms may include hypertension, muscle weakness, fatigue, and frequent urination.*
>
> ➤ *Treatment involves medications to control blood pressure, potassium supplements, and in some cases, surgery to remove the affected adrenal gland.*

Symptoms:

- Hypertension: High blood pressure (hypertension) is the most common symptom of hyperaldosteronism. It may be resistant to antihypertensive medications.

- Hypokalemia: Low potassium levels in the blood (hypokalemia) may lead to symptoms such as muscle weakness, fatigue, cramps, and palpitations.

- Polyuria and Polydipsia: Increased urination (polyuria) and thirst (polydipsia) may occur due to urinary potassium wasting and associated electrolyte imbalances.

- Muscle Weakness: Weakness and fatigue may result from hypokalemia and electrolyte disturbances.

- Headache: Some patients may experience headaches, although this symptom is nonspecific and can occur in many other conditions as well.

- Paralysis or Paresthesias: Severe hypokalemia may lead to muscle paralysis or abnormal sensations (paresthesias).

- Metabolic Alkalosis: Alkalosis (elevated blood pH) may occur due to urinary potassium and hydrogen ion excretion.

Causes and Risk Factors:

- Age: Hyperaldosteronism is more common in patients over the age of 40.

- Gender: Women are slightly more likely to develop hyperaldosteronism than men.

- Family History: There may be a genetic predisposition to hyperaldosteronism, although specific genetic mutations are relatively rare.

- Primary Aldosteronism: Conditions such as adrenal adenomas, adrenal hyperplasia, or adrenal carcinoma increase the risk of primary aldosteronism, the most common cause of hyperaldosteronism.
- Secondary Causes: Certain conditions such as renovascular disease, chronic kidney disease, or obstructive sleep apnea may lead to secondary hyperaldosteronism.

Epidemiology:
- The prevalence of primary hyperaldosteronism varies depending on the population studied and the diagnostic criteria used.
- Primary aldosteronism accounts for approximately 5-10% of cases of hypertension in patients referred to hypertension clinics.
- The condition is more common in patients with resistant hypertension, with estimates suggesting that up to 20% of patients with resistant hypertension may have primary aldosteronism.

Workup and Diagnosis:
- Aldosterone-Renin Ratio (ARR):

    The aldosterone-renin ratio (ARR) is a screening test for primary hyperaldosteronism. A high ARR (>30) suggests excess aldosterone production relative to renin levels.

- Confirmatory Tests:

    Confirmatory tests such as the saline infusion test or oral sodium loading test may be performed to confirm the diagnosis of primary hyperaldosteronism.

- Imaging Studies:

    Imaging studies such as computed tomography (CT) or magnetic resonance imaging (MRI) of the adrenal glands may be performed to identify adrenal adenomas or other structural abnormalities.

- Adrenal Vein Sampling:

    Adrenal vein sampling (AVS) is considered the gold standard for distinguishing unilateral (aldosterone-producing adenoma) from bilateral (idiopathic hyperaldosteronism) causes of primary hyperaldosteronism.

Treatment:

- Surgical Management:

    Surgical removal (adrenalectomy) of aldosterone-producing adenomas is the treatment of choice for unilateral primary hyperaldosteronism.

- Medical Therapy:

    For patients with bilateral adrenal hyperplasia or those who are not candidates for surgery, medical therapy with mineralocorticoid receptor antagonists (e.g., spironolactone, eplerenone) is the mainstay of treatment.

- Blood Pressure Control:

    Antihypertensive medications may be prescribed to control blood pressure and reduce the risk of cardiovascular complications.

- Potassium Supplementation:

    Oral potassium supplementation may be necessary to correct hypokalemia in patients with primary hyperaldosteronism.

- Regular Monitoring:

    Regular monitoring of blood pressure, serum potassium levels, and renal function is essential to assess treatment response and monitor for complications.

7.15. Congenital Adrenal Hyperplasia

> ➤ *Congenital adrenal hyperplasia (CAH) is a genetic disorder where enzymes necessary for cortisol production are deficient, leading to abnormal adrenal gland function.*
>
> ➤ *Symptoms vary based on the enzyme deficiency but may include ambiguous genitalia in females, salt wasting, and virilization in both sexes.*
>
> ➤ *Treatment involves hormone replacement therapy to manage cortisol deficiency and, in some cases, surgical correction of genital abnormalities.*

Symptoms:

- Ambiguous Genitalia: In females with CAH, excessive androgen production in utero may lead to ambiguous genitalia, with varying degrees of virilization of the external genitalia.

- Salt-Wasting Crisis: Some patients with CAH, particularly those with the salt-wasting form, may present in infancy with life-threatening salt-wasting crises characterized by dehydration, hyponatremia, hyperkalemia, and metabolic acidosis.
- Precocious Puberty: Excess androgens may lead to early onset of puberty in affected patients, manifesting as the development of secondary sexual characteristics at an abnormally young age.
- Virilization: In both males and females, excess androgens may lead to signs of virilization such as accelerated growth, deepening voice, increased body hair, and acne.
- Menstrual Irregularities: Adolescent and adult females with CAH may experience menstrual irregularities, including oligomenorrhea (infrequent menstruation) or amenorrhea (absence of menstruation).
- Infertility: Women with CAH may experience fertility issues due to irregular menstrual cycles and suboptimal ovarian function.
- Adrenal Crisis: Without proper management, patients with CAH are at risk of adrenal crisis, which can occur during times of stress or illness and is characterized by symptoms such as hypotension, vomiting, abdominal pain, and confusion.

Causes and Risk Factors:
- Genetic Factors: CAH is an autosomal recessive disorder caused by mutations in the genes encoding enzymes involved in cortisol and aldosterone biosynthesis, most commonly the CYP21A2 gene.
- Family History: patients with a family history of CAH or known carrier status are at increased risk of inheriting the condition.
- Ethnicity: CAH is more common in certain ethnic groups, particularly those of Ashkenazi Jewish, Mediterranean, or Hispanic descent.

Epidemiology:
- CAH is a relatively rare disorder, with an estimated incidence of 1 in 10,000 to 1 in 20,000 live births.
- The prevalence of CAH varies depending on the population studied and the specific genetic mutations involved.
- The salt-wasting form of CAH is the most severe and accounts for approximately 75% of cases, while the simple virilizing and non-classic forms are less common.

Workup and Diagnosis:
- Newborn Screening: CAH is included in newborn screening panels in many countries, allowing for early detection and intervention.

- <u>Hormone Testing:</u> Hormonal testing, including measurement of serum 17-hydroxyprogesterone (17-OHP) levels, is used to confirm the diagnosis of CAH.
- <u>Genetic Testing:</u> Genetic testing may be performed to identify specific mutations in the CYP21A2 gene or other genes associated with CAH.
- <u>Imaging Studies:</u>

    Imaging studies such as pelvic ultrasound or magnetic resonance imaging (MRI) may be performed to evaluate for internal reproductive organ abnormalities in females with CAH.

Treatment:

- <u>Glucocorticoid Replacement:</u>

    Glucocorticoid replacement therapy with oral hydrocortisone or cortisone acetate is the mainstay of treatment for CAH to replace deficient cortisol production and suppress excess adrenal androgen production.

- <u>Mineralocorticoid Replacement:</u>

    In patients with the salt-wasting form of CAH, mineralocorticoid replacement therapy with oral fludrocortisone is necessary to replace deficient aldosterone production and prevent salt-wasting crises.

- <u>Androgen Suppression:</u>

    Androgen suppression therapy with low-dose glucocorticoids may be used to suppress excess androgen production and reduce virilization in affected patients.

- <u>Monitoring and Supportive Care:</u>

    Regular monitoring of growth, development, hormone levels, and bone health is essential for patients with CAH. Supportive care measures such as salt supplementation, fluid management, and psychosocial support may also be necessary.

7.16. Pheochromocytoma

> ➤ *Pheochromocytoma is a rare tumor of the adrenal glands that produces excess catecholamines, leading to severe hypertension, headaches, sweating, and palpitations.*
>
> ➤ *Diagnosis involves biochemical testing for elevated catecholamine levels and imaging studies to locate the tumor.*
>
> ➤ *Treatment typically involves surgical removal of the tumor and management of blood pressure with medications preoperatively.*

Symptoms:

- Hypertension: Severe, episodic hypertension (high blood pressure) is the hallmark symptom of pheochromocytoma. These episodes may be paroxysmal, with blood pressure reaching hypertensive crisis levels.
- Headaches: Severe headaches, often described as throbbing or pounding, are common during hypertensive episodes.
- Palpitations: patients with pheochromocytoma may experience palpitations, rapid heart rate (tachycardia), or irregular heartbeats (arrhythmias) due to excess catecholamine release.
- Sweating: Profuse sweating (diaphoresis) may occur during hypertensive episodes, often accompanied by feelings of anxiety or nervousness.
- Tremors: Fine tremors or shaking of the hands may occur due to increased sympathetic nervous system activity.
- Pallor: Pallor (paleness of the skin) may occur during hypertensive crises, particularly in association with other symptoms such as sweating and palpitations.
- Abdominal Pain: Some patients with pheochromocytoma may experience abdominal pain or discomfort, which may mimic other gastrointestinal conditions.
- Weight Loss: Unexplained weight loss may occur in some cases, particularly if the tumor is secreting excess catecholamines.
- Other Symptoms: Other less common symptoms may include flushing of the skin, nausea, vomiting, constipation, and visual disturbances.

Causes and Risk Factors:

- Genetic Syndromes: Pheochromocytomas may occur as part of inherited genetic syndromes such as multiple endocrine neoplasia type 2 (MEN2), von Hippel-Lindau (VHL) disease, neurofibromatosis type 1 (NF1), and hereditary paraganglioma-pheochromocytoma syndrome.

- Family History: patients with a family history of pheochromocytoma or associated genetic syndromes are at increased risk of developing the condition.
- Age: Pheochromocytomas can occur at any age but are most commonly diagnosed in adults between the ages of 30 and 50 years.
- Sex: Pheochromocytomas affect both males and females equally.
- Previous Radiation Exposure: Previous radiation therapy to the abdomen or pelvis may increase the risk of developing pheochromocytoma.

Epidemiology:

- Pheochromocytomas are rare neuroendocrine tumors arising from chromaffin cells in the adrenal medulla or extra-adrenal paraganglia.
- The annual incidence of pheochromocytoma is estimated to be 0.8 to 1.3 per 100,000 patients.
- Approximately 10% of pheochromocytomas are malignant (metastatic), while the majority are benign (non-metastatic).

Workup and Diagnosis:

- Biochemical Testing:

    Measurement of plasma or urinary catecholamines (norepinephrine, epinephrine, dopamine) and their metabolites (metanephrines) is used for initial screening and diagnosis of pheochromocytoma.

- Imaging Studies:

    Radiological imaging studies such as computed tomography (CT) scan, magnetic resonance imaging (MRI), or metaiodobenzylguanidine (MIBG) scintigraphy may be performed to localize the tumor and evaluate for metastasis.

- Genetic Testing:

    Genetic testing may be indicated in patients with suspected hereditary forms of pheochromocytoma or a strong family history of the condition.

- Provocative Testing:

    Provocative testing with agents such as clonidine or glucagon may be used to confirm the diagnosis and assess catecholamine secretion in patients with equivocal biochemical results.

Treatment:
- Surgical Resection:

    Surgical removal (adrenalectomy) of the pheochromocytoma is the treatment of choice for localized tumors. Minimally invasive techniques such as laparoscopic adrenalectomy are often used when feasible.

- Preoperative Alpha-Blockade:

    Preoperative alpha-adrenergic blockade with medications such as phenoxybenzamine or doxazosin is essential to control hypertension and prevent intraoperative hypertensive crises.

- Beta-Blockade:

    Beta-adrenergic blockade with medications such as propranolol or metoprolol may be used adjunctively to control tachycardia and arrhythmias.

- Fluid and Electrolyte Management:

    Intravenous fluids and electrolyte supplementation may be necessary to correct volume depletion, electrolyte imbalances, and prevent hypotension during surgery.

- Postoperative Monitoring:

    Close postoperative monitoring of blood pressure, fluid status, and electrolyte levels is essential to detect and manage any postoperative complications such as hypotension or electrolyte abnormalities.

- Long-Term Surveillance:

    Long-term surveillance with periodic biochemical testing and imaging studies is recommended to monitor for recurrence or metastasis, particularly in patients with hereditary forms of pheochromocytoma or at increased risk of recurrence.

7.17. Multiple Endocrine Neoplasia Syndrome

> ➤ Multiple endocrine neoplasia (MEN) syndrome is a group of rare genetic disorders characterized by tumors in multiple endocrine glands, leading to hormone overproduction.
>
> ➤ Types include MEN1 (parathyroid, pancreas, pituitary tumors), MEN2 (thyroid, adrenal medulla tumors), and MEN3 (medullary thyroid carcinoma, pheochromocytoma).
>
> ➤ Management involves surveillance, tumor removal, and hormone replacement as necessary to prevent complications.

Symptoms:

MEN1 Syndrome:

- Parathyroid adenomas or hyperplasia leading to hyperparathyroidism.
- Pancreatic neuroendocrine tumors (e.g., gastrinomas, insulinomas).
- Pituitary adenomas causing hyperprolactinemia, acromegaly, or Cushing's disease.
- Non-endocrine tumors such as facial angiofibromas, collagenomas, and lipomas.

MEN2A Syndrome:

- Medullary thyroid carcinoma (MTC), often presenting as a palpable thyroid nodule.
- Pheochromocytoma, leading to episodic hypertension, palpitations, and sweating.
- Parathyroid hyperplasia or adenoma causing hyperparathyroidism.

MEN2B Syndrome:

- Medullary thyroid carcinoma (MTC) which tends to be more aggressive.
- Pheochromocytoma.
- Mucosal neuromas, particularly affecting the lips and tongue, leading to characteristic facial features (e.g., thickened lips, enlarged tongue).

Causes and Risk Factors:

- Genetic Mutations: MEN syndromes are inherited in an autosomal dominant pattern, with specific genetic mutations predisposing patients to develop tumors in multiple endocrine glands.

- Family History: patients with a family history of MEN syndrome or known genetic mutations associated with the condition are at increased risk of developing the disorder.
- Age: The age of onset and severity of symptoms may vary depending on the specific MEN subtype and genetic mutation involved.

Epidemiology:
- MEN syndromes are rare, with estimated prevalence rates ranging from 1 in 30,000 to 1 in 100,000 patients.
- The prevalence of specific MEN subtypes may vary geographically and among different populations.
- MEN1 syndrome is the most common subtype, accounting for approximately 80% of cases of MEN syndromes.

Workup and Diagnosis:
- Clinical Evaluation:

    Diagnosis of MEN syndrome requires a thorough clinical evaluation, including a detailed family history and physical examination to assess for signs and symptoms of endocrine tumors.

- Genetic Testing:

    Genetic testing may be performed to identify specific mutations associated with MEN syndromes, particularly in patients with a family history of the condition or those who meet clinical diagnostic criteria.

- Biochemical Testing:

    Measurement of hormone levels (e.g., calcitonin, parathyroid hormone, catecholamines) may be indicated to screen for associated endocrine abnormalities such as hyperparathyroidism or pheochromocytoma.

- Imaging Studies:

    Radiological imaging studies such as ultrasound, computed tomography (CT), or magnetic resonance imaging (MRI) may be performed to localize and characterize endocrine tumors in affected patients.

Treatment:
- Surgical Resection:

    Surgical removal of affected endocrine glands or tumors is the primary treatment approach for MEN syndromes, aimed at

- **Medication:**

    Pharmacological management may be used to control hormone excess or alleviate symptoms associated with endocrine tumors, such as calcium-lowering medications for hyperparathyroidism or alpha and beta-blockers for pheochromocytoma.

- **Lifelong Monitoring:**

    Lifelong surveillance and regular screening for tumor recurrence or metastasis are essential for patients with MEN syndromes, given the risk of developing multiple tumors over time.

- **Genetic Counseling:**

    Genetic counseling and testing should be offered to affected patients and their families to assess the risk of transmission, provide information about inheritance patterns, and offer guidance regarding family planning and screening recommendations.

7.18. Hypercalcemia

> ➢ *Hypercalcemia is a condition characterized by elevated levels of calcium in the blood, typically above 10.4 mg/dL.*
>
> ➢ *It can result from various causes, including hyperparathyroidism, malignancy, and excessive vitamin D intake, leading to symptoms such as weakness, confusion, constipation, and kidney stones.*
>
> ➢ *Treatment involves addressing the underlying cause, hydration, medications to lower calcium levels, and, in severe cases, intravenous bisphosphonates or calcitonin.*

Symptoms:

- Muscle Weakness: Weakness, fatigue, and lethargy are common symptoms of hypercalcemia.
- Bone Pain: Hypercalcemia can lead to bone pain, particularly in areas with increased bone turnover.
- Nausea and Vomiting: Gastrointestinal symptoms such as nausea, vomiting, constipation, and abdominal pain may occur.

- Polyuria and Polydipsia: Excessive urination (polyuria) and thirst (polydipsia) may result from impaired renal concentrating ability.
- Confusion and Cognitive Changes: Hypercalcemia can affect cognitive function, leading to confusion, memory impairment, and difficulty concentrating.
- Renal Symptoms: Renal symptoms may include nephrolithiasis (kidney stones), hematuria (blood in the urine), and renal impairment.
- Cardiac Symptoms: In severe cases, hypercalcemia can lead to cardiac arrhythmias, palpitations, and even cardiac arrest.
- Neuropsychiatric Symptoms: Neuropsychiatric manifestations such as depression, anxiety, and psychosis may occur, particularly in patients with severe hypercalcemia.

Causes and Risk Factors:
- Primary Hyperparathyroidism: The most common cause of hypercalcemia is primary hyperparathyroidism, typically due to a benign adenoma of the parathyroid gland.
- Malignancy: Hypercalcemia can occur as a paraneoplastic syndrome in various malignancies, including breast cancer, lung cancer, multiple myeloma, and lymphoma.
- Hyperthyroidism: Thyrotoxicosis, or hyperthyroidism, can lead to increased bone resorption and subsequent hypercalcemia.
- Medications: Certain medications such as thiazide diuretics, lithium, and calcium supplements can increase serum calcium levels.
- Immobilization: Prolonged immobilization or bed rest can lead to bone resorption and hypercalcemia.
- Hypercalcemia of Malignancy: Malignancy-associated hypercalcemia is more common in advanced cancer stages and may result from tumor production of parathyroid hormone-related protein (PTHrP), ectopic production of calcitriol (active vitamin D), or direct bone metastases.
- Chronic Kidney Disease: Impaired renal function can lead to decreased calcium excretion and subsequent hypercalcemia.

Epidemiology:
- The prevalence of hypercalcemia varies depending on the underlying cause, with primary hyperparathyroidism being the most common etiology.
- Hypercalcemia of malignancy is estimated to occur in 10% to 30% of cancer patients, particularly those with advanced disease.

- The incidence of hypercalcemia increases with age, with primary hyperparathyroidism being more common in postmenopausal women and malignancy-associated hypercalcemia more prevalent in older adults.

Workup and Diagnosis:

- Serum Calcium Levels: Hypercalcemia is defined as a serum calcium level greater than 10.4 mg/dL (2.6 mmol/L).

- Albumin Correction:

    Serum calcium levels should be corrected for hypoalbuminemia using the following formula: Corrected calcium (mg/dL) = Measured calcium (mg/dL) + 0.8 × (4 - serum albumin [g/dL]).

- Parathyroid Hormone (PTH) Levels:

    Measurement of intact PTH levels can help differentiate between hypercalcemia due to primary hyperparathyroidism (elevated PTH) and other causes such as malignancy (suppressed or normal PTH).

- Additional Laboratory Tests:

    Additional laboratory tests may include serum creatinine, phosphate, magnesium, 25-hydroxyvitamin D, and alkaline phosphatase levels to assess for underlying causes of hypercalcemia.

- Imaging Studies:

    Imaging studies such as neck ultrasound or sestamibi scan may be performed to localize parathyroid adenomas in cases of primary hyperparathyroidism.

Treatment:

- Hydration:

    Intravenous hydration with isotonic saline is the initial treatment for hypercalcemia to promote renal calcium excretion and prevent dehydration.

- Bisphosphonates:

    Intravenous bisphosphonates such as zoledronic acid or pamidronate inhibit bone resorption and are commonly used to lower serum calcium levels in hypercalcemia of malignancy.

- Calcitonin: Calcitonin can provide rapid but short-term reduction in serum calcium levels by inhibiting bone resorption.

- Corticosteroids:

    Glucocorticoids may be used in cases of granulomatous diseases or lymphoma-associated hypercalcemia to reduce intestinal absorption of calcium.

- Calcimimetics:

    Calcimimetic agents such as cinacalcet can lower serum calcium levels by increasing the sensitivity of the calcium-sensing receptor on parathyroid cells.

- Surgery:

    Parathyroidectomy is indicated in cases of severe primary hyperparathyroidism or symptomatic parathyroid adenomas that fail medical management.

7.19. Hypocalcemia

> - *Hypocalcemia is a condition characterized by low levels of calcium in the blood, typically below 8.5 mg/dL.*
> - *It can result from various causes, including hypoparathyroidism, vitamin D deficiency, or kidney disease, leading to symptoms such as muscle cramps, tingling sensations, seizures, and weakened bones.*
> - *Treatment involves calcium and vitamin D supplementation, addressing the underlying cause, and, in severe cases, intravenous calcium administration.*

Symptoms:

- Tingling and Numbness: Paresthesias, commonly described as tingling sensations or numbness, especially around the lips, fingers, and toes.
- Muscle Cramps: Spasms or cramps in the muscles, particularly in the hands, feet, and facial muscles.
- Twitching: Muscle twitching, especially in the face and extremities.
- Seizures: In severe cases, hypocalcemia can lead to seizures or convulsions.
- Cardiac Arrhythmias: Abnormal heart rhythms, such as bradycardia (slow heart rate) or ventricular arrhythmias, may occur.
- Chvostek's Sign: Facial muscle twitching elicited by tapping over the facial nerve, a clinical sign of neuromuscular irritability seen in hypocalcemia.

- Trousseau's Sign: Carpal spasm induced by inflating a blood pressure cuff above systolic pressure for a few minutes, another sign of neuromuscular irritability.

Causes and Risk Factors:
- Hypoparathyroidism: Hypocalcemia commonly occurs due to insufficient parathyroid hormone (PTH) secretion, either due to primary hypoparathyroidism or secondary to thyroid surgery or autoimmune destruction of the parathyroid glands.
- Vitamin D Deficiency: Inadequate vitamin D intake, impaired absorption, or impaired activation of vitamin D can lead to hypocalcemia, as vitamin D is essential for calcium absorption from the intestines.
- Chronic Kidney Disease: Impaired renal function can lead to decreased conversion of vitamin D to its active form, reduced calcium reabsorption, and increased phosphate retention, resulting in hypocalcemia.
- Malabsorption Syndromes: Conditions such as celiac disease, inflammatory bowel disease, or short bowel syndrome can impair calcium absorption from the intestines, leading to hypocalcemia.
- Medications: Certain medications such as bisphosphonates, calcimimetics, loop diuretics, antiepileptic drugs (e.g., phenytoin), and intravenous bisphosphonates can lower serum calcium levels.
- Alkalosis: Metabolic alkalosis can lead to hypocalcemia by reducing ionized calcium levels through increased protein binding.

Epidemiology:
- The prevalence of hypocalcemia varies depending on the underlying cause and population studied.
- Primary hypoparathyroidism is a rare disorder, with an estimated prevalence of 25 to 37 cases per 100,000 patients.
- Vitamin D deficiency is more prevalent in certain populations, including the elderly, patients with limited sun exposure, and those with malabsorption syndromes.

Workup and Diagnosis:
- <u>Serum Calcium Levels:</u> Hypocalcemia is defined as a serum calcium level less than 8.5 mg/dL (2.12 mmol/L).
- <u>Albumin Correction:</u>
    Serum calcium levels should be corrected for hypoalbuminemia using the following formula: Corrected calcium (mg/dL) = Measured calcium (mg/dL) + 0.8 × (4 - serum albumin [g/dL]).

- Parathyroid Hormone (PTH) Levels:

    Measurement of intact PTH levels can help differentiate between hypoparathyroidism (low or undetectable PTH) and other causes of hypocalcemia.

- Vitamin D Levels: Measurement of serum 25-hydroxyvitamin D levels can assess vitamin D deficiency, a common cause of hypocalcemia.

- Renal Function Tests:

    Assessment of renal function, including serum creatinine and estimated glomerular filtration rate (eGFR), is important to evaluate for chronic kidney disease as a potential cause of hypocalcemia.

Treatment:

- Calcium Supplementation:

    Oral calcium supplements, such as calcium carbonate or calcium citrate, may be prescribed to correct hypocalcemia and maintain serum calcium levels within the normal range.

- Active Vitamin D Analogues:

    Calcitriol (1,25-dihydroxyvitamin D) or other active vitamin D analogues may be used in cases of vitamin D deficiency or hypoparathyroidism to enhance intestinal calcium absorption.

- Magnesium Replacement:

    Hypomagnesemia should be corrected if present, as magnesium is essential for parathyroid hormone secretion and responsiveness to calcium.

- PTH Replacement Therapy: Recombinant human PTH (teriparatide) may be used in severe cases of hypoparathyroidism refractory to conventional therapy.

- Monitor and Treat Underlying Causes:

    Treatment of underlying conditions such as chronic kidney disease, malabsorption syndromes, or vitamin D deficiency is essential to correct hypocalcemia and prevent recurrence.

7.20. Mixed Hyperlipidemia

> ➤ *Mixed hyperlipidemia is a condition characterized by elevated levels of both cholesterol and triglycerides in the blood.*
>
> ➤ *It increases the risk of cardiovascular diseases such as heart attack and stroke.*
>
> ➤ *Management involves lifestyle changes, medication, and regular monitoring to reduce lipid levels and prevent complications.*

Symptoms:

- Xanthomas: Yellowish deposits of cholesterol under the skin, often found on the eyelids, elbows, knees, or buttocks.
- Xanthelasma: Yellowish plaques on the eyelids, which may be associated with elevated cholesterol levels.
- Arcus Senilis: A white or grayish ring around the cornea of the eye, caused by lipid deposition.
- Corneal Opacities: Clouding of the cornea, which may impair vision in severe cases.
- Pancreatitis: Severe abdominal pain, nausea, and vomiting due to inflammation of the pancreas, which can occur with extremely high triglyceride levels.
- Symptoms of Cardiovascular Disease: Mixed hyperlipidemia increases the risk of atherosclerosis, coronary artery disease, and other cardiovascular complications, which may manifest as chest pain (angina), shortness of breath, or heart attack.

Causes and Risk Factors:

- Genetics: Genetic factors play a significant role in mixed hyperlipidemia, with certain inherited lipid disorders (e.g., familial combined hyperlipidemia) predisposing patients to elevated LDL-C and TG levels.
- Diet: Consumption of a diet high in saturated fats, trans fats, and cholesterol can contribute to elevated LDL-C and TG levels.
- Obesity: Excess body weight, particularly abdominal obesity, is associated with dyslipidemia and increased cardiovascular risk.
- Physical Inactivity: Sedentary lifestyle and lack of regular exercise can lead to dyslipidemia and metabolic abnormalities.
- Diabetes: patients with diabetes mellitus, especially poorly controlled diabetes, are at increased risk of mixed hyperlipidemia and cardiovascular complications.

- Smoking: Tobacco use is associated with dyslipidemia and accelerates the progression of atherosclerosis.
- Alcohol Consumption: Excessive alcohol intake can elevate triglyceride levels and contribute to mixed hyperlipidemia.
- Certain Medications: Some medications, such as corticosteroids, diuretics, beta-blockers, antipsychotics, and immunosuppressants, can adversely affect lipid levels.

Epidemiology:
- Mixed hyperlipidemia is a common lipid disorder, with prevalence rates varying depending on population demographics and diagnostic criteria.
- The prevalence of mixed hyperlipidemia tends to increase with age and is more common in patients with other metabolic risk factors such as obesity, diabetes, and hypertension.
- It is estimated that mixed hyperlipidemia is present in approximately 30% to 50% of patients with established coronary artery disease.

Workup and Diagnosis:
- Lipid Profile:

    Diagnosis of mixed hyperlipidemia is based on laboratory testing of fasting lipid levels, including total cholesterol, LDL-C, HDL-C, and triglycerides.
- Criteria: Mixed hyperlipidemia is characterized by elevated levels of both LDL-C and triglycerides, along with decreased HDL-C levels.
- Other Tests:

    Additional tests may include measurement of apolipoprotein B (apoB) levels, lipoprotein (a) [Lp(a)], and non-HDL cholesterol, which provide additional information about cardiovascular risk.

Treatment:
- Lifestyle Modification:

    Dietary changes, regular exercise, weight management, and smoking cessation are fundamental components of managing mixed hyperlipidemia and reducing cardiovascular risk.
- Medications:

    Pharmacological therapy may be indicated to lower LDL-C and triglyceride levels and increase HDL-C. Treatment options include statins, fibrates, niacin, ezetimibe, and omega-3 fatty acids.

- Combination Therapy:

    In severe cases or when monotherapy is insufficient, combination therapy with multiple lipid-lowering agents may be used to achieve target lipid levels.

- Monitoring:

    Regular monitoring of lipid levels, liver function tests, and other relevant parameters is essential to assess treatment response and safety.

- Secondary Prevention:

    Patients with established cardiovascular disease or other high-risk conditions may require more aggressive lipid-lowering therapy to reduce the risk of recurrent events.

7.21. Metabolic syndrome

> ➤ *Metabolic syndrome is a cluster of conditions including high blood pressure, high blood sugar, excess body fat around the waist, and abnormal cholesterol or triglyceride levels.*
>
> ➤ *It increases the risk of heart disease, stroke, and type 2 diabetes.*
>
> ➤ *Management involves lifestyle changes such as diet and exercise, along with medication if necessary, to reduce risk factors and improve overall health.*

Symptoms:

Metabolic syndrome is a cluster of metabolic abnormalities that may not present with specific symptoms on their own.

However, patients with metabolic syndrome may experience symptoms associated with the underlying conditions contributing to the syndrome, such as:

- Abdominal obesity: Increased waist circumference, characterized by excess fat accumulation around the waist, is a central feature of metabolic syndrome.

- Insulin resistance: patients with metabolic syndrome may experience elevated blood sugar levels (hyperglycemia) due to insulin resistance, which can lead to symptoms such as increased thirst, frequent urination, fatigue, and blurred vision.

- Dyslipidemia: Abnormal lipid levels, including elevated triglycerides, low high-density lipoprotein (HDL) cholesterol, and elevated low-density lipoprotein (LDL) cholesterol, may increase the risk of

cardiovascular disease and its associated symptoms such as chest pain (angina), shortness of breath, and palpitations.
- Hypertension: High blood pressure, another component of metabolic syndrome, may not cause noticeable symptoms in the early stages but can lead to complications such as headaches, dizziness, blurred vision, and chest pain in severe cases.

Causes and Risk Factors:
- Obesity: Excess body weight, particularly central obesity (abdominal fat accumulation), is a major risk factor for metabolic syndrome.
- Physical inactivity: Lack of regular physical activity or sedentary lifestyle increases the risk of metabolic syndrome.
- Unhealthy diet: Diets high in refined carbohydrates, sugars, saturated fats, and processed foods contribute to the development of metabolic syndrome.
- Insulin resistance: patients with insulin resistance, prediabetes, or type 2 diabetes are at increased risk of metabolic syndrome.
- Age: The prevalence of metabolic syndrome increases with age, particularly in patients over 40 years old.
- Genetics: Family history of metabolic disorders, cardiovascular disease, or type 2 diabetes increases the risk of developing metabolic syndrome.
- Ethnicity: Certain ethnic groups, including Hispanic/Latino, African American, and Asian populations, have a higher prevalence of metabolic syndrome.
- Hormonal factors: Hormonal imbalances, such as polycystic ovary syndrome (PCOS) in women or low testosterone levels in men, may contribute to metabolic syndrome.
- Smoking: Tobacco use is associated with metabolic abnormalities and an increased risk of metabolic syndrome and cardiovascular disease.
- Sleep disorders: Conditions such as sleep apnea or insufficient sleep duration may increase the risk of metabolic syndrome.

Epidemiology:

Metabolic syndrome is a global public health concern, with a significant prevalence worldwide. Its prevalence varies depending on the population studied, diagnostic criteria used, and regional differences in lifestyle and dietary habits. In the United States, approximately one-third of adults are estimated to have metabolic syndrome, with higher rates observed in older adults and certain ethnic groups.

Workup and Diagnosis:

The diagnosis of metabolic syndrome is based on the presence of at least three of the following criteria, as defined by various international organizations such as the National Cholesterol Education Program (NCEP) Adult Treatment Panel III (ATP III) and the International Diabetes Federation (IDF):

- Abdominal obesity (waist circumference ≥ 102 cm in men or ≥ 88 cm in women)
- Elevated triglyceride levels (≥ 150 mg/dL or on medication for elevated triglycerides)
- Low HDL cholesterol levels (< 40 mg/dL in men or < 50 mg/dL in women or on medication for low HDL cholesterol)
- Elevated blood pressure (≥ 130/85 mmHg or on antihypertensive medication)
- Elevated fasting glucose levels (≥ 100 mg/dL or on medication for elevated blood glucose)

Treatment:

- Lifestyle modifications:

    Lifestyle interventions focusing on weight loss, regular physical activity, and dietary modifications are the cornerstone of metabolic syndrome management.

- Healthy diet:

    Emphasizing a balanced diet rich in fruits, vegetables, whole grains, lean proteins, and healthy fats while limiting intake of processed foods, sugars, and saturated fats.

- Regular exercise:

    Engaging in regular aerobic exercise, such as brisk walking, cycling, or swimming, for at least 150 minutes per week, along with strength training exercises.

- Smoking cessation: Encouraging smoking cessation for patients who smoke or use tobacco products to reduce cardiovascular risk factors.

- Medications:

    In some cases, medications may be prescribed to manage patient components of metabolic syndrome, such as antihypertensive medications, lipid-lowering agents (statins), or glucose-lowering medications for diabetes management.

References

- American Diabetes Association. (2021). Standards of medical care in diabetes. Diabetes Care, 44(Suppl 1), S1-S232.
- American Diabetes Association. (2021). Standards of medical care in diabetes. Diabetes Care, 44(Suppl 1), S1-S232.
- Garber, J. R., Cobin, R. H., & et al. (2012). Clinical practice guidelines for hypothyroidism in adults: Cosponsored by the American Association of Clinical Endocrinologists and the American Thyroid Association. Endocrine Practice, 18(6), 988-1028.
- Ross, D. S., Burch, H. B., & et al. (2016). American Thyroid Association guidelines for diagnosis and management of hyperthyroidism and other causes of thyrotoxicosis. Thyroid, 26(10), 1343-1421.
- Haugen, B. R., Alexander, E. K., & et al. (2016). American Thyroid Association management guidelines for adult patients with thyroid nodules and differentiated thyroid cancer: The American Thyroid Association guidelines task force on thyroid nodules and differentiated thyroid cancer. Thyroid, 26(1), 1-133.
- Garber, J. R., Cobin, R. H., & et al. (2012). Clinical practice guidelines for hypothyroidism in adults: Cosponsored by the American Association of Clinical Endocrinologists and the American Thyroid Association. Endocrine Practice, 18(6), 988-1028.
- Bornstein, S. R., Allolio, B., & et al. (2016). Diagnosis and treatment of primary adrenal insufficiency: An endocrine society clinical practice guideline. Journal of Clinical Endocrinology & Metabolism, 101(2), 364-389.
- Nieman, L. K., Biller, B. M., & et al. (2015). Treatment of Cushing's syndrome: An Endocrine Society clinical practice guideline. Journal of Clinical Endocrinology & Metabolism, 100(8), 2807-2831.
- Teede, H. J., Misso, M. L., & et al. (2018). Recommendations from the international evidence-based guideline for the assessment and management of polycystic ovary syndrome. Clinical Endocrinology, 89(3), 251-268.
- Bilezikian, J. P., Brandi, M. L., & et al. (2016). Guidelines for the management of asymptomatic primary hyperparathyroidism: Summary statement from the Fourth International Workshop. Journal of Clinical Endocrinology & Metabolism, 102(1), 106-107.
- Brandi, M. L., Bilezikian, J. P., & et al. (2016). Management of hypoparathyroidism: Summary statement and guidelines. Journal of Clinical Endocrinology & Metabolism, 101(6), 2273-2283.
- Freda, P. U., Beckers, A. M., & et al. (2011). Pituitary incidentaloma: An endocrine society clinical practice guideline. Journal of Clinical Endocrinology & Metabolism, 96(4), 894-904.

- Fleseriu, M., Hashim, I. A., & et al. (2016). Hormonal replacement in hypopituitarism in adults: An Endocrine Society clinical practice guideline. Journal of Clinical Endocrinology & Metabolism, 101(11), 3888-3921.
- Molitch, M. E., Clemmons, D. R., & et al. (2011). Evaluation and treatment of adult growth hormone deficiency: An Endocrine Society clinical practice guideline. Journal of Clinical Endocrinology & Metabolism, 96(6), 1587-1609.
- Funder, J. W., Carey, R. M., & et al. (2016). The management of primary aldosteronism: Case detection, diagnosis, and treatment: An Endocrine Society clinical practice guideline. Journal of Clinical Endocrinology & Metabolism, 101(5), 1889-1916.
- Speiser, P. W., Arlt, W., & et al. (2018). Congenital adrenal hyperplasia due to steroid 21-hydroxylase deficiency: An Endocrine Society clinical practice guideline. Journal of Clinical Endocrinology & Metabolism, 103(11), 4043-4088.
- Lenders, J. W., Duh, Q. Y., & et al. (2014). Pheochromocytoma and paraganglioma: An Endocrine Society clinical practice guideline. Journal of Clinical Endocrinology & Metabolism, 99(6), 1915-1942.
- Thakker, R. V., Newey, P. J., & et al. (2012). Clinical practice guidelines for multiple endocrine neoplasia type 1 (MEN1). Journal of Clinical Endocrinology & Metabolism, 97(9), 2990-3011.
- Bilezikian, J. P., Brandi, M. L., & et al. (2014). Management of asymptomatic primary hyperparathyroidism: Proceedings of the Fourth International Workshop. Journal of Clinical Endocrinology & Metabolism, 99(10), 3561-3569.
- Shoback, D. M., Bilezikian, J. P., & et al. (2016). Hypoparathyroidism in adults: Epidemiology, patient, and resource utilization in the real-world setting. Endocrine Practice, 22(4), 395-405.
- Grundy, S. M., Stone, N. J., & et al. (2018). 2018 AHA/ACC/AACVPR/AAPA/ABC/ACPM/ADA/AGS/APhA/ASPC/NLA/PCNA guideline on the management of blood cholesterol: Executive summary. Journal of the American College of Cardiology, 73(24), 3168-3209.
- Grundy, S. M., Brewer Jr, H. B., & et al. (2004). Definition of metabolic syndrome: Report of the National Heart, Lung, and Blood Institute/American Heart Association conference on scientific issues related to definition. Circulation, 109(3), 433-438.

Chapter 8. Infectious Disorders

Reviewed by
Vinh-Quan Nguyen, MD, PhD

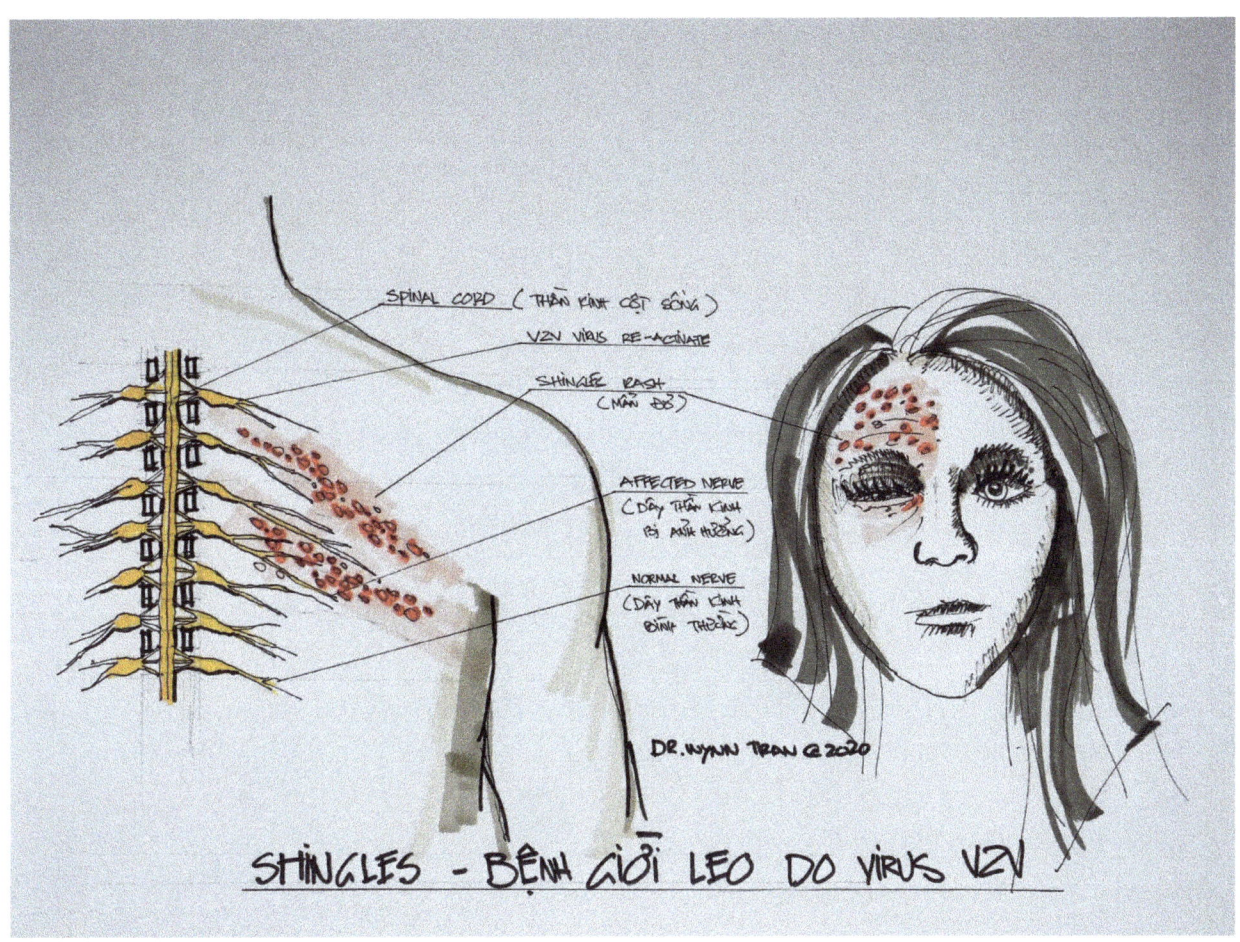

The APh should be familiar with the presentation, diagnosis, and management of these common infectious disorders to provide appropriate care and referral to the infectious disease physician when necessary.

8.1. Urinary Tract Infections

> ➤ *A urinary tract infection (UTI) is a bacterial infection affecting any part of the urinary system, including the bladder, kidneys, ureters, or urethra.*
>
> ➤ *Common symptoms include frequent urination, burning sensation during urination, and cloudy or bloody urine.*
>
> ➤ *Treatment typically involves antibiotics and increased fluid intake to flush out the bacteria.*

Symptoms:

- Urinary Urgency: Feeling the need to urinate urgently, often with little urine passed.
- Frequency: Increased frequency of urination, with small amounts of urine passed each time.
- Dysuria: Pain or burning sensation during urination.
- Hematuria: Presence of blood in the urine, which may be visible or detected only under a microscope.
- Cloudy or Foul-Smelling Urine: Urine may appear cloudy or have a strong odor.
- Pelvic Pain: Discomfort or pressure in the lower abdomen or pelvic region.
- Flank Pain: Pain or discomfort in the sides or back, indicating possible kidney involvement.
- Fever and Chills: Systemic symptoms may occur in more severe cases, indicating the presence of a kidney infection (pyelonephritis).

Causes and Risk Factors:

- Female Gender: Women are at higher risk due to their shorter urethra, which facilitates bacterial entry into the bladder.
- Sexual Activity: Sexual intercourse can introduce bacteria into the urinary tract, increasing the risk of infection.
- Urinary Catheterization: Presence of a urinary catheter provides a direct pathway for bacteria to enter the bladder.
- Anatomy: Structural abnormalities of the urinary tract, such as vesicoureteral reflux or urinary tract obstruction, increase susceptibility to UTIs.
- Menopause: Decreased estrogen levels in postmenopausal women can lead to changes in vaginal flora, increasing the risk of UTIs.

- Pregnancy: Hormonal changes and pressure on the bladder during pregnancy can predispose women to UTIs.
- Diabetes: Poorly controlled diabetes can impair immune function and increase the risk of UTIs.
- Immunosuppression: Conditions or medications that weaken the immune system, such as HIV/AIDS or corticosteroids, increase susceptibility to infections.
- Older Age: Elderly patients may have urinary retention, incontinence, or other factors contributing to UTI risk.

Epidemiology:
- UTIs are among the most common bacterial infections, affecting millions of patients worldwide each year.
- Women are more susceptible to UTIs than men, with approximately 50% of women experiencing at least one UTI during their lifetime.
- Recurrent UTIs are common, especially in women, with approximately 20-30% experiencing a recurrence within 6 months.

Workup and Diagnosis:
- Urinalysis: Examination of a urine sample for the presence of white blood cells, red blood cells, bacteria, and other abnormalities.
- Urine Culture: Identification of the causative bacteria and determination of antibiotic susceptibility.
- Clinical Evaluation: Assessment of symptoms, medical history, and risk factors to guide diagnosis and treatment decisions.
- Imaging Studies:
    In cases of complicated UTIs or recurrent infections, imaging tests such as ultrasound or CT scan may be performed to evaluate for structural abnormalities.

Treatment:
- Antibiotics: Empirical antibiotic therapy is often initiated based on clinical presentation and local antimicrobial resistance patterns.
- Specific Antibiotics:
    Choice of antibiotic depends on factors such as the suspected organism, local resistance patterns, and patient factors such as allergies and comorbidities.
- Duration: Treatment duration varies depending on the type and severity of the infection, typically ranging from 3 to 14 days.

- **Fluid Intake:** Encouraging increased fluid intake helps flush bacteria from the urinary tract and may help alleviate symptoms.
- **Pain Management:**

    Analgesics such as nonsteroidal anti-inflammatory drugs (NSAIDs) or urinary tract analgesics may be used to relieve pain and discomfort.
- **Preventive Measures:**

    Strategies to prevent UTIs may include urinating after intercourse, maintaining good genital hygiene, avoiding spermicides or irritants, and increasing cranberry juice consumption (although evidence is mixed).

8.2. Pyelonephritis

> ➤ *Pyelonephritis is a type of urinary tract infection (UTI) that specifically affects the kidneys. It often occurs when bacteria from the bladder travel up the ureters to the kidneys.*
>
> ➤ *Symptoms include fever, flank pain, nausea, and vomiting.*
>
> ➤ *Treatment involves antibiotics and adequate hydration, sometimes requiring hospitalization for severe cases.*

Symptoms:
- Fever: Often high-grade, accompanied by chills and rigors.
- Flank Pain: Pain or tenderness in the lower back or sides (flank), typically on one side.
- Costovertebral Angle Tenderness: Tenderness elicited upon palpation of the area overlying the kidneys at the costovertebral angle.
- Urinary Symptoms: Similar to lower UTI symptoms, including dysuria, urgency, frequency, and hematuria.
- Nausea and Vomiting: Gastrointestinal symptoms may occur, sometimes leading to dehydration.
- Systemic Symptoms: Malaise, fatigue, and generalized weakness may be present, indicating systemic infection.

Causes and Risk Factors:
- Female Gender: Women are at higher risk due to their anatomical predisposition to UTIs.

- Urinary Tract Abnormalities: Structural abnormalities such as vesicoureteral reflux, urinary tract obstruction, or urinary retention increase susceptibility.
- Urinary Tract Procedures: Recent urinary catheterization, cystoscopy, or instrumentation can introduce bacteria into the urinary tract.
- Pregnancy: Physiological changes during pregnancy increase the risk of urinary stasis and UTIs.
- Recurrent UTIs: patients with a history of recurrent UTIs are more prone to developing pyelonephritis.
- Immune Suppression: Conditions such as diabetes mellitus, HIV/AIDS, or immunosuppressive therapy weaken the immune system and predispose to infections.
- Urologic Conditions: Conditions such as kidney stones or benign prostatic hyperplasia (in men) can obstruct urinary flow and promote bacterial growth.
- Sexual Activity: Recent sexual intercourse, especially in women, can introduce bacteria into the urinary tract.
- Age: Infants, elderly patients, and those with impaired bladder emptying are at increased risk.

Epidemiology:
- Pyelonephritis is more common in women than men, with a female-to-male ratio of approximately 3:1.
- It is estimated that 1-2% of women will experience at least one episode of acute pyelonephritis in their lifetime.
- Incidence rates vary with age, with peaks in young adulthood and older age groups.
- Recurrent pyelonephritis is common in patients with predisposing factors such as urinary tract abnormalities or immunosuppression.

Workup and Diagnosis:
- <u>Clinical Presentation:</u> Symptoms suggestive of upper urinary tract infection, including fever, flank pain, and urinary symptoms.
- <u>Urinalysis:</u> Presence of leukocytes, nitrites, and bacteria in the urine, indicative of urinary tract infection.
- <u>Urine Culture:</u> Identification of the causative organism and determination of antibiotic susceptibility.
- <u>Blood Tests:</u> Complete blood count (CBC) may reveal leukocytosis, and inflammatory markers such as C-reactive protein (CRP) may be elevated.

- **Imaging Studies:** Ultrasound, CT scan, or MRI may be performed to assess for structural abnormalities, obstruction, or complications such as abscess formation.

Treatment:

- **Antibiotics:** Empirical antibiotic therapy is initiated based on local resistance patterns and severity of infection.
- **Hospitalization:**

    Severe cases, immunocompromised patients, or those with complicating factors may require hospitalization for intravenous antibiotics and supportive care.

- **Fluids:** Adequate hydration is important to maintain renal perfusion and facilitate antibiotic clearance.
- **Pain Management:** Analgesics may be prescribed to alleviate flank pain and discomfort.
- **Follow-up:**

    Close monitoring of symptoms, response to treatment, and resolution of infection is essential. Repeat urine cultures may be performed to ensure eradication of the infection.

8.3. Chlamydia

> *Chlamydia is a common sexually transmitted infection (STI) caused by the bacterium Chlamydia trachomatis.*
>
> *Often asymptomatic, it can lead to serious complications if left untreated, such as infertility or pelvic inflammatory disease.*
>
> *Diagnosis involves testing urine or genital swabs, and treatment typically consists of antibiotics.*

Symptoms:

- Genital Discharge: Clear or cloudy discharge from the penis or vagina.
- Painful Urination: Burning sensation or pain during urination (dysuria).
- Pelvic Pain: Pain in the lower abdomen or pelvic region, particularly in women.
- Rectal Symptoms: Anal itching, discharge, or pain, if the infection occurs in the rectum.
- Testicular Pain: Pain or swelling in the testicles (epididymitis) in men.

- Vaginal Bleeding: Abnormal vaginal bleeding, particularly after intercourse, in women.

Causes and Risk Factors:
- Unprotected Sex: Engaging in unprotected vaginal, anal, or oral sex with an infected partner.
- Multiple Sexual Partners: Having multiple sexual partners increases the risk of exposure to chlamydia and other sexually transmitted infections (STIs).
- Young Age: patients aged 15 to 24 years are at higher risk of chlamydia infection.
- Previous STIs: History of previous chlamydia or other STIs increases susceptibility to reinfection.
- Inconsistent Condom Use: Inconsistent or incorrect use of condoms during sexual activity increases the risk of transmission.
- Sexual Activity: Early initiation of sexual activity and high frequency of sexual encounters increase the risk of chlamydia infection.

Epidemiology:
- Chlamydia trachomatis is one of the most common bacterial STIs worldwide.
- It affects both men and women, with a higher prevalence in sexually active young adults.
- Incidence rates vary by region and population, with higher rates observed in certain demographic groups, including adolescents and young adults.
- Chlamydia infection is often asymptomatic, leading to underreporting and underdiagnosis.

Workup and Diagnosis:
- <u>Nucleic Acid Amplification Tests (NAATs):</u>
    Highly sensitive and specific tests that detect the genetic material of Chlamydia trachomatis in urine, vaginal, cervical, rectal, or throat swabs.
- <u>Urinalysis:</u> Examination of a urine sample may reveal white blood cells or other signs of inflammation, indicating a possible urinary tract infection.
- <u>Physical Examination:</u> Pelvic examination in women may reveal abnormal vaginal discharge or signs of inflammation.
- <u>Rectal Examination:</u> Digital rectal examination or anoscopy may be performed in patients with suspected rectal chlamydia infection.

- **Sexual History:** Assessment of sexual history and risk factors is essential for identifying patients at risk of chlamydia and other STIs.

Treatment:

- **Antibiotics:** Oral antibiotics such as azithromycin or doxycycline are commonly prescribed for the treatment of chlamydia infection.
- **Partner Treatment:** Sexual partners of patients diagnosed with chlamydia should also be treated to prevent reinfection and transmission.
- **Follow-Up:**

    Follow-up testing is recommended 3 months after treatment to ensure eradication of the infection, particularly in patients with high-risk sexual behaviors or those with persistent symptoms.

8.4. Gonorrhea

> *Gonorrhea is a sexually transmitted infection (STI) caused by the bacterium Neisseria gonorrhoeae.*
>
> *Symptoms may include painful urination, abnormal discharge, and genital itching, though many cases are asymptomatic.*
>
> *Untreated gonorrhea can lead to serious complications such as pelvic inflammatory disease and infertility.*

Symptoms:

- Genital Discharge: Yellowish or greenish discharge from the penis or vagina.
- Painful Urination: Burning sensation or pain during urination (dysuria).
- Rectal Symptoms: Anal itching, discharge, or pain, if the infection occurs in the rectum.
- Sore Throat: Pharyngeal gonorrhea may cause sore throat, particularly after oral sex.
- Painful or Swollen Testicles: In men, gonorrhea may cause epididymitis, resulting in testicular pain or swelling.
- Vaginal Bleeding: Abnormal vaginal bleeding, particularly after intercourse, in women.

Causes and Risk Factors:

- Unprotected Sex: Engaging in unprotected vaginal, anal, or oral sex with an infected partner.

- Multiple Sexual Partners: Having multiple sexual partners increases the risk of exposure to gonorrhea and other sexually transmitted infections (STIs).
- Young Age: patients aged 15 to 24 years are at higher risk of gonorrhea infection.
- Previous STIs: History of previous gonorrhea or other STIs increases susceptibility to reinfection.
- Inconsistent Condom Use: Inconsistent or incorrect use of condoms during sexual activity increases the risk of transmission.
- Sexual Activity: Early initiation of sexual activity and high frequency of sexual encounters increase the risk of gonorrhea infection.

Epidemiology:
- Neisseria gonorrhoeae, the bacterium that causes gonorrhea, is a common sexually transmitted pathogen worldwide.
- Gonorrhea affects both men and women, with a higher prevalence in sexually active young adults.
- Incidence rates vary by region and population, with higher rates observed in certain demographic groups, including adolescents and young adults.
- Gonorrhea infection is often asymptomatic, leading to underreporting and underdiagnosis.

Workup and Diagnosis:
- <u>Nucleic Acid Amplification Tests (NAATs):</u>

    Highly sensitive and specific tests that detect the genetic material of Neisseria gonorrhoeae in urine, vaginal, cervical, rectal, or throat swabs.

- <u>Culture:</u>

    Culture-based tests may be performed on specimens collected from the infected site, although they are less sensitive and require specialized laboratory facilities.

- <u>Physical Examination:</u>

    Genital, rectal, or pharyngeal examination may reveal signs of inflammation, discharge, or other abnormalities suggestive of gonorrhea infection.

- <u>Sexual History:</u> Assessment of sexual history and risk factors is essential for identifying patients at risk of gonorrhea and other STIs.

Treatment:

- Antibiotics:

    Oral antibiotics such as ceftriaxone or cefixime, often in combination with azithromycin, are commonly prescribed for the treatment of gonorrhea infection.

- Partner Treatment: Sexual partners of patients diagnosed with gonorrhea should also be treated to prevent reinfection and transmission.

- Follow-Up:

    Follow-up testing is recommended to ensure eradication of the infection, particularly in patients with high-risk sexual behaviors or those with persistent symptoms.

8.5. Syphilis

> ➤ *Syphilis is a sexually transmitted infection (STI) caused by the bacterium Treponema pallidum.*
>
> ➤ *It progresses through stages, starting with painless sores on the genitals and mouth, followed by a rash, and potentially leading to severe complications affecting the heart, brain, and nervous system if left untreated.*
>
> ➤ *Diagnosis involves blood tests, and treatment consists of antibiotics.*

Symptoms:

Primary Stage:

- Chancre: A painless sore or ulcer at the site of infection (genitals, mouth, or anus), appearing 10 to 90 days after exposure. The chancre heals spontaneously within 3 to 6 weeks.

Secondary Stage:

- Rash: A non-itchy, red or reddish-brown rash may appear on the palms of the hands, soles of the feet, or other parts of the body.
- Fever: Low-grade fever, fatigue, headache, and swollen lymph nodes may occur.
- Mucocutaneous Lesions: Lesions may develop in the mouth, throat, or genital area.

Latent Stage:
- Asymptomatic stage without any visible symptoms, which may last for years.

Tertiary Stage:
- Neurosyphilis: Infection of the central nervous system, leading to neurological symptoms such as dementia, stroke, or sensory deficits.
- Cardiovascular Syphilis: Involvement of the cardiovascular system, leading to aortic aneurysm, aortic regurgitation, or other cardiovascular complications.
- Gummatous Syphilis: Formation of granulomatous lesions (gummas) in various organs, including skin, bone, and liver.

Causes and Risk Factors:
- Unprotected Sexual Activity: Engaging in unprotected vaginal, anal, or oral sex with an infected partner.
- Multiple Sexual Partners: Having multiple sexual partners increases the risk of exposure to syphilis and other sexually transmitted infections (STIs).
- Men Who Have Sex With Men (MSM): MSM are at higher risk of syphilis infection due to increased sexual risk behaviors and higher prevalence of STIs within the community.
- HIV Infection: patients infected with HIV are at increased risk of acquiring syphilis due to shared risk factors and immunosuppression.
- Sex Worker: patients involved in commercial sex work or transactional sex are at higher risk of syphilis infection.
- Previous STIs: History of previous syphilis or other STIs increases susceptibility to reinfection.

Epidemiology:
- Syphilis is caused by the bacterium Treponema pallidum and is a globally distributed sexually transmitted infection.
- Incidence rates vary by region and population, with higher rates observed in certain demographic groups, including men who have sex with men (MSM) and patients living in urban areas.
- Syphilis infection rates have been increasing in recent years in many parts of the world, including the United States and Europe.

Workup and Diagnosis:

- Serological Tests:
    - Non-Treponemal Tests: Venereal Disease Research Laboratory (VDRL) and Rapid Plasma Reagin (RPR) tests detect antibodies against non-specific antigens released by the host in response to syphilis infection.
    - Treponemal Tests: Enzyme immunoassays (EIAs) and fluorescent treponemal antibody absorption (FTA-ABS) tests detect antibodies against specific Treponema pallidum antigens.
- Darkfield Microscopy:

    Examination of lesion exudate under darkfield microscopy may reveal the presence of motile Treponema pallidum spirochetes in the primary stage of infection.

- PCR Testing:

    Polymerase chain reaction (PCR) testing may be used to detect Treponema pallidum DNA in clinical samples, although it is less commonly used for routine diagnosis.

Treatment:

- Penicillin:

    Penicillin G is the preferred treatment for syphilis infection, administered as intramuscular injections for early and latent syphilis or intravenous infusion for late and tertiary syphilis.

- Alternative Antibiotics:

    In patients with penicillin allergy, alternative antibiotics such as doxycycline or ceftriaxone may be used, although efficacy may be lower.

- Follow-Up:

    Regular follow-up and serological testing are recommended to monitor treatment response and detect potential treatment failure or reinfection.

8.6. Genital Herpes

> ➢ *Genital herpes is a sexually transmitted infection (STI) caused by the herpes simplex virus (HSV), typically HSV-1 or HSV-2.*
> ➢ *Symptoms include painful sores or blisters on the genitals, buttocks, or anus, along with flu-like symptoms.*
> ➢ *While antiviral medications can manage outbreaks, there is no cure, and the virus can remain dormant and recur periodically.*

Symptoms:

- Lesions: Painful, fluid-filled blisters or sores on the genitals, buttocks, or anal area.
- Pain and Itching: Discomfort, burning, or itching in the affected area, often preceding the appearance of lesions.
- Ulcers: Blisters may rupture, forming ulcers that eventually crust over and heal.
- Flu-like Symptoms: Fever, headache, muscle aches, and swollen lymph nodes may accompany the initial outbreak or subsequent recurrences.
- Vaginal Discharge: Women may experience abnormal vaginal discharge or irritation.

Causes and Risk Factors:

- Unprotected Sexual Activity: Engaging in unprotected vaginal, anal, or oral sex with an infected partner increases the risk of genital herpes transmission.
- Multiple Sexual Partners: Having multiple sexual partners or a history of sexually transmitted infections (STIs) increases susceptibility to genital herpes.
- Previous Herpes Infection: patients with a history of genital herpes or oral herpes (cold sores) caused by herpes simplex virus (HSV) are at risk of recurrent outbreaks and transmission.
- Immunocompromised Status: Weakened immune system due to conditions such as HIV/AIDS, cancer, or immunosuppressive therapy increases the risk of severe or recurrent herpes outbreaks.
- Pregnancy: Pregnant women with genital herpes may transmit the virus to their newborn during childbirth, leading to neonatal herpes infection, which can have serious consequences.

Epidemiology:
- Genital herpes is caused by herpes simplex virus type 1 (HSV-1) or herpes simplex virus type 2 (HSV-2).
- HSV-2 is the most common cause of genital herpes, while HSV-1 is typically associated with oral herpes (cold sores).
- Genital herpes is a globally prevalent sexually transmitted infection, with millions of new cases reported annually.
- Incidence rates vary by region and population, with higher rates observed in sexually active patients, particularly young adults.

Workup and Diagnosis:
- Viral Culture: Sample collection from active lesions for viral culture to isolate and identify herpes simplex virus.
- Polymerase Chain Reaction (PCR) Test:
    Highly sensitive molecular diagnostic test to detect herpes simplex virus DNA in clinical samples, including swabs from active lesions or cerebrospinal fluid (CSF) in cases of suspected herpes encephalitis.
- Serological Testing:
    Blood tests to detect antibodies against herpes simplex virus, including type-specific IgG antibodies, to determine past exposure or current infection.
- Clinical Evaluation: Physical examination and assessment of symptoms, including characteristic genital lesions, for clinical diagnosis of genital herpes.

Treatment:
- Antiviral Medications:
    Oral antiviral drugs such as acyclovir, valacyclovir, and famciclovir are commonly prescribed for the treatment of genital herpes.
- Suppressive Therapy:
    Long-term use of antiviral medication to reduce the frequency and severity of recurrent herpes outbreaks and decrease the risk of transmission to sexual partners.
- Pain Management:
    Over-the-counter pain relievers such as ibuprofen or acetaminophen may be used to alleviate discomfort associated with genital herpes lesions.

- Patient Education:

    Counseling on safer sexual practices, including condom use and disclosure of herpes status to sexual partners, to prevent transmission of genital herpes.

8.7. Lyme Disease

> ➤ *Lyme disease is a bacterial infection transmitted through the bite of infected ticks, primarily the black-legged tick.*
> ➤ *Symptoms include fever, headache, fatigue, and a characteristic bull's-eye rash.*
> ➤ *Early diagnosis and antibiotic treatment are crucial to prevent long-term complications affecting the joints, heart, and nervous system.*

Symptoms:
- Erythema Migrans (EM) Rash: A characteristic bull's-eye rash that expands over time, typically appearing within 3 to 30 days after a tick bite.
- Flu-like Symptoms: Fever, chills, headache, fatigue, muscle and joint aches, and swollen lymph nodes may accompany the rash.
- Neurological Symptoms: Facial paralysis (Bell's palsy), meningitis, numbness or tingling in the hands or feet (peripheral neuropathy), and cognitive impairment (memory problems, difficulty concentrating).
- Cardiac Symptoms: Heart palpitations, chest pain, and shortness of breath due to Lyme carditis, a rare complication affecting the heart.
- Arthritis: Recurrent episodes of joint pain and swelling, particularly in large joints such as the knees, may occur weeks to months after infection.

Causes and Risk Factors:
- Outdoor Activities: Engaging in outdoor activities such as hiking, camping, or gardening in wooded or grassy areas where ticks are prevalent increases the risk of Lyme disease transmission.
- Tick Exposure: Exposure to black-legged ticks (Ixodes scapularis or Ixodes pacificus), particularly in regions with high tick populations, increases the risk of Lyme disease.
- Tick Bites: Being bitten by an infected black-legged tick carrying the bacterium Borrelia burgdorferi increases susceptibility to Lyme disease transmission.

- Seasonal Variation: Lyme disease incidence peaks during the spring and summer months when ticks are most active and outdoor activities are common.
- Geographic Location: Living or spending time in regions with high rates of Lyme disease transmission, such as the northeastern United States, upper Midwest, and Pacific coast, increases the risk of exposure.

Epidemiology:
- Lyme disease is the most common tick-borne illness in the Northern Hemisphere, primarily affecting regions with suitable tick habitats.
- In the United States, Lyme disease is endemic in the northeastern and north-central states, including areas of New England, the Mid-Atlantic, and the upper Midwest.
- Incidence rates vary by geographic region and fluctuate over time, influenced by factors such as tick population dynamics, climate conditions, and human behavior.
- Lyme disease is a reportable infectious disease in many countries, allowing for surveillance and monitoring of incidence trends.

Workup and Diagnosis:
- Clinical Evaluation: Assessment of symptoms, medical history, and potential tick exposure to guide diagnostic evaluation.
- Laboratory Testing:
    - Serological Testing: Enzyme-linked immunosorbent assay (ELISA) followed by Western blot assay to detect antibodies against Borrelia burgdorferi in blood samples.
    - Polymerase Chain Reaction (PCR): Molecular diagnostic test to detect Borrelia burgdorferi DNA in clinical specimens such as blood, cerebrospinal fluid (CSF), or joint fluid.
- Diagnostic Criteria: Clinical diagnosis based on compatible symptoms, history of tick exposure, and laboratory confirmation of infection.

Treatment:
- Antibiotics:

    Oral antibiotics such as doxycycline, amoxicillin, or cefuroxime are commonly prescribed for the treatment of early-stage Lyme disease.

- Duration of Treatment:

    The duration of antibiotic therapy varies depending on the stage of Lyme disease and the presence of complications such as neurologic or cardiac involvement.

- Supportive Care:

    Symptomatic treatment to alleviate pain, fever, and other symptoms may be recommended, including nonsteroidal anti-inflammatory drugs (NSAIDs) or analgesics.

- Follow-Up:

    Regular monitoring of symptoms and follow-up serological testing may be performed to assess treatment response and guide further management.

8.8. Hepatitis A

> ➤ *Hepatitis A is a highly contagious liver infection caused by the hepatitis A virus (HAV), often transmitted through contaminated food or water or close contact with an infected person.*
> ➤ *Symptoms may include fatigue, nausea, abdominal pain, and jaundice.*
> ➤ *Vaccination and good hygiene practices are key for prevention.*

Symptoms:
- Flu-like Symptoms: Fever, fatigue, malaise, and loss of appetite are common initial symptoms.
- Nausea and Vomiting: Some patients may experience nausea, vomiting, and abdominal discomfort.
- Jaundice: Yellowing of the skin and eyes may develop a few days after initial symptoms, along with dark urine and pale stools.
- Clay-Colored Stools: Discolored stools may occur due to impaired bile flow.
- Itchy Skin: Pruritus may occur in some cases.

Causes and Risk Factors:
- Poor Sanitation: Hepatitis A is commonly transmitted through the fecal-oral route, often due to inadequate sanitation and hygiene practices.
- Contaminated Food and Water: Consumption of contaminated food or water, particularly in areas with poor sanitation or during travel to endemic regions, increases the risk of hepatitis A transmission.

- Close Contact: Close contact with an infected patient, including household members or sexual partners, increases susceptibility to hepatitis A infection.
- Occupational Exposure: Healthcare workers, childcare providers, and patients working in settings with poor hygiene practices may be at higher risk of hepatitis A transmission.
- Injection Drug Use: Sharing needles or other injection drug equipment increases the risk of hepatitis A transmission among patients who inject drugs.

Epidemiology:
- Hepatitis A is a viral liver infection caused by the hepatitis A virus (HAV).
- Hepatitis A is endemic in many parts of the world, with varying rates of incidence and endemicity based on socioeconomic factors, sanitation standards, and vaccination coverage.
- Outbreaks of hepatitis A may occur in communities or populations with poor sanitation, crowded living conditions, or inadequate access to clean water and sanitation facilities.
- Hepatitis A incidence has declined in many developed countries following the introduction of routine childhood vaccination programs and improvements in sanitation and hygiene practices.

Workup and Diagnosis:
- <u>Serological Testing:</u>

    Detection of specific antibodies against hepatitis A virus (anti-HAV IgM and IgG) in blood samples using serological assays such as enzyme-linked immunosorbent assay (ELISA).
- <u>Liver Function Tests:</u>

    Assessment of liver function tests, including alanine aminotransferase (ALT) and aspartate aminotransferase (AST) levels, to evaluate liver function and assess for evidence of hepatocellular injury.
- <u>Clinical Evaluation:</u>

    Physical examination and assessment of symptoms, medical history, and potential risk factors for hepatitis A infection.

Treatment:
- <u>Supportive Care:</u>

    Supportive treatment to relieve symptoms and promote recovery, including rest, hydration, and adequate nutrition.

- Avoidance of Hepatotoxic Substances:

    Avoidance of hepatotoxic substances such as alcohol and certain medications that may exacerbate liver injury.

- Vaccination:

    Hepatitis A vaccine is highly effective in preventing hepatitis A infection and is recommended for patients at increased risk of exposure, including travelers to endemic regions, certain occupational groups, and patients with underlying liver disease.

- Post-Exposure Prophylaxis:

    Hepatitis A vaccine or immune globulin (IG) may be administered as post-exposure prophylaxis to patients exposed to hepatitis A virus, depending on the timing of exposure and patient risk factors.

8.9. Hepatitis B

> ➢ *Hepatitis B is a viral infection affecting the liver, caused by the hepatitis B virus (HBV), primarily transmitted through blood or bodily fluids during sex, childbirth, or sharing needles.*
>
> ➢ *Symptoms range from mild flu-like symptoms to chronic liver disease and liver cancer.*
>
> ➢ *Vaccination is crucial for prevention, and treatment may involve antiviral medications and monitoring.*

Symptoms:

- Asymptomatic: Many patients with hepatitis B infection remain asymptomatic or have mild, nonspecific symptoms.
- Acute Hepatitis Symptoms: Symptoms of acute hepatitis B infection may include fatigue, nausea, vomiting, abdominal pain, loss of appetite, and low-grade fever.
- Jaundice: Yellowing of the skin and eyes (jaundice) may develop in some cases, along with dark urine and pale stools.
- Chronic Hepatitis: Chronic hepatitis B infection may lead to progressive liver damage, liver cirrhosis, and increased risk of hepatocellular carcinoma (liver cancer) over time.

Causes and Risk Factors:

- Vertical Transmission: Transmission of hepatitis B virus (HBV) from an infected mother to her newborn during childbirth (perinatal

transmission) is a common mode of transmission, particularly in endemic regions.
- Horizontal Transmission: Transmission through exposure to infected blood or body fluids, such as unprotected sexual activity, sharing needles or syringes, and accidental needlesticks or healthcare-related exposures.
- Injection Drug Use: Sharing needles or other injection drug equipment increases the risk of hepatitis B transmission among patients who inject drugs.
- Occupational Exposure: Healthcare workers, laboratory personnel, and patients working in settings with potential exposure to blood or body fluids are at increased risk of hepatitis B infection.
- Unprotected Sexual Activity: Engaging in unprotected sexual activity with an infected partner increases susceptibility to hepatitis B transmission, particularly among men who have sex with men (MSM) and patients with multiple sexual partners.

Epidemiology:
- Hepatitis B is a viral liver infection caused by the hepatitis B virus (HBV).
- Hepatitis B is endemic in many parts of the world, with varying rates of prevalence and transmission based on geographic region, population demographics, and vaccination coverage.
- Chronic hepatitis B infection affects an estimated 240 million patients worldwide, with the highest prevalence observed in regions such as sub-Saharan Africa, Southeast Asia, and the Western Pacific.
- Hepatitis B incidence has declined in many developed countries following the implementation of universal vaccination programs and improvements in blood safety measures.

Workup and Diagnosis:
- <u>Serological Testing:</u>

    Detection of specific antibodies and antigens associated with hepatitis B virus infection in blood samples using serological assays such as enzyme-linked immunosorbent assay (ELISA) and chemiluminescent immunoassays (CLIA).

- <u>Liver Function Tests:</u>

    Assessment of liver function tests, including alanine aminotransferase (ALT), aspartate aminotransferase (AST), and bilirubin levels, to evaluate liver function and assess for evidence of hepatocellular injury.

- **HBV DNA Testing:**

    Measurement of hepatitis B virus DNA levels in blood samples using molecular diagnostic tests such as polymerase chain reaction (PCR) to quantify viral load and assess disease activity.

- **Liver Biopsy:**

    Invasive procedure to obtain liver tissue samples for histological examination and assessment of liver damage and fibrosis in cases of chronic hepatitis B infection.

Treatment:

- **Antiviral Therapy:**

    Oral antiviral medications such as nucleoside/nucleotide analogues (e.g., tenofovir, entecavir) are the mainstay of treatment for chronic hepatitis B infection.

- **Interferon Therapy:**

    Injectable interferon-alpha may be used as an alternative or adjunctive therapy for chronic hepatitis B, particularly in patients with contraindications to or resistance to antiviral agents.

- **Liver Monitoring:**

    Regular monitoring of liver function tests, hepatitis B virus DNA levels, and liver imaging studies to assess disease progression, treatment response, and risk of complications such as liver cirrhosis and hepatocellular carcinoma.

- **Liver Transplantation:**

    Liver transplantation may be considered for patients with advanced liver disease or liver failure due to chronic hepatitis B infection.

8.10. Hepatitis C

> ➤ *Hepatitis C is a viral infection of the liver caused by the hepatitis C virus (HCV), commonly transmitted through contaminated blood, often via injection drug use or unsafe medical practices.*
>
> ➤ *Symptoms can range from mild to severe liver damage, leading to cirrhosis or liver cancer.*
>
> ➤ *Treatment involves antiviral medications, and early detection can help prevent long-term complications.*

Symptoms:
- Asymptomatic: Many patients with hepatitis C infection remain asymptomatic or have mild, nonspecific symptoms.
- Acute Hepatitis Symptoms: Symptoms of acute hepatitis C infection may include fatigue, nausea, vomiting, abdominal pain, loss of appetite, and low-grade fever.
- Chronic Hepatitis: Chronic hepatitis C infection may lead to progressive liver damage, liver cirrhosis, and increased risk of hepatocellular carcinoma (liver cancer) over time.
- Jaundice: Yellowing of the skin and eyes (jaundice) may develop in some cases, along with dark urine and pale stools.
- Complications: Chronic hepatitis C infection can lead to extrahepatic manifestations, including cryoglobulinemia, glomerulonephritis, and dermatologic manifestations such as porphyria cutanea tarda.

Causes and Risk Factors:
- Injection Drug Use: Sharing needles or other injection drug equipment increases the risk of hepatitis C transmission among patients who inject drugs.
- Blood Transfusions: Receipt of blood transfusions or blood products before the implementation of blood screening measures for hepatitis C virus (HCV) increases the risk of infection.
- Healthcare-Related Exposures: Occupational exposure to infected blood or body fluids, such as needlestick injuries or accidental exposure during medical procedures, increases the risk of hepatitis C transmission among healthcare workers.
- Unsafe Medical Practices: Unsafe medical practices, such as reuse of needles or syringes, inadequate sterilization of medical equipment, and tattooing or body piercing performed with unsterile instruments, increase the risk of hepatitis C transmission.
- Vertical Transmission: Transmission of hepatitis C virus from an infected mother to her newborn during childbirth (perinatal transmission) is a less common but possible mode of transmission.

Epidemiology:
- Hepatitis C is a viral liver infection caused by the hepatitis C virus (HCV).
- Chronic hepatitis C infection affects an estimated 71 million patients worldwide, with the highest prevalence observed in regions such as North Africa, the Middle East, and Central and East Asia.

- Hepatitis C incidence has declined in many developed countries following the implementation of blood screening measures, harm reduction strategies, and improvements in infection control practices.
- In recent years, an increase in hepatitis C incidence has been observed among certain populations, including young adults who inject drugs and patients with high-risk sexual behaviors.

Workup and Diagnosis:
- Serological Testing:

    Detection of specific antibodies against hepatitis C virus (anti-HCV) in blood samples using serological assays such as enzyme-linked immunosorbent assay (ELISA) and chemiluminescent immunoassays (CLIA).

- HCV RNA Testing:

    Measurement of hepatitis C virus RNA levels in blood samples using molecular diagnostic tests such as polymerase chain reaction (PCR) or nucleic acid amplification testing (NAAT) to confirm active infection and quantify viral load.

- Liver Function Tests:

    Assessment of liver function tests, including alanine aminotransferase (ALT), aspartate aminotransferase (AST), and bilirubin levels, to evaluate liver function and assess for evidence of hepatocellular injury.

- Liver Biopsy:

    Invasive procedure to obtain liver tissue samples for histological examination and assessment of liver damage, fibrosis, and inflammation in cases of chronic hepatitis C infection.

Treatment:
- Direct-Acting Antiviral (DAA) Therapy:

    Oral antiviral medications known as direct-acting antivirals (DAAs), including sofosbuvir, ledipasvir, glecaprevir, pibrentasvir, and others, are the standard of care for the treatment of chronic hepatitis C infection.

- Combination Therapy:

    DAAs are often used in combination regimens to target different stages of the hepatitis C virus life cycle and achieve sustained virological response (SVR), indicating cure of hepatitis C infection.

- Duration of Treatment:

    The duration of DAA therapy varies depending on factors such as HCV genotype, prior treatment history, presence of liver cirrhosis, and patient comorbidities.

- Liver Monitoring:

    Regular monitoring of liver function tests, hepatitis C virus RNA levels, and liver imaging studies to assess treatment response, liver fibrosis regression, and risk of hepatocellular carcinoma recurrence.

8.11. Hepatitis D

> ➤ *Hepatitis D, also known as delta hepatitis, is a viral infection that only occurs in people who are already infected with the hepatitis B virus (HBV).*
>
> ➤ *It can lead to more severe liver disease than HBV alone and is transmitted through contact with infected blood or body fluids.*
>
> ➤ *Prevention involves HBV vaccination and avoiding behaviors that increase the risk of HBV transmission.*

Symptoms:

- Similar to Hepatitis B: Symptoms of hepatitis D (HDV) infection are similar to those of hepatitis B (HBV) infection, as HDV requires HBV for replication. They may include fatigue, nausea, vomiting, abdominal pain, loss of appetite, and jaundice (yellowing of the skin and eyes).

- Increased Severity: Hepatitis D infection may lead to more severe liver disease compared to hepatitis B infection alone, including a higher risk of liver cirrhosis and liver failure.

Causes and Risk Factors:

- HBV Infection: Hepatitis D virus (HDV) requires hepatitis B virus (HBV) for its replication. Therefore, patients who are already infected with HBV are at risk of acquiring HDV infection.

- Injection Drug Use: Sharing needles or other injection drug equipment increases the risk of both HBV and HDV transmission.

- Unprotected Sexual Activity: Engaging in unprotected sexual activity with an infected partner increases the risk of HBV and HDV transmission.

- Occupational Exposure: Healthcare workers and patients with occupational exposure to blood or body fluids are at increased risk of HBV and HDV infection through needlestick injuries or other accidental exposures.
- Vertical Transmission: Transmission of HBV and HDV from an infected mother to her newborn during childbirth (perinatal transmission) is a less common but possible mode of transmission.

Epidemiology:
- Hepatitis D is caused by the hepatitis D virus (HDV), which is a defective virus that requires the presence of hepatitis B virus (HBV) to replicate.
- HDV infection is relatively rare compared to HBV infection and is most commonly found in regions where HBV is endemic, such as parts of Africa, Asia, and the Mediterranean basin.
- The prevalence of HDV infection varies geographically and is highest in areas with high rates of HBV infection and inadequate healthcare infrastructure.
- In recent years, hepatitis D incidence has declined in many developed countries following the implementation of HBV vaccination programs and improvements in blood safety measures.

Workup and Diagnosis:
- Serological Testing:

    Detection of specific antibodies against hepatitis D virus (anti-HDV) in blood samples using serological assays such as enzyme-linked immunosorbent assay (ELISA) and chemiluminescent immunoassays (CLIA).

- Hepatitis B Testing:

    Testing for hepatitis B surface antigen (HBsAg) and hepatitis B core antibody (anti-HBc) to confirm concurrent HBV infection, as HDV requires HBV for its replication.

- Liver Function Tests:

    Assessment of liver function tests, including alanine aminotransferase (ALT), aspartate aminotransferase (AST), and bilirubin levels, to evaluate liver function and assess for evidence of hepatocellular injury.

- Liver Biopsy:

    Invasive procedure to obtain liver tissue samples for histological examination and assessment of liver damage, fibrosis, and inflammation in cases of chronic hepatitis D infection.

Treatment:

- Interferon Therapy:

    Injectable interferon-alpha is the mainstay of treatment for chronic hepatitis D infection. Interferon therapy may help suppress HDV replication and improve liver function in some patients.

- Antiviral Therapy:

    There are currently no approved antiviral medications specifically targeting hepatitis D virus. However, antiviral agents such as nucleoside/nucleotide analogues used in the treatment of hepatitis B may be considered in some cases to suppress HBV replication and reduce the risk of HDV superinfection.

- Liver Monitoring:

    Regular monitoring of liver function tests, HDV RNA levels, and liver imaging studies to assess treatment response, liver disease progression, and risk of liver-related complications such as cirrhosis and hepatocellular carcinoma.

8.12. Hepatitis E

> ➤ *Hepatitis E is a viral liver infection caused by the hepatitis E virus (HEV), often transmitted through contaminated water or food in areas with poor sanitation.*
>
> ➤ *Symptoms typically include jaundice, fatigue, nausea, and abdominal pain.*
>
> ➤ *While most cases resolve on their own, pregnant women and those with underlying liver disease are at higher risk of severe complications.*

Symptoms:

- Acute Hepatitis: Symptoms of acute hepatitis E infection are similar to those of other types of viral hepatitis and may include fatigue, nausea, vomiting, abdominal pain, loss of appetite, and low-grade fever.

- Jaundice: Yellowing of the skin and eyes (jaundice) may develop in some cases, along with dark urine and pale stools.

- Flu-like Symptoms: Some patients may experience flu-like symptoms such as muscle aches, joint pain, and headache.
- Chronic Infection: Chronic hepatitis E infection is rare but may occur in immunocompromised patients, pregnant women, and patients with underlying liver disease.

Causes and Risk Factors:
- Contaminated Water: Consumption of contaminated water, particularly in developing countries with poor sanitation infrastructure, is a common mode of hepatitis E transmission.
- Contaminated Food: Consumption of undercooked or raw pork products, shellfish, and other foods contaminated with hepatitis E virus (HEV) may increase the risk of infection.
- Travel to Endemic Areas: Travel to regions with high rates of hepatitis E transmission, such as parts of Asia, Africa, and the Middle East, increases the risk of exposure to the virus.
- Immunocompromised Status: patients with compromised immune systems, such as organ transplant recipients, HIV/AIDS patients, and patients undergoing chemotherapy, are at increased risk of chronic hepatitis E infection and severe disease.
- Pregnancy: Pregnant women, particularly those in the third trimester, are at increased risk of severe complications from hepatitis E infection, including liver failure and mortality.

Epidemiology:
- Hepatitis E is caused by the hepatitis E virus (HEV), which is primarily transmitted through the fecal-oral route via contaminated water or food.
- Hepatitis E is endemic in many parts of the world, particularly in developing countries with inadequate sanitation infrastructure and limited access to clean water.
- In industrialized countries, sporadic cases of hepatitis E infection may occur through consumption of contaminated food products, zoonotic transmission from infected animals (particularly pigs), or travel to endemic areas.
- The incidence of hepatitis E varies geographically and seasonally, with outbreaks often associated with flooding, natural disasters, and environmental contamination.
- Hepatitis E infection is typically self-limiting in healthy patients but may lead to severe complications, particularly in pregnant women and patients with underlying liver disease.

Workup and Diagnosis:
- Serological Testing:

    Detection of specific antibodies against hepatitis E virus (anti-HEV IgM and IgG) in blood samples using serological assays such as enzyme-linked immunosorbent assay (ELISA) and chemiluminescent immunoassays (CLIA).

- Molecular Testing:

    Detection of hepatitis E virus RNA in blood or stool samples using molecular diagnostic tests such as polymerase chain reaction (PCR) to confirm active infection and quantify viral load.

- Liver Function Tests:

    Assessment of liver function tests, including alanine aminotransferase (ALT), aspartate aminotransferase (AST), and bilirubin levels, to evaluate liver function and assess for evidence of hepatocellular injury.

Treatment:
- Supportive Care:

    Most cases of acute hepatitis E infection are self-limiting and do not require specific treatment. Supportive care measures such as adequate hydration, rest, and symptomatic relief of nausea and vomiting may be recommended.

- Avoidance of Alcohol and Hepatotoxic Substances:

    Patients with hepatitis E infection should avoid alcohol and hepatotoxic substances to prevent exacerbation of liver damage.

- Management of Complications:

    Pregnant women and patients with severe or fulminant hepatitis E infection may require hospitalization and supportive care, including monitoring for liver failure and management of complications such as coagulopathy and hepatic encephalopathy.

- Ribavirin Therapy:

    In cases of chronic hepatitis E infection or severe disease in immunocompromised patients, treatment with the antiviral medication ribavirin may be considered under medical supervision.

8.13. Chickenpox

> ➢ *Chickenpox, caused by the varicella-zoster virus, is a highly contagious viral infection characterized by an itchy rash with small, fluid-filled blisters.*
> ➢ *Symptoms include fever, headache, and fatigue.*
> ➢ *Vaccination provides effective prevention against chickenpox and its complications.*

Symptoms:
- Rash: The hallmark symptom of chickenpox is a pruritic (itchy) rash that typically starts on the face, scalp, and trunk before spreading to other parts of the body.
- Fever: Many patients with chickenpox develop a low-grade fever before the onset of the rash.
- Malaise: Feelings of fatigue, malaise, and general discomfort may precede the appearance of the rash.
- Fluid-Filled Blisters: The rash progresses from red spots to fluid-filled blisters (vesicles), which eventually crust over and form scabs as they heal.
- Other Symptoms: Other symptoms may include headache, sore throat, cough, and abdominal pain.

Causes and Risk Factors:
- Non-immunity: patients who have not been vaccinated against chickenpox and have not previously had the infection are at risk of developing chickenpox.
- Close Contact: Close contact with an infected person, particularly exposure to respiratory droplets from coughing or sneezing, increases the risk of chickenpox transmission.
- Age: Chickenpox is more common in children, but adults who have not had chickenpox or been vaccinated are also susceptible to infection.
- Immune Suppression: patients with weakened immune systems, such as those undergoing chemotherapy or organ transplantation, are at increased risk of severe chickenpox infection and complications.

Epidemiology:
- Chickenpox is caused by the varicella-zoster virus (VZV), which is highly contagious and primarily spreads through respiratory droplets and direct contact with fluid from chickenpox blisters.
- Before the introduction of the varicella vaccine, chickenpox was a common childhood illness worldwide, with seasonal peaks occurring in late winter and early spring.
- Routine vaccination against chickenpox has led to a significant decline in the incidence of chickenpox in many countries where vaccination programs have been implemented.
- Outbreaks of chickenpox may occur in settings such as schools, daycare centers, and households where susceptible patients are in close contact with an infected person.

Workup and Diagnosis:
- Clinical Presentation:

    Diagnosis of chickenpox is often based on the characteristic clinical presentation of the rash, along with a history of fever and other symptoms.

- Laboratory Testing:

    Laboratory tests such as polymerase chain reaction (PCR) or serological assays may be used to confirm the diagnosis of chickenpox in cases where the clinical presentation is atypical or uncertain.

Treatment:
- Supportive Care: Treatment of chickenpox is primarily supportive and focuses on relieving symptoms such as fever and itching.
- Antiviral Medications:

    Antiviral medications such as acyclovir, valacyclovir, or famciclovir may be prescribed in certain cases, particularly for patients at high risk of severe complications or those with severe or atypical presentations of chickenpox.

- Antipyretics: Over-the-counter medications such as acetaminophen or ibuprofen may be used to reduce fever and alleviate discomfort.
- Topical Treatments: Calamine lotion or oatmeal baths may help soothe itching and promote healing of chickenpox lesions.
- Preventive Measures:

Prevention of secondary bacterial infections through proper wound care and hygiene practices is important to prevent complications associated with chickenpox.

8.14. Measles

> ➢ *Measles is a highly contagious viral infection caused by the measles virus (MeV), presenting with fever, cough, runny nose, and a characteristic rash.*
> ➢ *Complications can be severe, including pneumonia and encephalitis, particularly in unvaccinated individuals.*
> ➢ *Vaccination with the measles, mumps, and rubella (MMR) vaccine is highly effective for prevention.*

Symptoms:
- Fever: Measles typically begins with a high fever, often exceeding 101°F (38.3°C).
- Cough: A persistent cough is a common symptom of measles and may be accompanied by nasal congestion.
- Conjunctivitis: Inflammation of the eyes (conjunctivitis) leads to redness, irritation, and excessive tearing.
- Rash: A characteristic rash appears 2-4 days after the onset of symptoms, starting on the face and spreading downward to the trunk and extremities. The rash consists of small red spots that may coalesce into larger patches.
- Koplik Spots: Small white spots with bluish centers, known as Koplik spots, may appear on the inside of the cheeks a day or two before the rash develops.

Causes and Risk Factors:
- Unvaccinated patients: patients who have not received the measles vaccine or who have not had measles previously are at risk of infection.
- Close Contact: Close contact with an infected person, particularly exposure to respiratory droplets from coughing or sneezing, increases the risk of measles transmission.
- Travel to Endemic Areas: Travel to regions with ongoing measles outbreaks or low vaccination coverage increases the risk of exposure to the virus.

- Immune Suppression: patients with weakened immune systems, such as those with HIV/AIDS or undergoing chemotherapy, are at increased risk of severe measles infection and complications.

Epidemiology:

- Measles is caused by the measles virus, a highly contagious virus that spreads through respiratory droplets and direct contact with infected patients.
- Measles remains a significant public health concern worldwide, particularly in regions with inadequate vaccination coverage and ongoing transmission.
- While measles incidence has declined significantly in countries with robust vaccination programs, outbreaks may still occur in communities with pockets of unvaccinated patients.
- Measles outbreaks often occur in settings such as schools, childcare facilities, and communities with low vaccination rates, where the virus can spread rapidly among susceptible patients.

Workup and Diagnosis:

- Clinical Presentation:

    Diagnosis of measles is often based on the characteristic clinical presentation of fever, cough, conjunctivitis, and rash, particularly in patients with a history of potential exposure to measles.

- Laboratory Testing:

    Laboratory tests such as polymerase chain reaction (PCR) or serological assays may be used to confirm the diagnosis of measles by detecting measles virus RNA or specific antibodies in blood or throat swab samples.

Treatment:

- Supportive Care: Treatment of measles is primarily supportive and focuses on relieving symptoms such as fever and cough.
- Antipyretics: Over-the-counter medications such as acetaminophen or ibuprofen may be used to reduce fever and alleviate discomfort.
- Fluids and Rest: Adequate hydration and rest are important for patients with measles to support recovery and prevent dehydration.
- Isolation:

    Infected patients should be isolated to prevent the spread of measles to others, particularly those who are unvaccinated or at high risk of severe complications.

- Vitamin A Supplementation:

    Vitamin A supplementation may be recommended for children with measles to reduce the risk of complications such as pneumonia and blindness, particularly in regions where vitamin A deficiency is common.

8.15. Mumps

> ➢ *Mumps is a contagious viral infection caused by the mumps virus, characterized by swelling of the salivary glands, particularly the parotid glands.*
> ➢ *Symptoms include fever, headache, and muscle aches.*
> ➢ *Vaccination with the MMR vaccine is highly effective in preventing mumps and its complications.*

Symptoms:

- Parotitis: The hallmark symptom of mumps is swelling and tenderness of one or both parotid glands, which are located below and in front of the ears. Parotitis may cause facial swelling and pain, particularly when chewing or swallowing.
- Fever: Fever is common in patients with mumps and may precede the onset of parotitis.
- Malaise: Feelings of fatigue, malaise, and general discomfort are often reported by patients with mumps.
- Headache: Some patients with mumps may experience headache, particularly during the acute phase of the illness.
- Sialadenitis: In addition to parotitis, mumps may cause inflammation of other salivary glands, such as the submandibular and sublingual glands.

Causes and Risk Factors:

- Non-immunity: patients who have not been vaccinated against mumps or have not had mumps previously are at risk of infection.
- Close Contact: Close contact with an infected person, particularly exposure to respiratory droplets from coughing or sneezing, increases the risk of mumps transmission.
- Crowded Settings: Settings such as schools, childcare facilities, and dormitories where patients are in close proximity to one another increase the risk of mumps outbreaks.

- Age: Mumps is more common in children, but unvaccinated adults are also susceptible to infection.

Epidemiology:
- Mumps is caused by the mumps virus, a contagious virus that spreads through respiratory droplets and direct contact with infected patients.
- Mumps was once a common childhood illness worldwide, but widespread vaccination with the measles, mumps, and rubella (MMR) vaccine has led to a significant decline in mumps incidence in many countries.
- Despite vaccination efforts, mumps outbreaks may still occur in communities with pockets of unvaccinated patients or suboptimal vaccination coverage.
- Mumps outbreaks often occur in settings such as schools, colleges, and other congregate settings where close contact and shared living spaces facilitate transmission.

Workup and Diagnosis:
- Clinical Presentation:

    Diagnosis of mumps is often based on the characteristic clinical presentation of parotitis, particularly in patients with a history of potential exposure to mumps.

- Laboratory Testing:

    Laboratory tests such as polymerase chain reaction (PCR) or serological assays may be used to confirm the diagnosis of mumps by detecting mumps virus RNA or specific antibodies in blood or saliva samples.

Treatment:
- Supportive Care: Treatment of mumps is primarily supportive and focuses on relieving symptoms such as fever and parotitis.
- Pain Management:

    Over-the-counter pain relievers such as acetaminophen or ibuprofen may be used to reduce pain and fever associated with mumps.

- Fluids and Rest: Adequate hydration and rest are important for patients with mumps to support recovery and prevent dehydration.

- Isolation:

    Infected patients should be isolated to prevent the spread of mumps to others, particularly those who are unvaccinated or at high risk of complications.

- Complications Management:

    In some cases, mumps may lead to complications such as orchitis (inflammation of the testicles), meningitis, encephalitis, or deafness. Treatment of complications may require additional medical intervention and supportive care.

8.16. Shingles

> ➢ *Shingles, caused by the varicella-zoster virus (VZV), is a painful skin rash typically occurring in adults who previously had chickenpox.*
>
> ➢ *It manifests as a band or patch of red blisters, often on one side of the body, and can be accompanied by itching, burning, or tingling sensations.*
>
> ➢ *Vaccination with the shingles vaccine can reduce the risk of developing shingles and alleviate symptoms.*

Symptoms:

- Pain: The most common early symptom of shingles is localized pain, often described as burning, tingling, or shooting pain, usually on one side of the body or face.
- Rash: A characteristic rash typically appears after a few days of pain. The rash consists of fluid-filled blisters that develop in a band-like pattern along a nerve pathway. The rash may be accompanied by redness, swelling, and itching.
- Flu-like Symptoms: Some patients may experience flu-like symptoms such as fever, headache, fatigue, and malaise.
- Sensitivity to Touch: The affected area may become sensitive to touch or pressure, exacerbating the pain.
- Complications: In some cases, shingles can lead to complications such as postherpetic neuralgia (persistent pain lasting beyond the resolution of the rash), bacterial skin infections, or neurological complications if the virus affects the nerves supplying vital organs.

Causes and Risk Factors:

- Previous Chickenpox: Shingles occurs as a reactivation of the varicella-zoster virus (VZV), the same virus that causes chickenpox.

patients who have had chickenpox are at risk of developing shingles later in life.

- Age: The risk of shingles increases with age, particularly after the age of 50. Aging weakens the immune system, making older adults more susceptible to viral reactivation.
- Immune Suppression: Conditions or treatments that weaken the immune system, such as HIV/AIDS, cancer chemotherapy, or organ transplantation, increase the risk of shingles.
- Stress: Emotional or physical stress can trigger shingles reactivation in some patients.
- Certain Medications: Certain medications, such as corticosteroids or immunosuppressive drugs, can increase the risk of shingles.

Epidemiology:

- Shingles is caused by the reactivation of the varicella-zoster virus (VZV), which remains dormant in nerve cells after primary infection with chickenpox.
- Shingles is relatively common, particularly among older adults, with an estimated 1 in 3 patients developing shingles during their lifetime.
- The incidence of shingles increases with age, with the highest rates observed in patients over 50 years old.
- Shingles can occur in otherwise healthy patients but is more common and severe in those with weakened immune systems.

Workup and Diagnosis:

- Clinical Presentation:

    Diagnosis of shingles is often based on the characteristic clinical presentation of localized pain and rash, particularly when accompanied by a history of chickenpox.

- Laboratory Testing:

    Laboratory tests such as viral culture, polymerase chain reaction (PCR), or serological assays may be used to confirm the diagnosis of shingles by detecting VZV DNA or specific antibodies in blood or fluid from the rash.

Treatment:

- Antiviral Medications:

    Antiviral medications such as acyclovir, valacyclovir, or famciclovir are commonly prescribed to shorten the duration and severity of shingles symptoms, particularly if started within 72 hours of rash onset.

- Pain Management:

    Pain relievers such as acetaminophen or nonsteroidal anti-inflammatory drugs (NSAIDs) may be used to alleviate pain associated with shingles. In some cases, prescription pain medications or topical treatments may be necessary to manage severe pain.

- Antiviral Medications:

    Antiviral medications such as acyclovir, valacyclovir, or famciclovir are commonly prescribed to shorten the duration and severity of shingles symptoms, particularly if started within 72 hours of rash onset.

- Topical Treatments: Calamine lotion, colloidal oatmeal baths, or antihistamine creams may help soothe itching and promote healing of shingles blisters.

- Complications Management:

    Complications of shingles such as postherpetic neuralgia may require additional treatment, including prescription medications such as antidepressants, anticonvulsants, or topical lidocaine patches to manage persistent pain.

8.17. Dengue Fever

> ➢ Dengue fever is a mosquito-borne viral infection caused by the dengue virus, transmitted primarily by the Aedes mosquito.
> ➢ Symptoms include high fever, severe headache, joint and muscle pain, rash, and in severe cases, hemorrhagic fever or shock syndrome.
> ➢ Prevention focuses on mosquito control measures and avoiding mosquito bites, as there is currently no specific treatment or vaccine available for dengue fever.

Symptoms:

- High Fever: Dengue fever typically begins with a sudden onset of high fever, often exceeding 104°F (40°C).

- Severe Headache: Intense headache, often described as a "breakbone" or "behind-the-eyes" pain, is common in patients with dengue fever.

- Severe Joint and Muscle Pain: Dengue fever is characterized by severe joint and muscle pain, which can be debilitating and may give rise to its colloquial name, "breakbone fever."

- Rash: A characteristic rash may develop 2-5 days after the onset of fever, consisting of small red spots or patches.
- Nausea and Vomiting: Some patients with dengue fever experience nausea, vomiting, and abdominal pain.
- Bleeding: In severe cases, dengue fever may lead to bleeding manifestations such as nosebleeds, gum bleeding, or easy bruising.

Causes and Risk Factors:
- Mosquito Exposure: Dengue fever is transmitted by the Aedes mosquitoes, primarily *Aedes aegypti* and *Aedes albopictus*, which are active during the daytime.
- Travel to Endemic Areas: Travel to regions with ongoing dengue virus transmission increases the risk of exposure to infected mosquitoes.
- Lack of Mosquito Control Measures: Inadequate mosquito control measures, such as stagnant water accumulation in containers or improper waste disposal, increase the risk of mosquito breeding and dengue transmission.
- Previous Dengue Infection: patients who have had dengue fever in the past are at increased risk of severe dengue if infected with a different dengue virus serotype.

Epidemiology:
- Dengue fever is a mosquito-borne viral illness caused by the dengue virus, which belongs to the Flaviviridae family.
- Dengue fever is endemic in tropical and subtropical regions worldwide, particularly in Asia, the Pacific Islands, the Caribbean, and parts of Central and South America.
- Dengue fever incidence has increased dramatically in recent decades, with up to 400 million cases estimated annually worldwide.
- Dengue outbreaks may occur periodically in endemic regions, particularly during the rainy season when mosquito populations increase.

Workup and Diagnosis:
- <u>Clinical Presentation:</u>

    Diagnosis of dengue fever is often based on the characteristic clinical presentation of fever, severe headache, joint and muscle pain, and rash, particularly in patients with a history of potential exposure to dengue virus.

- Laboratory Testing:

    Laboratory tests such as reverse transcription-polymerase chain reaction (RT-PCR) or serological assays may be used to confirm the diagnosis of dengue fever by detecting dengue virus RNA or specific antibodies in blood samples.

Treatment:

- Fluid Replacement:

    Adequate hydration is essential for patients with dengue fever to prevent dehydration, particularly if experiencing vomiting or diarrhea. Oral rehydration solutions or intravenous fluids may be administered as needed.

- Fever Control:

    Acetaminophen is commonly used to reduce fever and alleviate pain associated with dengue fever. **Avoidance** of nonsteroidal anti-inflammatory drugs (NSAIDs) such as aspirin, ibuprofen, or naproxen is recommended due to the risk of bleeding complications.

- Monitoring for Complications:

    Patients with dengue fever should be closely monitored for signs of severe dengue, such as persistent vomiting, abdominal pain, mucosal bleeding, lethargy, restlessness, or rapid breathing. Prompt medical attention is essential if complications develop.

- Preventive Measures:

    Prevention of mosquito bites is crucial to reduce the risk of dengue fever. Measures such as using insect repellents, wearing protective clothing, and using mosquito nets or screens can help prevent mosquito bites. Additionally, community-based mosquito control measures such as vector surveillance, larval source reduction, and insecticide spraying may help reduce mosquito populations and dengue transmission in endemic areas.

8.18. Malaria

> ➢ Malaria is a life-threatening mosquito-borne disease caused by Plasmodium parasites.
>
> ➢ Symptoms include fever, chills, and flu-like illness, which can progress to severe complications and even death if left untreated.
>
> ➢ Prevention involves mosquito control measures and antimalarial medications for travelers to endemic areas.

Symptoms:

- Fever: Fever is typically the hallmark symptom of malaria, characterized by recurrent episodes of high fever, often accompanied by chills and sweating.
- Chills: patients with malaria may experience severe chills, shaking, and shivering during fever episodes.
- Headache: Headache is common in patients with malaria and may be severe and throbbing.
- Muscle and Joint Pain: Malaria can cause muscle and joint pain, which may be generalized or localized.
- Fatigue: Fatigue and weakness are common symptoms of malaria, particularly during and after fever episodes.
- Nausea and Vomiting: Some patients with malaria may experience nausea, vomiting, and abdominal pain.
- Anemia: Malaria can cause hemolysis, leading to anemia, which may manifest as fatigue, pale skin, and shortness of breath.
- Other Symptoms: Other symptoms of malaria may include cough, diarrhea, and confusion, particularly in severe cases.

Causes and Risk Factors:

- Mosquito Exposure: Malaria is transmitted through the bite of infected female *Anopheles* mosquitoes, which are active primarily during the night.
- Travel to Endemic Areas: Travel to regions with ongoing malaria transmission increases the risk of exposure to infected mosquitoes.
- Outdoor Activities: Outdoor activities such as camping, hiking, or fieldwork in malaria-endemic areas increase the risk of mosquito bites and malaria transmission.
- Lack of Mosquito Control Measures: Inadequate mosquito control measures, such as stagnant water accumulation and improper waste

disposal, increase the risk of mosquito breeding and malaria transmission.
- Immune Status: patients with weakened immune systems, such as young children, pregnant women, and patients with HIV/AIDS or other immunocompromising conditions, are at increased risk of severe malaria.

Epidemiology:
- Malaria is caused by *Plasmodium* parasites, which are transmitted through the bite of infected *Anopheles* mosquitoes.
- Malaria is endemic in tropical and subtropical regions worldwide, particularly in Africa, Southeast Asia, the Western Pacific, and parts of the Americas.
- Malaria incidence varies by geographic region and climatic conditions, with higher transmission rates in areas with warm temperatures, high humidity, and abundant mosquito vectors.
- Malaria remains a major global health concern, with an estimated 229 million cases and 409,000 deaths reported worldwide in 2019.

Workup and Diagnosis:
- Clinical Presentation:

    Diagnosis of malaria is often based on the characteristic clinical presentation of fever and other symptoms, particularly in patients with a history of potential exposure to malaria.

- Laboratory Testing:

    Laboratory tests such as microscopy or rapid diagnostic tests (RDTs) may be used to confirm the diagnosis of malaria by detecting Plasmodium parasites or specific antigens in blood samples.

Treatment:
- Antimalarial Medications:

    Treatment of malaria typically involves antimalarial medications to eliminate the Plasmodium parasites from the bloodstream. The choice of antimalarial medication depends on factors such as the species of Plasmodium, the severity of illness, and the geographic region of infection.

- Artemisinin-based Combination Therapies (ACTs):

    ACTs are the recommended first-line treatment for uncomplicated falciparum malaria, the most severe form of malaria. ACTs combine an artemisinin derivative with a partner drug to provide rapid and effective parasite clearance.

- Quinine-based Therapies:

    Quinine and quinidine are alternative medications used to treat severe malaria or cases of malaria caused by parasites resistant to other antimalarial drugs.

- Supportive Care:

    Supportive care measures such as hydration, fever control, and treatment of complications such as anemia or electrolyte imbalances may be necessary, particularly in severe cases of malaria.

8.19. HIV/AIDS

> ➢ *HIV/AIDS is a viral infection caused by the human immunodeficiency virus (HIV), transmitted through blood, sexual contact, or from mother to child during childbirth or breastfeeding.*
>
> ➢ *HIV weakens the immune system, leading to acquired immunodeficiency syndrome (AIDS), characterized by opportunistic infections and cancers.*
>
> ➢ *Prevention includes safe sex practices, needle exchange programs, HIV testing, and antiretroviral therapy to manage the virus.*

Symptoms:

- Acute Retroviral Syndrome: Some patients may experience flu-like symptoms, including fever, fatigue, sore throat, swollen lymph nodes, and rash, within 2-4 weeks after initial HIV infection.

- Asymptomatic Stage: Many patients with HIV infection do not experience any symptoms during the early stages of infection. Without treatment, HIV can remain asymptomatic for several years.

- Chronic Symptoms: As HIV progresses, patients may develop chronic symptoms such as persistent fever, fatigue, weight loss, diarrhea, night sweats, and recurrent infections.

- Opportunistic Infections: HIV weakens the immune system, making patients more susceptible to opportunistic infections such as tuberculosis (TB), fungal infections, pneumonia, and certain cancers.

- Neurological Symptoms: Advanced HIV infection can lead to neurological symptoms such as cognitive impairment, memory loss, neuropathy, and motor dysfunction.

- AIDS-Defining Illnesses: AIDS (Acquired Immunodeficiency Syndrome) is the most severe stage of HIV infection, characterized by the presence of opportunistic infections or certain cancers. AIDS-defining illnesses include Pneumocystis pneumonia (PCP), Kaposi's sarcoma, cryptococcal meningitis, and cytomegalovirus (CMV) retinitis.

Causes and Risk Factors:
- Unprotected Sexual Activity: Unprotected sexual intercourse, particularly anal or vaginal intercourse without condoms, is a significant risk factor for HIV transmission.

- Injection Drug Use: Sharing needles or syringes contaminated with HIV-infected blood increases the risk of HIV transmission among injection drug users.

- Mother-to-Child Transmission: Pregnant women with HIV can transmit the virus to their infants during pregnancy, childbirth, or breastfeeding.

- Occupational Exposure: Healthcare workers and others may be at risk of HIV transmission through accidental needle-stick injuries or exposure to HIV-infected blood or body fluids.

- Unprotected Blood Transfusions: Before the implementation of blood screening measures, transfusion of HIV-infected blood or blood products posed a risk of HIV transmission. However, modern blood screening practices have greatly reduced this risk.

Epidemiology:
- HIV/AIDS is a global pandemic caused by the human immunodeficiency virus (HIV), a retrovirus that attacks the immune system, specifically CD4+ T cells.

- According to the World Health Organization (WHO), approximately 37.7 million patients were living with HIV worldwide in 2020, with an estimated 1.5 million new infections and 680,000 deaths from AIDS-related illnesses.

- Sub-Saharan Africa remains the most affected region, accounting for the majority of new HIV infections and AIDS-related deaths. However, HIV/AIDS also affects populations in other regions, including Asia, Latin America, the Caribbean, and Eastern Europe.

- Certain populations are disproportionately affected by HIV/AIDS, including men who have sex with men, transgender patients, patients who inject drugs, sex workers, prisoners, and marginalized communities with limited access to healthcare.

Workup and Diagnosis:
- HIV Antibody Testing:

    HIV infection is typically diagnosed through serological tests that detect antibodies to HIV in blood samples. Common tests include enzyme immunoassays (EIAs) and rapid HIV antibody tests.

- Antigen/Antibody Combination Tests:

    Some diagnostic tests detect both HIV antibodies and p24 antigen, a viral protein produced during early HIV infection, allowing for earlier detection of HIV.

- Nucleic Acid Testing (NAT):

    Nucleic acid amplification tests (NAATs) can detect HIV RNA or DNA in blood samples, providing rapid and sensitive detection of HIV during the acute stage of infection.

Treatment:
- Antiretroviral Therapy (ART):

    The cornerstone of HIV/AIDS treatment is antiretroviral therapy, which consists of combinations of antiretroviral drugs that suppress viral replication, reduce HIV-related morbidity and mortality, and improve quality of life.

- Prevention of Opportunistic Infections:

    Patients with HIV/AIDS may receive prophylactic medications to prevent opportunistic infections such as PCP, TB, toxoplasmosis, and fungal infections.

- Management of Co-Morbidities:

    Treatment of HIV/AIDS includes management of co-morbidities such as cardiovascular disease, diabetes, mental health disorders, and substance abuse, which may complicate HIV management.

- Prevention of Mother-to-Child Transmission:

    Pregnant women with HIV receive antiretroviral medications to prevent mother-to-child transmission of HIV during pregnancy, childbirth, and breastfeeding.

- Pre-Exposure Prophylaxis (PrEP):

    PrEP involves the use of antiretroviral medications by HIV-negative patients at high risk of HIV acquisition to prevent HIV infection.

- Post-Exposure Prophylaxis (PEP):

    PEP involves the use of antiretroviral medications by HIV-negative patients after potential exposure to HIV to prevent HIV infection.

- Supportive Care:

    Patients with HIV/AIDS may require supportive care interventions such as nutritional support, mental health services, substance abuse treatment, and adherence support to optimize treatment outcomes and quality of life.

8.20. Norovirus Infection

> ➢ *Norovirus is a highly contagious virus causing gastroenteritis, often spread through contaminated food, water, or surfaces and person-to-person contact.*
>
> ➢ *Symptoms include vomiting, diarrhea, stomach cramps, and nausea, typically lasting 1-3 days.*
>
> ➢ *Prevention involves thorough handwashing, proper food handling, and disinfection of contaminated surfaces.*

Symptoms:

- Gastrointestinal Symptoms: Norovirus infection typically manifests as acute gastroenteritis, with symptoms including nausea, vomiting, diarrhea, and abdominal cramps.

- Vomiting: Vomiting is a hallmark symptom of norovirus infection and may be sudden and projectile in nature.

- Diarrhea: Diarrhea is common in norovirus infection and is often watery and frequent.

- Nausea: patients with norovirus infection may experience persistent nausea, sometimes accompanied by retching.

- Abdominal Cramps: Abdominal cramps or stomach pain may occur due to gastrointestinal inflammation.

- Fever: Some patients may develop low-grade fever or elevated body temperature during norovirus infection, although fever is less common.

- Malaise: Generalized malaise, fatigue, and weakness may accompany norovirus infection, particularly in severe cases.

- Dehydration: Prolonged vomiting and diarrhea can lead to dehydration, with symptoms such as dry mouth, decreased urine output, and dizziness.

Causes and Risk Factors:
- Close Contact: Norovirus is highly contagious and can spread easily through close contact with infected patients, contaminated surfaces, or contaminated food and water.
- Crowded Settings: Outbreaks of norovirus infection often occur in crowded settings such as healthcare facilities, cruise ships, schools, childcare centers, and restaurants.
- Poor Hygiene Practices: Lack of handwashing, improper food handling, and inadequate sanitation can contribute to norovirus transmission.
- Compromised Immunity: patients with weakened immune systems, such as young children, older adults, and patients with chronic illnesses, are at increased risk of norovirus infection and severe complications.
- Travel: Travel to regions with ongoing norovirus outbreaks or close quarters on transportation vehicles such as airplanes, trains, or buses can increase the risk of norovirus transmission.

Epidemiology:
- Norovirus is a leading cause of acute gastroenteritis worldwide, responsible for millions of cases of illness and outbreaks each year.
- Norovirus outbreaks occur year-round but are more common during the winter months in temperate climates.
- Norovirus is highly contagious, with the ability to spread rapidly in closed or semi-closed settings such as households, healthcare facilities, cruise ships, schools, and restaurants.
- The virus can be transmitted through multiple routes, including person-to-person contact, consumption of contaminated food or water, and contact with contaminated surfaces or objects.
- Norovirus affects patients of all ages and can cause significant morbidity and economic burden, particularly in vulnerable populations such as young children, older adults, and immunocompromised patients.

Workup and Diagnosis:
- Clinical Presentation:

    Diagnosis of norovirus infection is primarily based on the characteristic clinical presentation of acute gastroenteritis, including nausea, vomiting, diarrhea, and abdominal cramps, particularly in the setting of an outbreak.

- Laboratory Testing:

    Laboratory tests such as enzyme immunoassays (EIAs) or polymerase chain reaction (PCR) assays may be used to detect norovirus RNA or antigens in stool samples, particularly in outbreak settings or cases with severe illness requiring medical attention.

Treatment:

- Supportive Care:

    There is no specific antiviral treatment for norovirus infection. Treatment typically focuses on supportive care to alleviate symptoms and prevent complications.

- Fluid Replacement:

    Rehydration is essential to manage dehydration resulting from vomiting and diarrhea. Oral rehydration solutions (ORS) or intravenous fluids may be used to replenish lost fluids and electrolytes.

- Antiemetics:

    Antiemetic medications may be prescribed to control nausea and vomiting in severe cases, particularly in children or patients at risk of dehydration.

- Nutritional Support:

    Maintaining adequate nutrition is important during norovirus infection. Small, frequent meals and bland foods may help alleviate gastrointestinal symptoms.

- Infection Control Measures:

    Preventing the spread of norovirus infection is crucial to controlling outbreaks. Measures such as handwashing with soap and water, disinfection of contaminated surfaces, isolation of infected patients, and exclusion from high-risk settings may help reduce transmission.

8.21. Rabies

> ➢ Rabies is a deadly viral infection transmitted through the saliva of infected animals, commonly through bites or scratches.
>
> ➢ Symptoms include fever, headache, agitation, and eventually, paralysis and death if untreated.
>
> ➢ Prompt medical attention, including post-exposure prophylaxis with rabies vaccine, is crucial for prevention after suspected exposure.

Symptoms:

- Prodromal Phase: Initial symptoms of rabies may resemble flu-like symptoms, including fever, headache, malaise, and fatigue.
- Neurological Symptoms: As the disease progresses, patients may experience neurological symptoms such as agitation, anxiety, confusion, hallucinations, and delirium.
- Hydrophobia: One of the characteristic symptoms of rabies is hydrophobia, an irrational fear of water. patients with rabies may experience painful spasms of the throat muscles when attempting to swallow liquids.
- Aerophobia: Rabies may also cause aerophobia, an exaggerated fear of drafts of air or moving air, due to the painful spasms and difficulty breathing associated with the disease.
- Paralysis: Progressive paralysis may occur, starting with paralysis of the muscles around the bite site and eventually leading to paralysis of the respiratory muscles, which can result in respiratory failure and death.

Causes and Risk Factors:

- Animal Exposure: Rabies is primarily transmitted through the bite or scratch of an infected animal, particularly dogs, cats, bats, and wildlife such as raccoons, foxes, and skunks.
- High-Risk Activities: patients who work with animals or are involved in activities such as veterinary medicine, animal control, wildlife research, or spelunking (caving) may be at increased risk of rabies exposure.
- Travel to Endemic Areas: Travelers to regions where rabies is endemic, particularly in developing countries with inadequate rabies control measures, may be at risk of exposure to rabid animals.

- Unvaccinated Pets: Pets that are not vaccinated against rabies may contract the virus from wildlife or other infected animals and pose a risk of transmission to humans through bites or scratches.
- Outdoor Activities: Outdoor activities such as camping, hiking, or hunting may increase the risk of encountering rabid wildlife and sustaining bites or scratches.

Epidemiology:
- Rabies is a zoonotic viral disease caused by the rabies virus, which belongs to the Lyssavirus genus.
- Rabies is found worldwide, with the exception of Antarctica, but is more prevalent in regions with large populations of stray dogs and inadequate animal control measures.
- Dogs are the primary reservoir and source of human rabies deaths in many countries, particularly in Asia and Africa, where canine rabies remains a significant public health concern.
- Wildlife, including bats, raccoons, skunks, foxes, and coyotes, also serve as reservoirs for rabies virus transmission in certain regions.
- Human rabies cases are relatively rare, but the disease is almost always fatal once symptoms develop, underscoring the importance of prevention and timely post-exposure prophylaxis.

Workup and Diagnosis:
- Clinical Presentation:

    Diagnosis of rabies is primarily based on clinical symptoms and history of animal exposure, particularly bites or scratches from animals suspected of being rabid.

- Laboratory Testing:

    Laboratory tests such as reverse transcription-polymerase chain reaction (RT-PCR) assays or direct fluorescent antibody (DFA) tests may be performed on samples of saliva, cerebrospinal fluid, or brain tissue to detect rabies virus antigens or RNA.

Treatment:
- Post-Exposure Prophylaxis (PEP):

    Post-exposure prophylaxis with rabies vaccine and rabies immune globulin (RIG) is highly effective in preventing rabies if administered promptly after exposure to a potentially rabid animal. PEP consists of a series of rabies vaccine doses administered over a 28-day period, along with a single dose of RIG administered at the site of the bite or scratch.

- Symptomatic Treatment:

    Once symptoms of rabies develop, there is no specific treatment available, and the disease is almost invariably fatal. Supportive care measures may be provided to alleviate symptoms and ensure comfort in terminal stages of the disease.

8.22. Leprosy

> ➢ *Leprosy, also known as Hansen's disease, is a chronic infectious disease caused by the bacterium Mycobacterium leprae, primarily affecting the skin, nerves, and mucous membranes.*
>
> ➢ *Symptoms vary from skin lesions and nerve damage to deformities and loss of sensation.*
>
> ➢ *Early diagnosis and multidrug therapy are effective in treating leprosy and preventing disability.*

Symptoms:

- Skin Lesions: Leprosy primarily affects the skin and peripheral nerves, leading to the development of skin lesions. These lesions may vary in appearance and may be hypopigmented, erythematous, or nodular.

- Nerve Damage: Leprosy can cause nerve damage, resulting in sensory loss, muscle weakness, and paralysis. Numbness or loss of sensation in the skin, particularly in the hands and feet, is a common early symptom.

- Thickened Nerves: In some cases, affected nerves may become thickened and tender, leading to visible nerve enlargement or nodules, particularly in the face (facial nerve involvement is characteristic of lepromatous leprosy).

- Eye Problems: Leprosy can affect the eyes, leading to dryness, redness, corneal ulcers, and blindness if left untreated.

- Musculoskeletal Symptoms: Advanced leprosy may cause musculoskeletal complications such as joint pain, stiffness, and deformities, particularly in the hands and feet.

- Systemic Symptoms: In some cases, leprosy may cause systemic symptoms such as fever, fatigue, weight loss, and malaise.

Causes and Risk Factors:
- Close Contact: Leprosy is primarily transmitted through prolonged close contact with untreated patients who have active leprosy infection.
- Household Contacts: patients living in close proximity to untreated leprosy patients, particularly family members or household contacts, are at increased risk of contracting the disease.
- Poor Socioeconomic Conditions: Leprosy is more prevalent in areas with poor socioeconomic conditions, inadequate sanitation, and limited access to healthcare services.
- Genetic Susceptibility: Genetic factors may play a role in susceptibility to leprosy, with certain genetic polymorphisms increasing the risk of infection or development of leprosy-related complications.
- Immune Status: Immunosuppression, whether due to HIV infection, immunosuppressive therapy, or other factors, can increase the risk of developing active leprosy disease in patients exposed to the bacterium.

Epidemiology:
- Leprosy, also known as Hansen's disease, is caused by infection with the bacterium Mycobacterium leprae.
- Leprosy is found primarily in tropical and subtropical regions, particularly in South Asia, Southeast Asia, Africa, and Latin America.
- The global burden of leprosy has declined significantly over the past few decades, but the disease remains endemic in certain regions, with new cases reported each year.
- Leprosy transmission occurs through respiratory droplets from untreated patients with active leprosy infection, although the exact mechanisms of transmission are not fully understood.
- Leprosy is not highly contagious, and most patients exposed to M. leprae do not develop clinical disease. However, some patients may develop active leprosy infection months to years after exposure, particularly if they have genetic susceptibility or other risk factors.

Workup and Diagnosis:
- <u>Clinical Evaluation:</u>
    Diagnosis of leprosy is primarily based on clinical evaluation, including the presence of characteristic skin lesions, nerve involvement, and musculoskeletal symptoms.

- Skin Biopsy:

    Skin biopsy may be performed to obtain tissue samples for histopathological examination and detection of acid-fast bacilli (AFB) using special stains such as Fite or Wade-Fite stain.

- Slit Skin Smear:

    Slit skin smear examination may be performed to detect acid-fast bacilli in skin lesions, although this method has lower sensitivity and specificity compared to skin biopsy.

- Nerve Biopsy:

    Nerve biopsy may be indicated in cases of suspected neural involvement to confirm the presence of M. leprae and assess nerve damage.

Treatment:

- Multidrug Therapy (MDT):

    Multidrug therapy is the standard treatment for leprosy and consists of a combination of antibiotics to eradicate the M. leprae bacteria and prevent disease progression. The World Health Organization (WHO) recommends multidrug therapy regimens based on the classification of leprosy as paucibacillary (PB) or multibacillary (MB) disease.

- Paucibacillary (PB) Leprosy: Paucibacillary leprosy is treated with a combination of rifampicin and dapsone for six months.

- Multibacillary (MB) Leprosy: Multibacillary leprosy is treated with a combination of rifampicin, dapsone, and clofazimine for 12 months.

- Management of Complications:

    In addition to antibiotics, management of leprosy may involve supportive care, treatment of complications such as nerve damage and musculoskeletal deformities, and rehabilitation services to improve function and quality of life.

- Prevention of Disability:

    Early diagnosis and treatment of leprosy are essential for preventing permanent disability and deformities associated with advanced disease.

8.23. Respiratory Syncytial Virus

> ➢ *Respiratory syncytial virus (RSV) is a common respiratory virus causing infections ranging from mild cold-like symptoms to severe respiratory illness, particularly in infants and older adults.*
>
> ➢ *Symptoms include coughing, wheezing, fever, and difficulty breathing.*
>
> ➢ *Prevention involves good hygiene practices, especially around infants, and in severe cases, supportive care may be necessary.*

Symptoms:

- Mild Respiratory Symptoms: RSV infection typically presents with mild respiratory symptoms similar to the common cold, including runny nose, nasal congestion, cough, and mild fever.
- Severe Respiratory Symptoms: In some cases, particularly in infants and young children, RSV infection may lead to more severe respiratory symptoms such as wheezing, difficulty breathing, rapid breathing, and coughing.
- Bronchiolitis: RSV is a common cause of bronchiolitis, an inflammatory condition of the small airways in the lungs, characterized by wheezing, coughing, and difficulty breathing.
- Pneumonia: Severe RSV infection can progress to pneumonia, particularly in high-risk patients such as infants, young children, older adults, and patients with weakened immune systems.

Causes and Risk Factors:

- Age: Infants and young children, particularly premature infants and those with underlying medical conditions, are at increased risk of severe RSV infection and complications.
- Prematurity: Premature infants, especially those born before 35 weeks of gestation, are at higher risk of severe RSV infection and may require hospitalization.
- Chronic Lung Disease: Children with chronic lung diseases such as asthma or bronchopulmonary dysplasia (BPD) are more susceptible to severe RSV infection and may experience more severe respiratory symptoms.
- Weakened Immune System: patients with weakened immune systems, including those with HIV/AIDS, cancer, or receiving immunosuppressive therapy, are at increased risk of severe RSV infection and complications.

Epidemiology:
- RSV is a common respiratory virus that circulates worldwide, causing seasonal outbreaks of respiratory illness, particularly in the fall and winter months.
- RSV is highly contagious and spreads through respiratory droplets when an infected person coughs or sneezes or by direct contact with contaminated surfaces.
- RSV infection occurs in all age groups, but infants, young children, older adults, and patients with underlying medical conditions are at higher risk of severe disease and complications.
- RSV is a leading cause of respiratory illness in infants and young children, accounting for a significant proportion of hospitalizations and healthcare utilization in this population.

Workup and Diagnosis:
- <u>Clinical Evaluation:</u> Diagnosis of RSV infection is primarily based on clinical symptoms and history of exposure to patients with respiratory illness.
- <u>Laboratory Testing:</u>

    Laboratory tests such as rapid antigen detection tests (RADTs) or nucleic acid amplification tests (NAATs) may be performed on respiratory specimens (e.g., nasopharyngeal swabs, nasal washes, or aspirates) to detect RSV viral antigens or nucleic acids.

Treatment:
- <u>Supportive Care:</u>

    Treatment of RSV infection is primarily supportive and includes measures to alleviate symptoms and ensure adequate hydration and nutrition.

- <u>Bronchodilators:</u>

    Bronchodilators such as albuterol may be used to relieve wheezing and improve breathing in patients with bronchiolitis or reactive airway disease.

- <u>Oxygen Therapy:</u> Supplemental oxygen may be administered to patients with severe respiratory distress or hypoxemia.
- <u>Antiviral Therapy:</u>

    Antiviral medications such as ribavirin may be considered for severe RSV infection in hospitalized infants and young children or immunocompromised patients, although their efficacy is limited and they are not routinely recommended for uncomplicated RSV infection.

- Prevention:

    Prevention of RSV infection relies primarily on infection control measures such as hand hygiene, respiratory etiquette (e.g., covering coughs and sneezes), avoiding close contact with patients with respiratory illness, and vaccination for high-risk groups (e.g., infants born prematurely or with certain medical conditions).

References

- Gupta, K., Hooton, T. M., & et al. (2011). International clinical practice guidelines for the treatment of acute uncomplicated cystitis and pyelonephritis in women: A 2010 update by the Infectious Diseases Society of America and the European Society for Microbiology and Infectious Diseases. Clinical Infectious Diseases, 52(5), e103-e120.
- Biswas, B., & Bhagat, M. (2020). Pyelonephritis. In StatPearls [Internet]. StatPearls Publishing.
- Workowski, K. A., & Bolan, G. A. (2015). Sexually transmitted diseases treatment guidelines, 2015. MMWR. Recommendations and Reports, 64(RR-03), 1-137.
- Workowski, K. A., & Bolan, G. A. (2015). Sexually transmitted diseases treatment guidelines, 2015. MMWR. Recommendations and Reports, 64(RR-03), 1-137.
- Workowski, K. A., & Bolan, G. A. (2015). Sexually transmitted diseases treatment guidelines, 2015. MMWR. Recommendations and Reports, 64(RR-03), 1-137.
- Kimberlin, D. W., Rouse, D. J., & et al. (2013). Neonatal herpes simplex virus infections. Clinical Microbiology Reviews, 26(4), 723-735.
- Stanek, G., Wormser, G. P., & et al. (2012). Lyme borreliosis: Clinical case definitions for diagnosis and management in Europe. Clinical Microbiology and Infection, 17(1), 69-79.
- Centers for Disease Control and Prevention. (2019). Hepatitis A questions and answers for health professionals. Retrieved from https://www.cdc.gov/hepatitis/hav/havfaq.htm
- Terrault, N. A., Lok, A. S. F., & et al. (2018). Update on prevention, diagnosis, and treatment of chronic hepatitis B: AASLD 2018 hepatitis B guidance. Hepatology, 67(4), 1560-1599.
- American Association for the Study of Liver Diseases and Infectious Diseases Society of America. (2018). HCV guidance: Recommendations for

- testing, managing, and treating hepatitis C. Retrieved from https://www.hcvguidelines.org/
- Rizzetto, M., & Canese, M. G. (2019). Treatment of chronic delta hepatitis. Gastroenterology, 156(5), 1380-1382.
- Dalton, H. R., Kamar, N., & et al. (2018). Hepatitis E virus and neurological injury. Nature Reviews Neurology, 14(2), 96-103.
- Marin, M., & Leung, J. (2016). Prevention of varicella: Recommendations of the Advisory Committee on Immunization Practices (ACIP). MMWR. Recommendations and Reports, 45(RR-6), 1-36.
- Centers for Disease Control and Prevention. (2019). Measles (rubeola) questions and answers for health professionals. Retrieved from https://www.cdc.gov/measles/hcp/index.html
- Patel, M., Lee, A. D., & et al. (2018). National update on measles cases and outbreaks—United States, January 1-October 1, 2018. MMWR. Morbidity and Mortality Weekly Report, 67(44), 1246.
- Harpaz, R., Ortega-Sanchez, I. R., & et al. (2008). Prevention of herpes zoster: Recommendations of the Advisory Committee on Immunization Practices (ACIP). MMWR. Recommendations and Reports, 57(RR-5), 1-30.
- World Health Organization. (2009). Dengue: Guidelines for diagnosis, treatment, prevention, and control. Retrieved from https://www.who.int/denguecontrol/9789241547871/en/
- World Health Organization. (2015). Guidelines for the treatment of malaria. Retrieved from https://www.who.int/malaria/publications/atoz/9789241549127/en/
- Panel on Antiretroviral Guidelines for Adults and Adolescents. (2020). Guidelines for the use of antiretroviral agents in adults and adolescents with HIV. Retrieved from https://clinicalinfo.hiv.gov/sites/default/files/guidelines/documents/AdultandAdolescentGL.pdf
- Hall, A. J., Wikswo, M. E., & et al. (2013). Vital signs: Foodborne norovirus outbreaks—United States, 2009-2012. MMWR. Morbidity and Mortality Weekly Report, 62(35), 739.
- World Health Organization. (2018). Rabies vaccines: WHO position paper, April 2018. Weekly Epidemiological Record, 93(16), 201-220.
- World Health Organization. (2020). Weekly epidemiological record. Geneva: World Health Organization.
- American Academy of Pediatrics. (2014). Respiratory syncytial virus. In Red book: 2015 report of the Committee on Infectious Diseases (pp. 686-696). American Academy of Pediatrics.

Chapter 9. Neurologic and Psychiatric Disorders

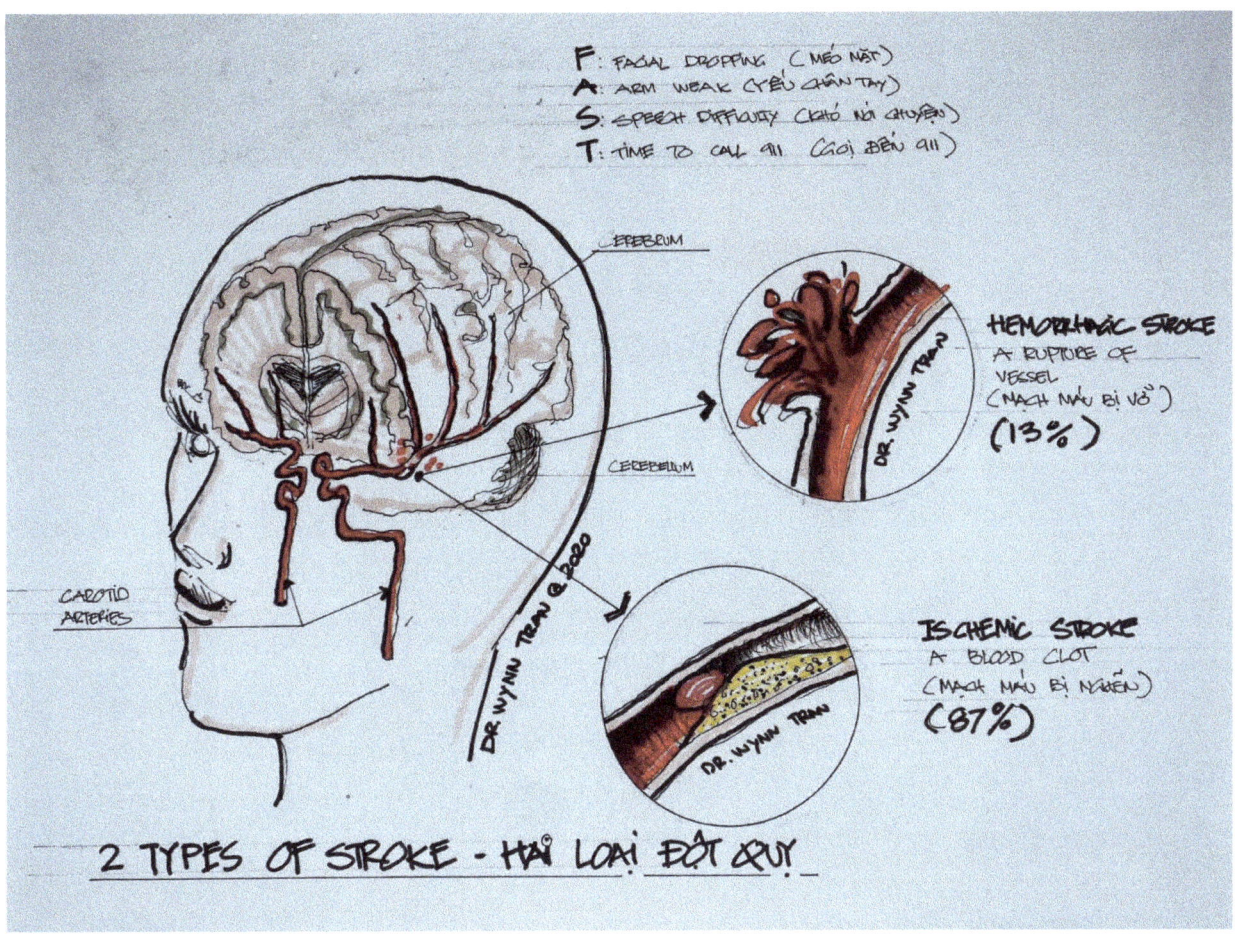

The APh should be familiar with the presentation, diagnosis, and management of these common neurologic disorders to provide appropriate care and referral to the neurologist/psychiatrist when necessary.

9.1. General Headache

> ➤ *General headaches can stem from various causes such as stress, dehydration, or muscle tension.*
>
> ➤ *Symptoms often include dull, achy pain, pressure, or tightness in the head.*
>
> ➤ *Treatment usually involves rest, hydration, and over-the-counter pain medications. Addressing underlying triggers is also important.*

Symptoms:

- Pain: Headache is characterized by pain or discomfort in the head or neck region.
- Location: Headache pain may be localized to a specific area or may involve the entire head.
- Intensity: Headache severity can range from mild to severe, affecting daily activities and quality of life.
- Duration: Headaches may last for a **few minutes to several hours or even days**, depending on the underlying cause.
- Associated Symptoms: Headaches may be accompanied by other symptoms such as nausea, vomiting, sensitivity to light or sound, and visual disturbances.

Risk Factors:

- Genetics: Family history of headaches or migraine can increase the risk of developing headaches.
- Gender: Women are more prone to headaches, particularly migraines, compared to men.
- Age: Headaches can occur at any age, but certain types such as tension-type headaches tend to peak during middle age.
- Hormonal Changes: Hormonal fluctuations, such as those occurring during menstruation, pregnancy, or menopause, can trigger headaches in susceptible patients.

Epidemiology:

- Headaches are one of the most common medical complaints worldwide, affecting patients of all ages, races, and socioeconomic backgrounds.
- The prevalence of headaches varies depending on the type and population studied.

- Tension-type headaches are the most common type of primary headache disorder, followed by migraines and cluster headaches.
- Migraine affects approximately 12% of the population globally, with a higher prevalence among women.
- Headaches can occur sporadically or chronically, with some patients experiencing frequent or daily headaches that significantly impact their quality of life.

Diagnosis:
- Clinical Evaluation: Diagnosis of headaches is primarily based on clinical history and physical examination.
- Headache Diary: Keeping a headache diary to track the frequency, duration, severity, and associated symptoms of headaches can help Advanced Pharmacist Practitioners make an accurate diagnosis.
- Diagnostic Criteria: Specific diagnostic criteria, such as those outlined in the International Classification of Headache Disorders (ICHD), may be used to classify headaches into primary or secondary types.
- Laboratory Tests and Imaging: In some cases, laboratory tests (e.g., blood tests) or imaging studies (e.g., MRI, CT scan) may be ordered to rule out underlying medical conditions causing secondary headaches.

Treatment:
- Acute Treatment
    - Over-the-counter pain relievers such as acetaminophen, ibuprofen, or aspirin may be used to alleviate mild to moderate headaches.
    - For more severe headaches, prescription medications such as triptans or ergotamines may be prescribed.
- Preventive Treatment
    - For patients with frequent or chronic headaches, preventive medications such as beta-blockers, tricyclic antidepressants, antiepileptic drugs, or botulinum toxin injections may be recommended to reduce the frequency and severity of headaches.
- Lifestyle Modifications
    - Lifestyle changes such as maintaining a regular sleep schedule, staying hydrated, managing stress, and avoiding known triggers (e.g., certain foods, environmental factors) can help prevent headaches.

- Complementary Therapies
    - Relaxation techniques, biofeedback, acupuncture, physical therapy, and cognitive-behavioral therapy may be used as adjunctive treatments for headache management.
- Patient Education
    - Educating patients about their headache triggers, treatment options, and self-management strategies are essential for empowering them to effectively manage their condition and improve their quality of life.

9.2. Migraine

> *Migraine is a neurological condition characterized by recurrent episodes of severe headache. Triggers include hormonal changes, certain foods, and environmental factors.*
>
> *Migraines can significantly impact daily life and quality of life. Symptoms include headache, aura, nausea, vomiting, and sensitivity to light and sound.*
>
> *Treatment includes medications to relieve symptoms and prevent attacks, lifestyle modifications, and stress management techniques.*

Symptoms:

- Headache: Migraine headaches typically present as moderate to severe pulsating or throbbing pain, often unilateral and aggravated by routine physical activity.
- Aura: Some patients may experience aura symptoms before or during the migraine headache, including visual disturbances (such as flashing lights or blind spots), sensory changes (such as tingling or numbness), or motor symptoms (such as weakness or difficulty speaking).
- Nausea and Vomiting: Nausea, vomiting, or abdominal discomfort commonly accompany migraine headaches.
- Sensitivity to Light and Sound: Many patients with migraines are sensitive to light (photophobia) and sound (phonophobia) during an attack.
- Duration and Frequency: Migraine attacks typically last **4 to 72 hours** if untreated and may occur episodically (less than 15 days per month) or chronically (15 or more days per month)

Risk Factors:
- Family History: Migraine tends to run in families, suggesting a genetic predisposition to the condition.
- Gender: Migraine is more prevalent in women, particularly during reproductive years, suggesting hormonal influences.
- Hormonal Factors: Fluctuations in estrogen levels, such as those occurring during menstrual cycles, pregnancy, or menopause, can trigger migraines in susceptible patients.
- Environmental Triggers: Certain environmental factors, such as stress, sleep disturbances, sensory stimuli (e.g., bright lights, loud noises), weather changes, or dietary factors (e.g., alcohol, caffeine, aged cheeses), can trigger migraine attacks.
- Medical Conditions: Underlying medical conditions such as depression, anxiety, sleep disorders, and other pain disorders (e.g., fibromyalgia) are associated with an increased risk of migraine.
- Certain medications: Including hormonal contraceptives, vasodilators, and some over-the-counter medications, can trigger migraines in susceptible patients.

Epidemiology:
- Migraine is a common neurological disorder, affecting approximately 12% of the population worldwide.
- Migraine prevalence varies by age, gender, and geographic region, with higher rates observed in women, patients aged 18-44 years, and those living in high-income countries.
- Migraine prevalence peaks in mid-adulthood and declines with advancing age.
- Migraine is a leading cause of disability and contributes to significant healthcare utilization and economic burden globally.

Diagnosis:
- Clinical Evaluation: Diagnosis of migraine is primarily based on clinical history and characteristic symptoms, including the pattern and duration of headaches, associated symptoms (e.g., aura, nausea), and response to treatment.
- Diagnostic Criteria: Migraine is diagnosed according to criteria established by the International Classification of Headache Disorders (ICHD), which specifies the presence of specific symptoms and features to distinguish migraine from other types of headaches.
- Differential Diagnosis: Other primary headache disorders (such as tension-type headache and cluster headache) and secondary

headaches (caused by underlying medical conditions or medications) should be considered in the differential diagnosis.

Treatment:
- Acute Treatment
    - Acute migraine attacks are typically managed with medications to alleviate pain and associated symptoms.
    - Options include nonsteroidal anti-inflammatory drugs (NSAIDs), triptans (e.g., sumatriptan, rizatriptan), ergotamine derivatives, and antiemetics for nausea and vomiting.
- Preventive Treatment
    - Patients with frequent or severe migraine attacks may benefit from preventive medications to reduce the frequency and severity of headaches.
    - Options include beta-blockers, calcium channel blockers, antidepressants, anticonvulsants, and botulinum toxin injections.
- Lifestyle Modifications
    - Lifestyle modifications, including stress management techniques, regular exercise, adequate hydration, healthy sleep habits, and dietary adjustments (e.g., avoiding trigger foods), may help reduce migraine frequency and severity.
- Acute Rescue Therapies
    - For refractory migraine attacks or those associated with severe nausea or vomiting, rescue medications such as intravenous fluids, corticosteroids, or intravenous dihydroergotamine (DHE) may be used in hospital settings.
- Patient Education
    - Patient education is essential to help patients understand their migraine triggers, recognize early warning signs, and optimize self-management strategies, including medication adherence and lifestyle modifications.

9.3. Tension Headache

> ➢ *Tension headaches are the most common type of headache. They are characterized by mild to moderate, diffuse pain resembling a band around the head.*
> ➢ *Common triggers include stress, poor posture, and eye strain.*
> ➢ *Treatment often includes over-the-counter pain relievers, relaxation techniques and addressing underlying factors like stress or posture.*

Symptoms:
- Headache: Tension-type headaches typically present as mild to moderate bilateral pressure or tightness around the head, often described as a "band-like" sensation.
- Duration: Headaches may last from minutes to days, with a chronic pattern of episodic or frequent headaches.
- Location: Pain is usually diffuse and commonly involves the forehead, temples, or the back of the head and neck.
- Absence of Associated Symptoms: Unlike migraine headaches, tension-type headaches typically do not present with aura, nausea, vomiting, or sensitivity to light and sound.
- Mild to Moderate Intensity: Pain intensity is usually mild to moderate, although it may vary within and between episodes.

Risk Factors:
- Psychological Factors: Stress, anxiety, depression, and other psychological factors are strongly associated with tension-type headaches.
- Musculoskeletal Factors: Poor posture, muscle tension, and temporomandibular joint (TMJ) dysfunction may contribute to the development of tension-type headaches.
- Lifestyle Factors: Irregular sleep patterns, poor sleep quality, caffeine consumption, and skipping meals are potential triggers for tension-type headaches.
- Environmental Factors: Prolonged exposure to screens, noise, and bright lights, as well as work-related stress and environmental factors, may exacerbate tension-type headaches.
- Gender and Age: Tension-type headaches are more common in women and tend to peak during middle age.

Epidemiology:
- Tension-type headache is the most common primary headache disorder, affecting a large proportion of the global population.
- It is estimated that up to 80% of adults experience tension-type headaches at some point in their lives.
- Tension-type headaches have a relatively uniform global prevalence, occurring across all age groups and geographic regions.
- The prevalence of tension-type headaches tends to decrease with advancing age, particularly after middle age.

Diagnosis:
- Clinical Evaluation: Diagnosis of tension-type headache is primarily based on clinical history and examination.
- Diagnostic Criteria: The International Classification of Headache Disorders (ICHD) provides diagnostic criteria for tension-type headache, including duration, frequency, and characteristics of headache episodes.
- Differential Diagnosis: Tension-type headache should be differentiated from other primary headache disorders (such as migraine) and secondary headaches (caused by underlying medical conditions or medications).

Treatment:
- Acute Treatment: Mild to moderate tension-type headaches can often be managed with over-the-counter analgesics such as acetaminophen, nonsteroidal anti-inflammatory drugs (NSAIDs), or aspirin.
- Nonpharmacologic Therapies: Stress reduction techniques, relaxation exercises, biofeedback, cognitive-behavioral therapy, and physical therapy may help alleviate muscle tension and reduce headache frequency.
- Pharmacologic Therapies: For patients with frequent or severe tension-type headaches, prescription medications such as muscle relaxants, tricyclic antidepressants (e.g., amitriptyline), or selective serotonin reuptake inhibitors (SSRIs) may be considered for preventive treatment.
- Lifestyle Modifications: Regular exercise, adequate hydration, healthy sleep habits, stress management, and avoidance of headache triggers (e.g., caffeine, alcohol, poor posture) may help reduce headache frequency and severity.

- Combination Therapy: Some patients may benefit from a combination of pharmacologic and nonpharmacologic therapies to optimize headache management and improve quality of life.

9.4. Cluster Headache

> ➤ *Cluster headaches are severe, excruciating headaches that occur in clusters or cycles. They often strike suddenly and repeatedly around the same time each day.*
> ➤ *Cluster headaches typically cause intense pain on one side of the head. Other symptoms may include eye watering, nasal congestion, and restlessness.*
> ➤ *Treatment options include medications to alleviate symptoms and prevent attacks. Oxygen therapy and nerve stimulation techniques are sometimes used.*

Symptoms:
- Severe Pain
    - Cluster headaches are characterized by excruciating, unilateral pain typically located around one eye or temple.
    - The pain is often described as stabbing, piercing, or burning in nature.
- Duration
    - Cluster headaches have a distinct pattern of occurring in clusters or "attacks" lasting between **15 minutes to 3 hours**.
    - Attacks may occur multiple times a day, usually at the same time of day or night.
- Frequency: Cluster headache attacks may occur frequently for **weeks to months**, followed by periods of remission where no headaches occur.
- Autonomic Symptoms: Patients with cluster headaches often experience autonomic symptoms on the same side as the headache such as redness and tearing of the eye, nasal congestion or discharge, drooping eyelid (ptosis), and constriction of the pupil (miosis).
- Restlessness: During a cluster headache attack, patients may exhibit agitation or restlessness, pacing, or rocking movements in an attempt to alleviate the pain.

Risk Factors:
- Age and Gender: Cluster headaches are more common in males, with *onset typically* occurring between the ages of 20 and 40 years.
- Family History: A family history of cluster headaches or other primary headache disorders may increase the risk of developing cluster headaches.
- Smoking: Cigarette smoking is strongly associated with cluster headaches, with smokers having a higher prevalence compared to nonsmokers.
- Alcohol Consumption: Alcohol consumption, particularly during cluster periods, can trigger or exacerbate cluster headache attacks.
- Seasonal Variations: Some patients experience seasonal variations in cluster headache occurrence, with higher prevalence during certain times of the year.

Epidemiology:
- Cluster headaches are relatively rare compared to other primary headache disorders, with a prevalence of approximately 0.1% to 0.4% in the general population.
- The male-to-female ratio is approximately **3:1**.
- Cluster headaches tend to occur in clusters or "bouts," typically lasting several weeks to months, followed by periods of remission lasting months to years.

Diagnosis:
- Clinical Evaluation: Diagnosis of cluster headache is primarily based on clinical history and characteristic symptoms, including the pattern, severity, and duration of headache attacks.
- Diagnostic Criteria: The International Classification of Headache Disorders (ICHD) provides diagnostic criteria for cluster headache, including the presence of specific features such as unilateral pain, autonomic symptoms, and regularity of attacks.
- Differential Diagnosis: Cluster headaches should be differentiated from other primary headache disorders (such as migraine and tension-type headache) and secondary headaches (caused by underlying medical conditions or medications).

Treatment:
- Acute Treatment: Acute cluster headache attacks are typically managed with high-flow oxygen therapy and triptan medications (e.g., sumatriptan), which can be administered subcutaneously or intranasally to stop the attack.

- **Preventive Treatment**: For patients with frequent or severe cluster headache bouts, preventive medications such as verapamil, lithium, corticosteroids, or antiepileptic drugs (e.g., topiramate) may be used to reduce the frequency and severity of attacks.
- **Invasive Procedures:** Invasive procedures such as occipital nerve stimulation, deep brain stimulation, or sphenopalatine ganglion (SPG) blockade may be considered for refractory cases or patients who do not respond to conventional treatments.
- **Lifestyle Modifications**: Avoiding triggers such as alcohol, cigarette smoke, and high-altitude environments may help reduce the frequency and severity of cluster headache attacks.
- **Patient Education**: Patient education is essential to help patients understand their condition, recognize early warning signs of cluster headaches, and optimize treatment adherence and lifestyle modifications.

9.5. Transient Ischemic Attack

> ➢ *Transient ischemic attack (TIA) is a brief episode of neurological dysfunction due to temporary disruption in brain blood flow. It is often a warning sign of an impending stroke.*
> ➢ *Symptoms resemble a stroke, including sudden weakness or numbness on one side of the body, difficulty speaking or understanding speech, and temporary vision loss.*
> ➢ *Prompt medical evaluation is crucial to prevent a full-blown stroke.*

Symptoms:
- Sudden Onset: TIAs typically present with sudden onset neurological symptoms that resolve within 24 hours.
- Focal Neurological Deficits: Symptoms vary based on the affected brain area and can include weakness or paralysis on one side of the body, numbness or tingling, visual disturbances like blurred vision or loss of vision in one eye, slurred speech, difficulty understanding speech, dizziness, and loss of balance or coordination.
- Transient Nature: TIAs usually last for a few minutes to hours, with symptoms completely resolving within 24 hours without leaving permanent neurological deficits.
- Warning Sign: TIAs are often considered warning signs of an impending stroke and require urgent medical evaluation and intervention.

Risk Factors:
- Hypertension: High blood pressure is the most significant risk factor for TIAs and strokes.
- Atrial Fibrillation: Irregular heart rhythm increases the risk of blood clots forming in the heart and traveling to the brain, leading to a TIA or stroke.
- Diabetes: Poorly controlled diabetes can damage blood vessels and increase the risk of atherosclerosis and clot formation.
- High Cholesterol: Elevated levels of cholesterol in the blood can contribute to the buildup of plaque in the arteries, leading to narrowing and reduced blood flow.
- Smoking: Tobacco use is a major risk factor for cardiovascular disease, including TIAs and strokes.
- Age: Risk of TIAs increases with age, particularly after 55 years old.
- Family History: Patients with a family history of stroke or TIA are at higher risk.
- Previous Stroke or TIA: Patients who have had a previous stroke or TIA are at increased risk of having another one.

Epidemiology:
- TIAs are common, with an estimated annual incidence of around 240,000 to 500,000 cases in the United States.
- The incidence of TIAs increases with age, with the highest rates observed in patients over 65 years old.
- Men are slightly more likely to experience TIAs than women.
- TIAs are considered medical emergencies and require prompt evaluation and treatment to prevent progression to a full-blown stroke.

Diagnosis:
- <u>Clinical Evaluation:</u> Diagnosis of TIA is primarily based on clinical history, including the sudden onset and transient nature of neurological symptoms.
- <u>Physical Examination:</u> Neurological examination may reveal focal neurological deficits corresponding to the affected area of the brain.
- <u>Imaging Studies:</u> Imaging studies such as MRI or CT scans may be performed to rule out other potential causes of symptoms and assess for evidence of acute ischemic changes in the brain.
- <u>Laboratory Tests:</u> Blood tests may be ordered to assess for risk factors such as high cholesterol, diabetes, and clotting disorders.

Treatment:

- Immediate Medical Evaluation: Patients suspected of having a TIA should seek immediate medical attention to determine the underlying cause and appropriate management.
- Antiplatelet Therapy: Aspirin or other antiplatelet medications may be prescribed to reduce the risk of blood clot formation and stroke recurrence.
- Anticoagulant Therapy: In cases where atrial fibrillation or other cardiac conditions are identified as the underlying cause, anticoagulant medications such as warfarin or direct oral anticoagulants (DOACs) may be prescribed.
- Lifestyle Modifications: Lifestyle changes such as smoking cessation, healthy diet, regular exercise, weight management, and blood pressure control are essential for reducing the risk of future TIAs and strokes.
- Medication Management: Management of underlying risk factors such as hypertension, diabetes, and high cholesterol with appropriate medications and monitoring.
- Surgery or Interventional Procedures: In some cases, surgical or interventional procedures may be recommended to improve blood flow to the brain or reduce the risk of stroke, such as carotid endarterectomy or angioplasty with stenting.

9.6. Epilepsy

> ➤ *Epilepsy is a neurological disorder characterized by recurrent seizures, caused by abnormal electrical activity in the brain.*
> ➤ *Seizure types vary, ranging from brief moments of confusion to convulsions.*
> ➤ *Treatment involves antiepileptic medications, lifestyle modifications, and sometimes surgery for refractory cases.*

Symptoms:

- Seizures: The hallmark symptom of epilepsy, seizures can manifest in various forms, including convulsions, loss of consciousness, staring spells, muscle stiffness, and repetitive movements.
- Aura: Some patients may experience warning signs or sensations (auras) before a seizure occurs, such as strange smells, tastes, or visual disturbances.

- Loss of awareness: During certain types of seizures, patients may lose awareness of their surroundings or experience altered consciousness.

Risk Factors:

- Genetic factors: Family history of epilepsy or certain genetic syndromes increases the risk of developing epilepsy.
- Brain injuries: Traumatic brain injuries, strokes, brain tumors, infections, and other brain conditions can increase the risk of epilepsy.
- Developmental disorders: Conditions such as autism spectrum disorder and cerebral palsy are associated with an increased risk of epilepsy.
- Brain abnormalities: Structural abnormalities in the brain present from birth or acquired later in life can predispose patients to epilepsy.
- Neurological conditions: Certain neurological disorders, such as Alzheimer's disease and stroke, are associated with an increased risk of epilepsy.

Epidemiology:

- Epilepsy is one of the most common neurological disorders, affecting patients of all ages worldwide.
- It is estimated that approximately 1% of the global population has epilepsy.
- Epilepsy can develop at any age, but it is most commonly diagnosed in childhood or in patients over the age of 65.
- The prevalence of epilepsy varies by region, with higher rates reported in low- and middle-income countries.

Diagnosis:

- Clinical evaluation: Diagnosis is based on a thorough medical history, physical examination, and description of seizure events by the patient or witnesses.
- EEG (electroencephalogram): EEG is a key diagnostic test that records the electrical activity of the brain and can help identify abnormal patterns associated with epilepsy.
- Imaging studies: MRI (magnetic resonance imaging) or CT (computed tomography) scans may be performed to identify structural abnormalities or lesions in the brain that could be causing seizures.

Treatment:
- Antiseizure medications (antiepileptic drugs or AEDs)
  - The primary treatment for epilepsy involves medication to control seizures.
  - The choice of medication depends on the type of seizures, patient patient factors, and potential side effects.
- Surgery
  - In cases where seizures are not well controlled with medication, surgery may be considered to remove or disconnect the part of the brain responsible for causing seizures.
- Vagus Nerve Stimulation (VNS)
  - VNS therapy involves implanting a device that stimulates the vagus nerve, which can help reduce the frequency and severity of seizures.
- Ketogenic diet
  - A high-fat, low-carbohydrate diet may be recommended for some patients with epilepsy, particularly children, when medications are ineffective.

9.7. Peripheral Neuropathy

> ➢ *Peripheral neuropathy is a condition resulting from damage to the peripheral nerves, leading to symptoms such as numbness, tingling, weakness, and pain, typically in the hands and feet.*
> ➢ *Causes include diabetes, infections, autoimmune disorders, and exposure to toxins.*
> ➢ *Treatment aims to manage symptoms, address underlying causes, and may include medications, physical therapy, and lifestyle changes.*

Symptoms:
- Numbness or reduced sensation: Patients may experience numbness, tingling, or a "pins and needles" sensation, particularly in the hands or feet.
- Pain: Peripheral neuropathy can cause sharp, stabbing, burning, or throbbing pain, often described as shooting or electric-like sensations.

- Muscle weakness: Weakness or difficulty moving the affected limbs may occur, leading to difficulties with balance and coordination.
- Sensory changes: Some patients may have difficulty detecting temperature changes, experiencing sensitivity to touch, or feeling as if they are wearing gloves or socks when they are not.
- Motor symptoms: In advanced cases, peripheral neuropathy can lead to muscle wasting, loss of reflexes, and impaired motor function.

Risk Factors:
- Diabetes: Diabetic neuropathy is one of the most common causes of peripheral neuropathy, affecting patients with poorly controlled diabetes.
- Age: The risk of peripheral neuropathy increases with age, with older adults being more susceptible to nerve damage.
- Chronic diseases: Conditions such as diabetes, autoimmune disorders, kidney disease, liver disease, and certain infections (e.g., HIV, hepatitis) can increase the risk of neuropathy.
- Alcohol abuse: Excessive alcohol consumption can lead to nutritional deficiencies and nerve damage, contributing to peripheral neuropathy.
- Medications: Some medications, including certain chemotherapy drugs, antiretroviral drugs, and certain antibiotics, can cause peripheral neuropathy as a side effect.
- Trauma: Physical injury, repetitive stress, or compression of nerves due to trauma or accidents can lead to neuropathic symptoms.
- Genetics: Certain genetic factors may predispose patients to peripheral neuropathy.

Epidemiology:
- Peripheral neuropathy is a common neurological disorder, with prevalence increasing with age.
- It is estimated that approximately 20 million Americans have peripheral neuropathy.
- The prevalence of peripheral neuropathy is higher among patients with diabetes, affecting up to 50% of diabetic patients.
- Other common causes of peripheral neuropathy include alcoholism, chemotherapy-induced neuropathy, and autoimmune disorders.

Diagnosis:
- <u>Clinical evaluation</u>: Diagnosis is based on a comprehensive medical history, physical examination, and neurological assessment.

- Nerve conduction studies (NCS) and electromyography (EMG): These tests measure the electrical activity and function of peripheral nerves and muscles, helping to diagnose and assess the severity of neuropathy.
- Blood tests: Laboratory tests may be performed to evaluate underlying medical conditions such as diabetes, vitamin deficiencies, autoimmune disorders, and infections.
- Imaging studies: MRI or CT scans may be ordered to identify structural abnormalities or compression of nerves.

Treatment:
- Management of underlying conditions: Treating underlying medical conditions such as diabetes, autoimmune disorders, and vitamin deficiencies is essential for managing peripheral neuropathy.
- Medications: Pharmacological treatment options may include pain relievers (e.g., gabapentin, pregabalin), antidepressants (e.g., amitriptyline, duloxetine), and antiseizure medications (e.g., carbamazepine).
- Physical therapy: Exercises and physical therapy techniques can help improve strength, flexibility, and coordination, as well as reduce pain and discomfort.
- Lifestyle modifications: Avoiding alcohol consumption, maintaining a healthy weight, managing blood sugar levels, and practicing proper foot care are important for preventing further nerve damage and managing symptoms

9.8. Multiple Sclerosis

> ➤ *Multiple sclerosis (MS) is a chronic autoimmune disease affecting the central nervous system, leading to inflammation, demyelination, and neurological dysfunction.*
> ➤ *Symptoms vary widely but commonly include fatigue, weakness, numbness, and difficulty with coordination and balance.*
> ➤ *Treatment focuses on managing symptoms, slowing disease progression, and improving quality of life through medications, physical therapy, and lifestyle adjustments.*

Symptoms:
- Fatigue: The common symptom of MS, which can significantly impact daily activities and quality of life.

- Motor symptoms: Weakness, muscle stiffness, tremors, spasticity, and difficulty with coordination and balance are common motor symptoms.
- Sensory symptoms: Numbness, tingling, burning sensations, and pain in various parts of the body can occur.
- Visual disturbances: Blurred vision, double vision (diplopia), optic neuritis (inflammation of the optic nerve), and loss of vision may occur.
- Cognitive changes: MS can affect cognitive function, leading to problems with memory, concentration, and decision-making.
- Emotional changes: Mood swings, depression, anxiety, and irritability are common emotional symptoms.
- Bladder and bowel dysfunction: MS can cause urinary urgency, frequency, incontinence, and constipation or diarrhea.

Risk Factors:
- Autoimmune factors: MS is believed to occur when the immune system mistakenly attacks the myelin sheath, leading to inflammation and damage to nerve fibers.
- Genetic factors: Certain genetic variations are associated with an increased risk of developing MS, although genetics alone are not sufficient to cause the disease.
- Environmental factors: Factors such as vitamin D deficiency, smoking, and exposure to certain viruses (e.g., Epstein-Barr virus) may increase the risk of developing MS.
- Gender and age: MS is more common in women than men and typically develops between the ages of 20 and 40, although it can occur at any age.

Epidemiology:
- MS is one of the most common neurological disorders affecting young adults, with an estimated 2.8 million patients affected worldwide.
- The prevalence of MS varies by geographic region, with higher rates reported in temperate climates and northern latitudes.
- MS is more common in patients of European descent, but it can affect patients of all ethnic backgrounds.
- The incidence of MS appears to be increasing, particularly in regions where it was previously less common.

Diagnosis:

- Clinical evaluation: Diagnosis is based on a comprehensive medical history, physical examination, and neurological assessment.
- MRI scans: Detect characteristic lesions (plaques) in the brain and spinal cord that are indicative of MS.
- Lumbar puncture: Analysis of cerebrospinal fluid can reveal elevated levels of immune cells and proteins associated with MS.
- Evoked potentials: These tests measure the electrical activity of the brain in response to sensory stimuli and can help assess nerve function.

Treatment:

- Disease-modifying therapies (DMTs): DMTs are medications that can help reduce the frequency and severity of MS relapses, slow disease progression, and manage symptoms.
- Symptomatic treatment: Medications and therapies may be prescribed to manage specific symptoms such as fatigue, muscle spasticity, pain, and bladder dysfunction.
- Rehabilitation: Physical therapy, occupational therapy, speech therapy, and other rehabilitation services can help improve mobility, strength, coordination, and cognitive function.
- Lifestyle modifications: Maintaining a healthy lifestyle, including regular exercise, balanced nutrition, stress management, and adequate rest, can help manage MS symptoms and improve overall well-being.

9.9. Parkinson's Disease

> ➤ *Parkinson's disease is a progressive neurological disorder characterized by tremors, stiffness, slow movements, and impaired balance and coordination.*
> ➤ *It results from the loss of dopamine-producing neurons in the brain.*
> ➤ *Treatment typically involves medications to manage symptoms, physical therapy, and sometimes surgery for advanced cases.*

Symptoms:

- Bradykinesia: Slowness of movement and difficulty initiating and controlling voluntary movements.
- Tremor: Typically a resting tremor that affects the hands, fingers, or other limbs.

- Muscle rigidity: Stiffness and resistance to movement in the muscles, which can lead to decreased range of motion.
- Postural instability: Impaired balance and coordination, leading to difficulty maintaining an upright posture and an increased risk of falls.
- Other motor symptoms: Freezing of gait, reduced arm swing while walking, and difficulty with fine motor tasks such as writing or buttoning clothes.
- Non-motor symptoms: These may include cognitive impairment, mood changes (such as depression or anxiety), sleep disturbances, constipation, urinary problems, and changes in speech or swallowing.

Risk Factors:
- Age: The risk of Parkinson's disease increases with age, with most cases diagnosed after the age of 60.
- Gender: Men are slightly more likely to develop Parkinson's disease than women.
- Family history: Having a close relative with Parkinson's disease increases the risk of developing the condition.
- Environmental factors: Exposure to certain toxins or environmental pollutants may increase the risk of Parkinson's disease.
- Genetic factors: While most cases of Parkinson's disease are sporadic, certain genetic mutations have been linked to an increased risk of the disease.

Epidemiology:
- Parkinson's disease is the second most common neurodegenerative disorder after Alzheimer's disease, affecting approximately 1% of patients over the age of 60.
- The prevalence of Parkinson's disease increases with age, with estimates ranging from 1% to 2% in patients over 65 years of age.
- The incidence and prevalence of Parkinson's disease vary by geographic region and population demographics.
- While Parkinson's disease is more common in older adults, it can also affect younger patients, known as early-onset Parkinson's disease.

Diagnosis:
- Diagnosis of Parkinson's disease primarily based on clinical evaluation by a healthcare professional, typically a neurologist specializing in movement disorders.
- There is no single diagnostic test for Parkinson's disease, so diagnosis is based on the presence of characteristic motor symptoms

and the exclusion of other conditions that may mimic Parkinson's disease.
- Diagnostic criteria established by expert consensus, such as the UK Brain Bank criteria or the Movement Disorder Society (MDS) diagnostic criteria, may be used to guide diagnosis.

Treatment:
- Medications: Dopamine replacement therapy with **levodopa** and **dopamine agonists** are the mainstay of treatment for Parkinson's disease, helping to alleviate motor symptoms.
- Physical therapy: Exercises and physical therapy techniques can help improve mobility, balance, flexibility, and muscle strength.
- Occupational therapy: Occupational therapists can provide strategies to help patients with Parkinson's disease manage activities of daily living and maintain independence.
- Speech therapy: Speech therapists can help improve speech and swallowing difficulties commonly associated with Parkinson's disease.
- Deep brain stimulation (DBS): For patients with advanced Parkinson's disease who are not adequately controlled with medication, DBS surgery may be recommended to implant electrodes in the brain and modulate abnormal brain activity.

9.10. Alzheimer's Disease

> *Alzheimer's disease is a progressive neurodegenerative disorder leading to memory loss, cognitive decline, and impaired functioning.*
> *Characterized by the accumulation of abnormal protein plaques and tangles in the brain.*
> *Currently, there is no cure, but treatments aim to manage symptoms and slow disease progression.*

Symptoms:
- Memory loss: Difficulty remembering recently learned information and important dates or events.
- Cognitive decline: Impaired reasoning, judgment, and problem-solving abilities.
- Language difficulties in finding the right words, following conversations, and understanding written or spoken language.
- Disorientation: Confusion about time, place, and surroundings, leading to getting lost in familiar places.

- Changes in mood and behavior: Mood swings, irritability, anxiety, depression, and social withdrawal are common.
- Difficulty with daily tasks: Challenges with performing familiar tasks such as cooking, dressing, and managing finances.
- Progressive decline: Symptoms worsen over time, leading to severe impairment in memory, cognition, and function.

Risk Factors:

- Age is the greatest risk factor for Alzheimer's disease, with the risk increasing significantly after the age of 65.
- Genetics: Having a family history of Alzheimer's disease or carrying certain genetic mutations, such as mutations in the genes for amyloid precursor protein (APP), presenilin 1 (PSEN1), or presenilin 2 (PSEN2), increases the risk.
- Down syndrome: Patients with Down syndrome have an increased risk of developing Alzheimer's disease, particularly as they age.
- Cardiovascular risk factors: hypertension, diabetes, obesity, and high cholesterol may increase the risk.
- Traumatic brain injury: A history of severe head trauma, such as a concussion or traumatic brain injury, may increase the risk of developing Alzheimer's disease later in life.

Epidemiology:

- Alzheimer's disease is the most common cause of dementia in older adults, accounting for 60-80% of cases.
- The prevalence of Alzheimer's disease increases with age, with estimates suggesting that approximately 5-10% of patients over the age of 65 and up to 30-40% of patients over the age of 85 have Alzheimer's disease.
- The number of patients living with Alzheimer's disease is expected to increase significantly in the coming decades due to population aging.

Diagnosis:

- Diagnosis of Alzheimer's disease is based on a comprehensive medical history, physical examination, neurological assessment, and cognitive testing.
- Diagnostic criteria established by expert consensus, such as those from the *National Institute on Aging-Alzheimer's Association (NIA-AA)*, may be used to guide diagnosis.
- Imaging studies such as *magnetic resonance imaging (MRI)* and *positron emission tomography (PET)* may be used to assess brain

structure and function and rule out other causes of cognitive impairment.

Treatment:

- Medications: Cholinesterase Inhibitors (e.g. Donepezil, Rivastigmine, Galantamine) and memantine are approved by the Food and Drug Administration (FDA) for the treatment of Alzheimer's disease and may help improve cognitive symptoms and slow disease progression.
- Symptomatic treatment: Antidepressants, anti-anxiety medications, and antipsychotic medications may be prescribed to manage mood and behavioral symptoms associated with Alzheimer's disease.
- Supportive care: Caregiver support, counseling, and education are essential components of Alzheimer's disease management, helping patients and families cope with the challenges of the disease.

Alzheimer Biologic Treatment:

Lecanemab

Lecanemab received approval from the FDA in 2023 for the treatment of Alzheimer's disease following the successful completion of a randomized trial that demonstrated its clinical efficacy. Lecanemab works by targeting and reducing amyloid beta plaques in the brain, which are a hallmark feature of Alzheimer's disease.

Aducanumab

Aducanumab was the first amyloid beta-directed therapy to receive FDA approval for Alzheimer's disease treatment in 2021. Aducanumab is also designed to target amyloid beta plaques in the brain.

Both Lecanemab and Aducanumab represent significant advancements in Alzheimer's treatment, emphasizing targeting the disease's underlying pathology rather than just managing symptoms.

9.11. General Vertigo

> ➤ *Vertigo is characterized by the sensation of spinning or movement, often accompanied by nausea, balance problems, and nystagmus, usually resulting from inner ear disorders or neurological conditions.*
>
> ➤ *Diagnosis involves a detailed patient history, physical examination, and possibly imaging or vestibular testing.*
>
> ➤ *Treatment focuses on managing the underlying cause, with strategies ranging from repositioning maneuvers and medication to vestibular rehabilitation therapy.*

Symptoms:

- Spinning Sensation: Feeling like you or your surroundings are spinning or moving.
- Nausea and Vomiting: Often due to the disorienting sensations of movement.
- Balance Problems: Difficulty standing or walking, increased risk of falls.
- Nystagmus: Involuntary eye movements, often horizontal or rotational, observed during episodes.
- Hearing Loss or Tinnitus: In cases related to inner ear issues.

Risk Factors

- Inner Ear Infections: Such as labyrinthitis or vestibular neuritis.
- Meniere's Disease: Characterized by fluid buildup in the inner ear.
- Age: Older adults are more susceptible to conditions that cause vertigo.
- Head Injury: Trauma to the head can impact inner ear function.
- Migraine: Those with migraines may experience vertigo as a symptom.
- Certain Medications: That affect ear function or blood flow.

Epidemiology

- Vertigo is a common complaint, particularly in individuals over 65, affecting about 20% to 30% of the general population at some point in their lives.
- Females are slightly more likely to experience vertigo than males.

Diagnosis
- <u>Patient History:</u> Including symptom description, duration, and triggering factors.
- <u>Physical Examination</u>: Focused on ear, neurologic, and balance assessments.
- <u>Dix-Hallpike Maneuver or Roll Test</u>: To diagnose benign paroxysmal positional vertigo (BPPV).
- <u>Hearing Tests</u>: To identify related hearing loss issues.
- <u>Imaging Tests</u>: MRI or CT scans if a central cause is suspected, like a brain lesion or multiple sclerosis.
- <u>Vestibular Testing</u>: Including videonystagmography (VNG) or electronystagmography (ENG) to evaluate inner ear function and balance responses.

Treatment
- <u>Epley Maneuver:</u> A series of head movements to treat BPPV by moving dislodged ear crystals.
- <u>Medications</u>: Including antihistamines, anticholinergics, and benzodiazepines for acute episodes, and betahistine for Meniere's disease.
- <u>Vestibular Rehabilitation Therapy (VRT)</u>: Exercises to improve balance and reduce dizziness.

Specific Conditions
- <u>Meniere's Disease</u>: Treatment might include diuretics, dietary changes (low sodium diet), and, in severe cases, surgical interventions.
- <u>Vestibular Neuritis</u>: Corticosteroids may be prescribed to reduce inner ear inflammation.
- <u>Migraine-Associated Vertigo</u>: Preventive migraine medications and lifestyle modifications.

Lifestyle and Home Remedies
- <u>Stay Hydrated</u>: Especially if episodes are related to dehydration.
- <u>Safety Measures:</u> To prevent falls during vertigo episodes.
- <u>Avoid Triggers</u>: Such as sudden head movements or specific activities that provoke vertigo.

9.12. Peripheral Vertigo

> ➢ *Peripheral vertigo is a type of dizziness caused by problems in the inner ear or vestibular nerve, resulting in a false sensation of spinning or movement.*
>
> ➢ *Common causes include benign paroxysmal positional vertigo (BPPV), vestibular neuritis, and Meniere's disease.*
>
> ➢ *Treatment may involve vestibular rehabilitation exercises, medications, or maneuvers to reposition displaced inner ear crystals.*

Symptoms:

- Vertigo: A sensation of spinning or movement, often triggered by changes in head position.

- Nystagmus: Involuntary rhythmic eye movements, which may be horizontal, vertical, or rotary.

- Imbalance or unsteadiness: Feeling off-balance or like the world is tilting or swaying.

- Nausea and vomiting: Some patients may experience nausea or vomiting, particularly during severe vertigo episodes.

- Tinnitus: Ringing, buzzing, or roaring noises in the ears may accompany peripheral vertigo.

- Hearing loss: In some cases, peripheral vertigo may be associated with hearing loss, particularly if it is caused by inner ear disorders such as Ménière's disease.

Risk Factors:

- Inner ear disorders: Conditions such as benign paroxysmal positional vertigo (BPPV), vestibular neuritis, Ménière's disease, and labyrinthitis are common causes of peripheral vertigo.

- Head trauma: Injuries to the head or neck can damage the inner ear structures and lead to vertigo.

- Aging: Age-related changes in the vestibular system, such as degeneration of vestibular hair cells, may increase the risk of peripheral vertigo.

- Medications: Certain medications, such as antibiotics, anticonvulsants, and antihypertensives, can cause vestibular dysfunction and vertigo as side effects.

- Migraine: Patients with migraine headaches may be more prone to experiencing episodes of peripheral vertigo.

Epidemiology:
- Peripheral vertigo is a common complaint encountered in primary care and otolaryngology clinics.
- The prevalence of specific causes of peripheral vertigo varies depending on factors such as age, sex, and geographic location.
- Benign paroxysmal positional vertigo (BPPV) is the most common cause of vertigo overall, particularly in older adults.

Diagnosis:
- Diagnosis of peripheral vertigo is based on a thorough medical history, physical examination, and vestibular function testing.
- The Dix-Hallpike maneuver and supine roll test can help diagnose benign paroxysmal positional vertigo (BPPV), while caloric testing, videonystagmography (VNG), or electronystagmography (ENG) may be used to assess vestibular function.
- Additional diagnostic tests, such as imaging studies (e.g., MRI) or blood tests, may be ordered to rule out other potential causes of vertigo.

Treatment:
- <u>Canalith repositioning maneuvers:</u> For benign paroxysmal positional vertigo (BPPV), maneuvers such as the Epley maneuver or Semont maneuver can help reposition displaced otoliths (calcium crystals) within the inner ear.
- <u>Medications:</u> Depending on the underlying cause of peripheral vertigo, medications such as vestibular suppressants (e.g., meclizine, diazepam) or antiemetics (e.g., promethazine, ondansetron) may be prescribed to relieve symptoms.
- <u>Vestibular rehabilitation therapy</u>: This specialized form of physical therapy involves exercises and maneuvers designed to improve balance, reduce dizziness, and promote vestibular compensation.
- <u>Surgical intervention</u>: In rare cases where peripheral vertigo is caused by structural abnormalities (e.g., vestibular schwannoma), surgical procedures such as vestibular nerve section or labyrinthectomy may be considered.

9.13. Benign Paroxysmal Positional Vertigo

> ➤ *Benign paroxysmal positional vertigo (BPPV) is a common inner ear disorder causing brief episodes of dizziness triggered by head movements.*
>
> ➤ *It occurs due to the displacement of small calcium crystals in the inner ear.*
>
> ➤ *Symptoms include sudden spinning sensations (vertigo) that typically last less than a minute and can be managed with specific positional maneuvers or medication.*

Symptoms:

- Vertigo: The primary symptom of BPPV is vertigo, a sensation that you or your surroundings are spinning or moving. These episodes can be mild or intense and are usually triggered by changes in head position.

- Nausea and Vomiting: The vertigo can be severe enough to cause nausea and sometimes vomiting.

- Nystagmus: An involuntary movement of the eyes, typically from side to side.

- Balance Issues: Difficulty in maintaining balance, especially during vertigo episodes.

- Dizziness: A lightheaded, floating sensation can also occur.

Risk Factors

- Age: BPPV is more common in people over the age of 50.
- Gender: Women are slightly more likely to develop BPPV than men.
- Head Injury: Any trauma to the head can increase the risk of BPPV.
- Osteoporosis: Conditions that affect bone health can be linked to BPPV.
- Viral Infections: Infections of the inner ear can lead to BPPV.
- Prolonged Bed Rest: Being immobile for extended periods can contribute to the development of BPPV.

Epidemiology

- BPPV is the most common cause of vertigo.
- It can affect people of any age but is more prevalent in older adults.
- The exact prevalence varies, but it is recognized as a common disorder in the general population.

- The condition can recur, with some individuals experiencing multiple episodes over their lifetime.

Diagnosis
- Physical Exam: Including the Dix-Hallpike test, where the patient's head is moved in specific ways to trigger vertigo while the doctor observes for nystagmus.
- Imaging Tests: Rarely used for BPPV diagnosis but may be employed to rule out other causes of vertigo.
- Other Tests: May include tests of inner ear function and balance.

Treatment
- Epley Maneuver: A series of specific head and body movements performed by a healthcare provider to move the calcium deposits out of the canal into an area of the inner ear where they will not cause vertigo.
- Medications: Sometimes used to relieve nausea and motion sickness, but they do not cure BPPV.
- Surgery: Rare, but may be considered in persistent cases that do not respond to other treatments.
- Home Care: Includes exercises that can be done at home to manage symptoms and reduce the risk of recurrence.

9.14. Ménière's Disease

> *Ménière's disease is a disorder of the inner ear characterized by episodes of vertigo, fluctuating hearing loss, tinnitus, and a feeling of fullness or pressure in the ear.*
>
> *Its exact cause is unclear but may involve fluid buildup in the inner ear.*
>
> *Treatment includes medication to manage symptoms, dietary changes, and in severe cases, surgical procedures to alleviate pressure in the inner ear.*

Symptoms:
- Vertigo: Intense episodes of spinning dizziness that can last for minutes to hours, often accompanied by nausea, vomiting, and sweating.
- Fluctuating hearing loss: Episodes of hearing loss or muffled hearing, usually affecting one ear initially but potentially progressing to both ears over time.

- Tinnitus: Ringing, buzzing, or roaring noises in the affected ear, which may fluctuate in intensity.
- Aural fullness: A sensation of pressure or fullness in the ear, similar to the feeling of having a plugged ear.
- Imbalance: Feeling unsteady or off-balance, particularly during or after vertigo attacks.

Risk Factors:
- Age: Ménière's disease typically affects patients between the ages of 20 and 50, with peak onset in the fourth and fifth decades of life.
- Genetics: There may be a genetic predisposition to Ménière's disease, as it tends to run in families.
- Autoimmune disorders: Some research suggests that autoimmune factors may contribute to the development of Ménière's disease in certain patients.
- Environmental factors: Exposure to certain environmental triggers such as stress, changes in barometric pressure, or dietary factors (e.g., high salt intake) may exacerbate symptoms in susceptible patients.

Epidemiology:
- Ménière's disease is relatively rare, with an estimated prevalence of 0.2-0.5% of the population.
- It affects both men and women, although some studies suggest a slightly higher prevalence in women.
- The exact cause of Ménière's disease remains unknown, but it is believed to involve a combination of factors, including abnormalities in fluid regulation within the inner ear.

Diagnosis:
- Diagnosis of Ménière's disease is primarily based on clinical history and symptom presentation.
- Diagnostic criteria include the presence of recurrent episodes of vertigo lasting at least 20 minutes, fluctuating sensorineural hearing loss, tinnitus or aural fullness, and exclusion of other potential causes of symptoms.
- Audiometric testing, such as pure-tone audiometry and tympanometry, may be used to assess hearing function and rule out other causes of hearing loss.
- Additional tests, such as vestibular function tests (e.g., caloric testing, videonystagmography) and imaging studies (e.g., MRI), may

be ordered to further evaluate vestibular and auditory function and rule out structural abnormalities.

Treatment:
- Symptomatic management: Treatment aims to alleviate symptoms and prevent or minimize the frequency and severity of vertigo attacks.
- Dietary modifications: Limiting salt intake and avoiding caffeine and alcohol may help reduce fluid retention and fluid pressure in the inner ear.
- Medications: Medications such as diuretics (e.g., hydrochlorothiazide) and vestibular suppressants (e.g., meclizine, diazepam) may be prescribed to control symptoms during vertigo attacks.
- Vestibular rehabilitation therapy: This specialized form of physical therapy involves exercises and maneuvers designed to improve balance and reduce dizziness.
- Invasive therapies: In severe cases of Ménière's disease that do not respond to conservative treatments, invasive therapies such as intratympanic injections of corticosteroids or gentamicin, or surgical procedures such as endolymphatic sac decompression or vestibular nerve section may be considered.

9.15. Hearing Loss

> ➢ *Hearing loss is a common condition characterized by a decreased ability to hear sounds, which can range from mild to profound severity.*
> ➢ *It can result from genetic causes, aging, exposure to loud noises, infections, and certain medical conditions.*
> ➢ *Treatment options vary and may include hearing aids, cochlear implants, and lifestyle modifications to manage the condition and improve quality of life.*

Symptoms:
- Difficulty understanding words, especially against background noise or in a crowd
- Frequently asking others to speak more slowly, clearly, and loudly
- Needing to turn up the volume of the television or radio
- Withdrawal from conversations
- Avoidance of some social settings

- Ringing in the ears (tinnitus) may also accompany hearing loss

Risk Factors and Causes:
- Aging: Natural deterioration of hearing over time is the most common cause among older adults.
- Exposure to Loud Noise: Occupational noise from machinery, as well as exposure to loud music or explosions, can damage hearing.
- Infections: Certain infections, such as meningitis, can lead to hearing loss.
- Ototoxic Medications: Some medications can damage the inner ear.
- Genetic Factors: Hereditary predisposition to hearing loss.
- Illnesses: Diseases that result in high fever, such as measles or mumps, can damage hearing.
- Head Injuries: Trauma to the head can affect the ears' ability to function properly.

Epidemiology
- Hearing loss is one of the most common conditions affecting older adults, with approximately one in three people in the United States between the ages of 65 and 74 having some degree of hearing loss.
- The prevalence increases with age, affecting about half of those older than 75.
- It also affects children and adults of all ages, with genetic factors, prenatal and postnatal infections, and environmental exposure to noise and ototoxic drugs being significant contributors.

Types of Hearing Loss:
- *Sensorineural Hearing Loss:* the most common type, resulting from damage to the inner ear or auditory nerve, often due to aging, noise exposure, genetic factors, or certain diseases. It's typically permanent and can be managed with hearing aids or cochlear implants.
- *Conductive Hearing Loss:* Caused by problems with the ear canal, eardrum, or middle ear structures. Common causes include infections, fluid in the middle ear, earwax blockage, and abnormalities of the ear structure.
- *Mixed Hearing Loss:* A combination of sensorineural and conductive hearing loss, indicating damage both in the outer or middle ear and in the inner ear or auditory nerve pathway. Treatment strategies may include those used for both sensorineural and conductive hearing losses, tailored to the individual's specific condition.

Workup and Diagnosis:
- Pure Tone Audiometry: To measure the faintest tones a person can hear at various pitches.
- Speech Audiometry: To measure speech reception threshold and speech discrimination.
- Tympanometry: To assess the functioning of the middle ear.
- Otoacoustic Emissions (OAEs): To test inner ear health by measuring sound emissions in response to a stimulus.

Treatment:
- Hearing Aids: Electronic devices that amplify sound for people with sensorineural hearing loss.
- Cochlear Implants: For those with profound hearing loss, bypassing the normal acoustic hearing process to stimulate the auditory nerve directly.
- Assistive Listening Devices (ALDs): For specific situations, like talking on the phone or watching TV.
- Surgical Procedures: For conductive hearing loss, depending on the cause.
- Communication Strategies and Lip-Reading Training: To improve understanding without relying solely on hearing.

9.16. Amyotrophic Lateral Sclerosis

> ➢ *Amyotrophic lateral sclerosis (ALS), also known as Lou Gehrig's disease, is a progressive neurodegenerative disorder affecting nerve cells in the brain and spinal cord.*
>
> ➢ *It leads to muscle weakness, paralysis, and eventually respiratory failure, with no known cure.*
>
> ➢ *Treatment focuses on managing symptoms, maintaining quality of life, and support from multidisciplinary care teams.*

Symptoms:
- Muscle weakness: Initial symptoms often involve weakness in the hands, arms, legs, or muscles of speech, swallowing, or breathing.
- Muscle twitching: Visible twitching or involuntary muscle contractions, particularly in the arms or legs.
- Spasticity: Stiff or tight muscles, often accompanied by exaggerated reflexes.

- Difficulty with speech and swallowing: Progressive difficulty in speaking clearly, chewing, or swallowing food and liquids.
- Muscle cramps and stiffness: Painful cramps and stiffness in affected muscles.
- Progressive paralysis: As the disease progresses, patients may experience increasing difficulty with mobility and may eventually become completely paralyzed, including respiratory muscles.

Risk Factors:

- Age: ALS most commonly affects patients between the ages of 40 and 70, with the average age of onset around 55.
- Genetics: Approximately **5-10%** of ALS cases are familial, meaning they are inherited from a family member who also had ALS. Mutations in genes such as C9orf72, SOD1, TARDBP, and FUS have been implicated in familial ALS.
- Environmental factors: Some studies suggest that exposure to certain environmental toxins or heavy metals may increase the risk of developing ALS, although the evidence is inconclusive.
- Smoking: Smoking has been identified as a potential risk factor for ALS, with smokers being at higher risk compared to non-smokers.

Epidemiology:

- ALS is relatively rare, with an estimated incidence of 1-2 cases per 100,000 patients per year.
- It affects patients of all races and ethnicities worldwide, although some studies suggest a slightly higher incidence in Caucasians.
- The exact cause of ALS is unknown, but it is thought to involve a complex interaction between genetic, environmental, and lifestyle factors.

Diagnosis:

- Diagnosis of ALS is primarily based on clinical presentation and exclusion of other possible causes of symptoms.
- Diagnostic criteria include progressive muscle weakness and atrophy in multiple regions of the body, along with evidence of upper and lower motor neuron dysfunction in neurological examination.
- Electromyography (EMG) and nerve conduction studies may be performed to assess electrical activity and function of muscles and nerves.
- Imaging studies such as MRI may be used to rule out other conditions that mimic ALS, such as spinal cord compression or tumors.

Treatment:
- There is currently no cure for ALS, and treatment focuses on managing symptoms, improving quality of life, and providing supportive care.
- Medications such as *Riluzole* and *Edaravone* may be prescribed to slow disease progression and alleviate symptoms.
- Physical therapy, occupational therapy, and speech therapy can help maintain mobility, independence, and communication abilities.
- Assistive devices such as wheelchairs, braces, and communication aids may be recommended to help patients with ALS adapt to their changing abilities.
- Palliative care and hospice services can provide comprehensive support for patients with advanced ALS and their families, focusing on comfort and symptom management.

9.17. Guillain-Barré Syndrome

> ➢ *Guillain-Barré Syndrome (GBS) is a rare autoimmune disorder where the immune system attacks the peripheral nerves, leading to muscle weakness, numbness, and in severe cases, paralysis.*
>
> ➢ *It often follows a viral or bacterial infection and can progress rapidly.*
>
> ➢ *Treatment involves supportive care, such as intravenous immunoglobulin (IVIG) or plasmapheresis, to reduce symptoms and aid recovery.*

Symptoms:
- Muscle weakness: GBS typically starts with weakness and tingling sensations in the legs, which may spread to the arms and upper body.
- Ascending paralysis:
  - Weakness usually begins in the feet and legs and gradually moves upward to the arms and trunk.
  - In severe cases, it can affect the muscles responsible for breathing, leading to respiratory failure.
- Sensory symptoms: Patients may experience numbness, tingling, or pain in the affected areas.
- Reflex loss: Reduced or absent reflexes, such as the knee-jerk reflex, may be observed.

- Autonomic dysfunction: GBS can also affect the autonomic nervous system, leading to symptoms such as fluctuations in blood pressure, heart rate abnormalities, and difficulty controlling bladder and bowel function.

Risk Factors:
- Infection:
    - GBS is often triggered by a preceding infection, most commonly gastrointestinal or respiratory infections caused by bacteria or viruses.
    - Campylobacter jejuni infection is the most commonly identified preceding infection.
- Other factors: Recent surgery, vaccination (rare), and certain medications have also been associated with an increased risk of GBS, although the exact mechanisms are not fully understood.

Epidemiology:
- GBS is relatively rare, with an estimated annual incidence of 1-2 cases per 100,000 patients.
- It can occur at any age, but it is more common in adults and older patients.
- GBS affects both genders equally and occurs worldwide.

Diagnosis:
- Clinical evaluation: Diagnosis of GBS is primarily based on clinical features, including the characteristic pattern of muscle weakness and sensory symptoms.
- Nerve conduction studies (NCS) and electromyography (EMG): These tests can help confirm the diagnosis by demonstrating characteristic findings such as slowed nerve conduction velocities and abnormal muscle electrical activity.
- Lumbar puncture: Analysis of cerebrospinal fluid (CSF) may show an elevated protein level without an increase in white blood cells (albuminocytologic dissociation), which is a typical finding in GBS.
- Imaging studies: MRIs are usually normal but may be performed to rule out other conditions that mimic GBS, such as spinal cord compression.

Treatment:
- Intravenous immunoglobulin (IVIG) and Plasma Exchange: The mainstays of treatment for GBS. These therapies help reduce the immune response and speed up recovery.

- **Supportive care**: Patients with severe weakness or respiratory involvement may require hospitalization and supportive measures such as mechanical ventilation, physical therapy, and pain management.
- **Monitoring**: Close monitoring of respiratory function, cardiac status, and autonomic function is essential, especially in severe cases.

9.18. Myasthenia Gravis

> ➢ *Myasthenia Gravis is an autoimmune disorder characterized by weakness and rapid fatigue of voluntary muscles, worsening with activity and improving with rest.*
> ➢ *It's caused by antibodies blocking or destroying nicotinic acetylcholine receptors at the neuromuscular junction.*
> ➢ *Treatment options include medications, thymectomy, and supportive therapies to manage symptoms and improve quality of life.*

Symptoms:
- Muscle Weakness: The most common symptom, which may worsen with activity and improve with rest.
- Weakness in Arms, Legs, Neck, and Fingers.
- Ptosis: Drooping of one or both eyelids.
- Diplopia: Double vision.
- Facial Paralysis: Difficulty in facial expressions like smiling or frowning.
- Dysphagia: Leading to choking or gagging.
- Dysarthria: Speech may be soft or nasal.
- Shortness of Breath: Due to weakness of the muscles that control breathing.

Causes and Risk Factors:
- Autoimmune disorder patients are at a higher risk.
- Thymus Gland Abnormalities: Such as thymoma or thymic hyperplasia.
- Gender and Age: Women under 40 and men over 60 are more commonly affected.
- Genetics: A family history of MG may increase risk.

Epidemiology
- MG can occur at any age, but it most commonly begins for women in their *20s and 30s* and for men in their *50s and 60s*.
- Its prevalence varies geographically, but it is estimated to affect about 20 per 100,000 people in the population.
- The condition does not discriminate by race or ethnicity.

Workup and Diagnosis
- Antibody Blood Tests: To check for antibodies that may be attacking the neurotransmitter acetylcholine or muscle-specific kinase (MuSK).
- Edrophonium Test: Injection of a drug that temporarily increases the levels of acetylcholine at the neuromuscular junction.
- Electromyography (EMG): To measure the electrical activity of muscles.
- Ice Pack Test: For patients with ptosis, applying an ice pack may temporarily improve muscle strength.
- Imaging Tests: Such as MRI or CT scans to check for thymoma.
- Pulmonary Function Tests: To evaluate the respiratory muscle strength.

Treatment
- Medications: Such as anticholinesterase agents (e.g., pyridostigmine) to improve neuromuscular transmission, and immunosuppressive drugs to decrease antibody production.
- Thymectomy: Surgical removal of the thymus gland, which may improve symptoms in some patients, especially those with a thymoma.
- Plasmapheresis and Intravenous Immunoglobulin (IVIG): These can be used for individuals in myasthenic crisis or as a rapid short-term treatment for severe symptoms.
- Lifestyle Changes and Support: Adjustments to daily activities, diet, and physical therapy can help manage symptoms.

9.19. Other Neuromuscular Disorders

> ➢ *Neuromuscular disorders encompass a broad range of conditions that affect the muscles and the nervous system that controls them, leading to muscle weakness, fatigue, and loss of muscle control.*
> ➢ *These disorders can be genetic or acquired, affecting people of all ages, and range from mild to life-threatening.*
> ➢ *Diagnosis and treatment vary depending on the specific condition, but may include medication, physical therapy, and surgical interventions.*

Symptoms:
- Muscle weakness:
    - Weakness in the limbs, face, or other muscle groups is a common symptom of neuromuscular disorders.
    - For example, progressive muscle weakness could be a symptom of Duchenne Muscular Dystrophy (DMD) or Becker Muscular Dystrophy
- Muscle atrophy: Progressive loss of muscle mass may occur in affected areas.
- Fasciculations: Visible twitching or spontaneous contractions of muscle fibers may be observed.
- Muscle cramps and stiffness: Painful cramps and stiffness may occur, particularly after exertion.
- Fatigue: Generalized fatigue and weakness may be present, especially with prolonged activity.
- Sensory symptoms: Some neuromuscular disorders may also involve sensory disturbances such as numbness, tingling, or pain.

Risk Factors:
- Genetic factors:
    - Many neuromuscular disorders have a genetic basis and may run in families.
    - Mutations in specific genes can predispose patients to these conditions.
- Environmental factors: Exposure to certain toxins, chemicals, or infections may increase the risk of developing some neuromuscular disorders.
- Age: Some neuromuscular disorders may have an onset in childhood or adolescence, while others may develop later in adulthood.

Epidemiology:
- The prevalence and incidence of neuromuscular disorders vary widely depending on the specific condition.
- Some neuromuscular disorders, such as Duchenne muscular dystrophy, are relatively rare, while others, such as peripheral neuropathy, are more common.
- Certain neuromuscular disorders may have a higher prevalence in specific populations or ethnic groups.

Diagnosis:
- Clinical evaluation: Diagnosis of a neuromuscular disorder typically involves a thorough medical history, physical examination, and assessment of symptoms.
- Electrophysiological studies: Tests such as electromyography (EMG) and nerve conduction studies (NCS) can help evaluate the function of nerves and muscles.
- Imaging studies: Imaging techniques such as MRI may be used to assess the structure of the nerves, muscles, and surrounding tissues.
- Genetic testing: Molecular genetic testing may be performed to identify specific gene mutations associated with inherited neuromuscular disorders.
- Laboratory tests: Blood tests may be conducted to assess levels of specific enzymes or proteins that can indicate muscle damage or dysfunction.

Treatment:
- Treatment of neuromuscular disorders varies depending on the underlying cause and specific symptoms.
- Medications: Some neuromuscular disorders may be treated with medications to manage symptoms, slow disease progression, or modify the immune response.
- Physical therapy: Exercise programs and physical therapy can help maintain muscle strength, flexibility, and function.
- Assistive devices: Devices such as braces, orthotics, wheelchairs, or mobility aids may be recommended to improve mobility and independence.
- Supportive care: Palliative care and supportive measures such as pain management, respiratory support, and nutritional support may be provided to improve quality of life and manage complications.

9.20. Neuralgia

> ➤ *Neuralgia refers to severe pain along the course of a nerve, due to nerve damage or irritation, manifesting as sharp, shooting, or burning sensations.*
>
> ➤ *It can be triggered by a variety of factors, including infections, diabetes, nerve pressure, or trauma.*
>
> ➤ *Treatment often involves medications for pain relief, nerve blocks, and addressing the underlying cause to prevent further nerve damage.*

Symptoms:
- Sharp, stabbing, or burning pain along the path of a nerve
- Sensitivity to touch or pressure in the affected area
- Pain that may be intermittent or constant
- Numbness or tingling sensations
- Muscle weakness or paralysis in severe cases

Risk Factors:
- Previous nerve injury or damage
- Certain medical conditions such as diabetes, multiple sclerosis, or postherpetic neuralgia.
- Aging, as neuralgia is more common in older adults
- Trauma or surgery affecting nerves
- Infections such as herpes zoster or Lyme disease

Epidemiology:
- Neuralgia can affect patients of any age, but it is more common in older adults.
- Certain types of neuralgia, such as trigeminal neuralgia, are more prevalent in females and patients over the age of 50.

Diagnosis:
- <u>Medical history and physical examination</u>: A detailed history of symptoms and a thorough physical examination can help diagnose neuralgia.
- <u>Imaging tests:</u> MRI or CT scans may be ordered to visualize the affected nerve and rule out other potential causes of pain, such as tumors or structural abnormalities.

- Nerve conduction studies (NCS) and electromyography (EMG): These tests may be performed to assess nerve function and identify areas of nerve damage or dysfunction.

Treatment:
- Medications:
    - *Anticonvulsants*: Drugs such as carbamazepine or gabapentin may help relieve nerve pain by stabilizing nerve cell membranes.
    - *Antidepressants*: Tricyclic antidepressants like amitriptyline or selective serotonin and norepinephrine reuptake inhibitors (SSNRIs) such as duloxetine may be prescribed to alleviate neuropathic pain.
    - *Topical agents*: Capsaicin cream or lidocaine patches applied to the affected area may provide relief.
- Nerve blocks: Local anesthetic injections may be administered around the affected nerve to temporarily block pain signals.
- Physical therapy: Techniques such as massage, stretching, and exercises may help improve muscle strength and reduce nerve-related pain.
- Surgery: In cases of severe or refractory neuralgia, surgical procedures such as microvascular decompression or nerve ablation may be considered to alleviate pressure on the affected nerve or interrupt pain signals.
- Lifestyle modifications:
    - Stress reduction techniques such as meditation or relaxation exercises may help manage neuralgia symptoms.
    - Avoiding triggers such as cold temperatures, certain foods, or activities that exacerbate pain can help minimize discomfort.

9.21. Carpal Tunnel Syndrome

> ➤ *Carpal Tunnel Syndrome (CTS) is a condition resulting from pressure on the median nerve in the wrist, leading to numbness, tingling, and weakness in the hand and arm.*
>
> ➤ *It's often caused by repetitive motions or anatomical differences that narrow the carpal tunnel.*
>
> ➤ *Treatment ranges from wrist splinting and anti-inflammatory medications to surgical intervention in severe cases.*

Symptoms:
- Numbness or tingling: Patients with CTS often experience numbness or tingling sensations, typically in the thumb, index finger, middle finger, and half of the ring finger.
- Pain or discomfort:
  - Pain may radiate from the wrist up the arm or down into the palm or fingers.
  - It may worsen at night or with certain activities that involve flexing or extending the wrist.
- Weakness: Weakness or clumsiness in the hand may occur due to muscle atrophy or impaired nerve function.
- Sensory changes: Some patients may experience a sensation of swelling or stiffness in the fingers, despite no actual swelling being present.

Risk Factors:
- Repetitive hand and wrist movements: Activities that involve repetitive hand and wrist movements, such as typing, assembly line work, or playing musical instruments, can increase the risk of CTS.
- Prolonged or forceful hand use: Jobs or hobbies that require prolonged or use of the hands or wrists may contribute to the development of CTS.
- Medical conditions: Certain medical conditions such as obesity, diabetes, rheumatoid arthritis, thyroid disorders, and pregnancy may increase the risk of CTS.
- Anatomy: Patients with smaller carpal tunnels or certain anatomical variations may be more prone to developing CTS.

Epidemiology:
- CTS is one of the most common nerve compression disorders, affecting millions of patients worldwide.
- It is more common in women than men, and the prevalence increases with age.
- Certain occupations that involve repetitive hand movements or use of vibrating tools have a higher incidence of CTS.

Workup and Diagnosis:
- <u>Clinical evaluation</u>: Diagnosis of CTS typically involves a detailed medical history, physical examination, and assessment of symptoms.
- <u>Nerve conduction studies (NCS) and electromyography (EMG)</u>: These tests measure the speed and strength of electrical signals traveling

along the median nerve and can help confirm the diagnosis of CTS and assess its severity.
- Tinel's sign and Phalen's maneuver: These physical tests may reproduce symptoms of CTS and aid in diagnosis.

Treatment:
- Conservative management:
  - *Wrist splinting*: Wearing a splint at night to keep the wrist in a neutral position can help relieve symptoms by reducing pressure on the median nerve.
  - *Activity modification*: Avoiding activities that exacerbate symptoms or taking frequent breaks can help reduce strain on the wrist.
  - *Nonsteroidal anti-inflammatory drugs (NSAIDs)*: Over-the-counter NSAIDs may help alleviate pain and inflammation.
- Corticosteroid injections: Injections of corticosteroids into the carpal tunnel can help reduce inflammation and relieve symptoms, although the effects are usually temporary.
- Surgical intervention:
  - *Carpal tunnel release surgery*: In cases of severe or persistent symptoms, surgical release of the transverse carpal ligament may be recommended to relieve pressure on the median nerve.

9.22. Restless Legs Syndrome

> ➤ *Restless Legs Syndrome (RLS) is a neurological disorder characterized by an irresistible urge to move the legs.*
> ➤ *Symptoms typically worsen during periods of inactivity or at night, leading to disrupted sleep and significant discomfort.*
> ➤ *Treatment options may include lifestyle changes, medications, and management of underlying conditions.*

Symptoms:
- Unpleasant sensations: such as crawling, tingling, itching, or burning in the legs, typically occurring in the evening or at night.
- Urge to move legs: These uncomfortable sensations provoke an irresistible urge to move the legs to alleviate the discomfort, which temporarily relieves the symptoms.

- Worsening with rest: Symptoms typically worsen during periods of rest or inactivity, such as sitting or lying down, and are often relieved by movement or activity.
- Disruption of sleep: RLS symptoms can significantly disrupt sleep, leading to insomnia and daytime fatigue.

Risk Factors:
- Family history: RLS tends to run in families, suggesting a genetic component to the disorder.
- Age: RLS can develop at any age but is more common in middle-aged and older adults, with symptoms often worsening with age.
- Gender: Women are more likely than men to develop RLS, particularly during pregnancy.
- Certain medical conditions: Conditions such as iron deficiency anemia, kidney failure, peripheral neuropathy, diabetes, and Parkinson's disease are associated with an increased risk of RLS.
- Medications: Certain medications, such as antipsychotics, antidepressants, antihistamines, and anti-nausea drugs, may worsen RLS symptoms.

Epidemiology:
- RLS is a relatively common disorder, with prevalence estimates varying depending on the population studied and diagnostic criteria used.
- It affects both men and women but is more common in women, particularly during pregnancy.
- The prevalence of RLS tends to increase with age.

Diagnosis:
- Diagnosis of RLS is typically based on clinical evaluation and the presence of specific criteria established by the International Restless Legs Syndrome Study Group (IRLSSG).
- The diagnosis is primarily clinical and based on a patient's description of symptoms and medical history.
- In some cases, additional tests such as blood tests to assess iron levels and ruling out other conditions may be performed.

Treatment:
- <u>Lifestyle modifications:</u> Strategies such as regular exercise, avoiding caffeine and alcohol, establishing a regular sleep schedule, and practicing relaxation techniques may help alleviate symptoms.

- **Medications**: Several medications may be prescribed to manage RLS symptoms, including dopaminergic agents (e.g., pramipexole, ropinirole), alpha-2-delta ligands (e.g., gabapentin, pregabalin), opioids, and benzodiazepines.
- <u>Iron supplementation</u>: For patients with iron deficiency anemia or low ferritin levels, iron supplementation may be recommended to improve symptoms.
- <u>Other therapies:</u> In some cases, treatments such as pneumatic compression devices, transcutaneous electrical nerve stimulation (TENS), or acupuncture may provide relief.

9.23. Essential Tremor

> ➤ *Essential Tremor (ET) is a common neurological disorder causing rhythmic shaking, typically affecting the hands but can involve other body parts.*
>
> ➤ *It often worsens with movement or stress, impacting daily tasks such as writing or eating.*
>
> ➤ *While medications and lifestyle adjustments can help manage symptoms, severe cases may require surgical interventions like deep brain stimulation.*

Symptoms:
- Involuntary shaking: The hallmark symptom of essential tremor is a rhythmic shaking movement, usually occurring during voluntary muscle contractions or when maintaining a particular posture.
- Tremor location: Essential tremor commonly affects the hands, causing trembling or shaking movements that may impair fine motor tasks such as writing, eating, or holding objects steady.
- Tremor severity:
    - The severity of tremor can vary widely among patients, ranging from mild to severe.
    - Tremor frequency may also fluctuate over time.
- Other potential symptoms: In addition to hand tremor, essential tremor may also affect the arms, head (including a "yes-yes" or "no-no" motion), voice (resulting in a shaky or quivering voice), legs, or other parts of the body.

Risk Factors:
- Genetic predisposition:

- Essential tremor often runs in families, suggesting a genetic component to the disorder.
  - Patients with a family history of essential tremor are at higher risk of developing the condition.
- Age: Essential tremor typically begins in middle age or later, although it can occur at any age.
- Other medical conditions: Certain medical conditions or factors may exacerbate essential tremor, including hyperthyroidism, Parkinson's disease, anxiety, caffeine consumption, and stress.

Epidemiology:
- Essential tremor is one of the most common movement disorders, affecting an estimated 0.4% to 5% of the population worldwide.
- It can occur at any age but is more common in older adults, with prevalence increasing with advancing age.
- Essential tremor affects both men and women, although some studies suggest a slightly higher prevalence in men.

Tremor Classification:
- Rest Tremor: Present when the affected body part is at rest and typically associated with Parkinson's disease.
- Action Tremor: Occurs during voluntary muscle contraction and can be further classified into subtypes such as:
  - *Postural Tremor:* Present when maintaining a position against gravity, like holding the arms outstretched.
  - *Kinetic Tremor*: Evident during voluntary movements, such as reaching for an object.
  - *Intention Tremor*: Occurs during precise movements towards a target, worsening as the target is approached.
- Task-Specific Tremor: Activated by specific tasks or activities, like writing or speaking.
- Physiological Tremor: A normal tremor that can be induced by factors such as fatigue, caffeine intake, or stress, and is not associated with any neurological disorder.

Diagnosis:
- Diagnosis of essential tremor is typically based on clinical evaluation, medical history, and physical examination.
- There are no specific diagnostic tests for essential tremor, but diagnostic criteria may include the presence of a bilateral action

tremor (i.e., tremor occurring during voluntary movement) affecting the arms or other body parts.
- Differential diagnosis: Essential tremor must be distinguished from other movement disorders such as Parkinson's disease, dystonia, or tremor associated with medications or other medical conditions.

Treatment:
- Medications: Medications such as beta-blockers (e.g., propranolol) and anticonvulsants (e.g., primidone) may be prescribed to reduce tremor severity in some patients.
- Deep brain stimulation (DBS): For patients with severe or disabling tremor that does not respond to medication, surgical options such as deep brain stimulation (DBS) may be considered.
- Lifestyle modifications: Strategies such as avoiding caffeine and other tremor-triggering substances, reducing stress, and getting adequate rest may help alleviate tremor symptoms.
- Occupational therapy: Occupational therapy techniques such as adaptive devices, ergonomic modifications, and assistive technology may help patients manage daily tasks affected by tremor.

9.24. Depression

> *Depression is a common mental health disorder characterized by persistent sadness, loss of interest in activities, and a range of physical and emotional problems.*
> *It significantly affects a person's daily life, including work and relationships.*
> *Treatment typically involves a combination of psychotherapy, medication, and lifestyle changes.*

Symptoms:
- Persistent Sadness or Low Mood: A deep, ongoing sense of sadness that does not lift.
- Loss of Interest or Pleasure: In activities that were once enjoyed.
- Changes in Appetite: Significant weight loss or gain unrelated to dieting.
- Sleep Disturbances: Insomnia or excessive sleeping.
- Fatigue or Loss of Energy: Feeling tired all the time.

- Feelings of Worthlessness or Excessive Guilt: Harsh criticism of perceived faults and mistakes.
- Difficulty Concentrating: Trouble focusing, making decisions, or remembering things.
- Physical Symptoms: Unexplained aches and pains.
- Thoughts of Death or Suicide: Frequent or recurrent thoughts of death, suicidal ideation, or suicide attempts.

Risk Factors:
- Genetics: Family history of depression.
- Brain Chemistry: Imbalances in neurotransmitters.
- Personality: Traits such as low self-esteem or being overly dependent, self-critical, or pessimistic.
- Environmental Factors: Continuous exposure to violence, neglect, abuse, or poverty.
- Life Events: Such as the death of a loved one, a difficult relationship, financial problems, or any stressful situation.
- Medical Conditions: Chronic illness, insomnia, chronic pain, or ADHD.
- Substance Use: Abuse of alcohol or drugs.

Epidemiology:
- Depression is a widespread condition affecting millions globally, making it one of the most common mental health disorders.
- It can occur at any age, but often begins in adulthood.
- Depression is more prevalent in women than in men.
- Various factors, including changes in societal roles and stress levels, contribute to its epidemiology.

Diagnosis:
- Clinical Evaluation: Per DSM-5 (Diagnostic and Statistical Manual of Mental Disorders, Fifth Edition) criteria, a patient must experience at least five of the following symptoms during the same 2-week period, and at least one of the symptoms should be either (1) depressed mood or (2) loss of interest or pleasure.
    - Depressed mood most of the day, nearly every day, as indicated by either subjective report.
    - Markedly diminished interest or pleasure in all, or almost all, activities most of the day, nearly every day.
    - Significant weight loss when not dieting or weight gain.
    - Insomnia or hypersomnia nearly every day.

- Psychomotor agitation or retardation nearly every day.
- Fatigue or loss of energy nearly every day.
- Feelings of worthlessness or excessive or inappropriate guilt (which may be delusional) nearly every day.
- Diminished ability to think or concentrate, or indecisiveness, nearly every day.
- Recurrent thoughts of death (not just fear of dying), recurrent suicidal ideation without a specific plan, or a suicide attempt or a specific plan for committing suicide.
- Screening Tools: Such as the Patient Health Questionnaire (PHQ-9), which is widely used.
- Physical Examination and Tests: To rule out other medical conditions that might cause similar symptoms.

Treatment:
- Psychotherapy: Cognitive Behavioral Therapy (CBT) and Interpersonal Therapy (IPT) are effective treatments.
- Medications: Antidepressants, such as SSRIs (Selective Serotonin Reuptake Inhibitors), can be effective in managing symptoms.
- Lifestyle Modifications: Regular exercise, a healthy diet, and adequate sleep can help manage symptoms.
- Support Groups: Offer emotional support and shared experiences.
- Electroconvulsive Therapy (ECT): For severe depression that does not respond to other treatments.
- Integrated Care: A combination of treatments tailored to the individual's condition, including monitoring and adjusting treatments as needed.

9.25. General Anxiety Disorder

> ➢ *Generalized Anxiety Disorder (GAD) is characterized by excessive, uncontrollable worry about everyday matters, leading to physical symptoms like restlessness, fatigue, and muscle tension.*
>
> ➢ *It affects daily functioning and can significantly impair social, occupational, and other important areas of life.*
>
> ➢ *Treatment typically involves psychotherapy, especially cognitive behavioral therapy, medication, and lifestyle changes.*

Symptoms:
- Excessive Worry: Chronic, exaggerated worry about everyday activities and events, often disproportionate to the actual source of stress.
- Restlessness or Feeling on Edge: Difficulty relaxing, feeling constantly tense.
- Fatigue: Easily tired despite low activity levels.
- Concentration Problems: Difficulty focusing or mind going blank.
- Irritability: More prone to agitation than usual.
- Muscle Tension: Persistent muscle aches or soreness.
- Sleep Disturbances: Trouble falling asleep, staying asleep, or unsatisfactory sleep.

Risk Factors:
- Genetics: Family history of anxiety or other mental health disorders.
- Brain Chemistry: Imbalances in neurotransmitters or differences in brain functioning.
- Personality: Traits of shyness or behavioral inhibition in childhood, low self-esteem, and increased sensitivity to stress.
- Life Events: Traumatic or negative experiences, especially in childhood, or a history of stressful or traumatic events in adulthood.
- Health Conditions: Chronic health conditions or other mental health disorders, such as depression.

Epidemiology:
- GAD affects millions worldwide and can occur at any age, though the risk is highest between childhood and middle age.
- It's more common in women than in men.
- Prevalence rates can vary by country and population, with lifetime prevalence estimates around 5-9% in more developed countries.

Diagnosis:
- <u>Clinical Assessment</u>: Diagnosis is based on patient history, symptomatology, and the exclusion of other mental health disorders. The DSM-5 criteria include excessive anxiety and worry on more days than not for at least six months, about a number of activities or events.
- <u>Psychological Questionnaires</u>: May be used to assess the severity of anxiety and to screen for other anxiety or mood disorders.

- **Physical Examination:** To rule out medical conditions that could mimic or worsen symptoms of anxiety.

Treatment:
- Psychotherapy: Cognitive-behavioral therapy (CBT) is highly effective, focusing on teaching specific skills to manage worry and anxiety.
- Medications: Antidepressants (SSRIs and SNRIs) are commonly used. Benzodiazepines may be used short-term for acute anxiety symptoms, but they are not recommended for long-term management due to the risk of dependence.
- Lifestyle Modifications: Includes stress management techniques, regular physical activity, adequate sleep, and reduction of caffeine and alcohol intake.
- Support Groups: Can provide additional emotional support and coping strategies.

9.26. Panic Disorder

> ➤ *Panic Disorder is marked by recurrent unexpected panic attacks—sudden periods of intense fear or discomfort, along with physical symptoms such as heart palpitations, sweating, and trembling.*
>
> ➤ *It often leads to persistent worry about future attacks and changes in behavior to avoid triggers.*
>
> ➤ *Treatment includes psychotherapy, particularly cognitive behavioral therapy, medication, and lifestyle modifications.*

Symptoms:
- Panic Attacks: Sudden episodes of intense fear or discomfort peaking within minutes, including palpitations, pounding heart, or accelerated heart rate.
- Sweating, Trembling, or Shaking: Physical symptoms that occur unexpectedly and without an obvious cause.
- Shortness of Breath or Smothering Sensations: Feeling as though you can't breathe deeply enough.
- Feelings of Choking: Sensation of choking without a physical blockage.
- Chest Pain or Discomfort: Often mistaken for a heart attack.
- Nausea or Abdominal Distress: Gastrointestinal discomfort.

- Dizziness, Lightheadedness, or Faintness: Feeling unsteady, dizzy, or faint.
- Fear of Losing Control or "Going Crazy"
- Fear of Dying: Intense fear that the attack will lead to death.
- Numbness or Tingling Sensations (Paresthesias)
- Chills or Hot Flashes

Risk Factors:
- Family History: Genetic predisposition to anxiety disorders.
- Stressful Life Events: Traumatic events or significant life changes.
- Temperament: Traits of sensitivity to stress or negative emotions.
- Other Mental Health Disorders: Co-occurring conditions such as depression.
- Substance Use: Abuse of drugs or alcohol can increase vulnerability.

Epidemiology:
- Panic disorder affects about 2-3% of adults in the United States each year, with women being twice as likely as men to have the disorder.
- It can begin in adolescence or early adulthood, but not everyone who experiences panic attacks will develop panic disorder.

Diagnosis:
- <u>Clinical Evaluation</u>: DSM-5 criteria require recurrent unexpected panic attacks and at least one of the attacks has been followed by one month (or more) of one or both of the following: persistent concern or worry about additional panic attacks or their consequences, a significant maladaptive change in behavior related to the attacks.
- <u>Rule Out Medical Conditions</u>: It's important to exclude medical conditions that can mimic panic disorder, such as thyroid disorders, through physical examination and possibly laboratory tests.

Treatment:
- <u>Psychotherapy</u>: Cognitive Behavioral Therapy (CBT) is the most effective form, focusing on changing the thoughts and behaviors that lead to panic attacks.
- <u>Medications</u>:
    - Selective Serotonin Reuptake Inhibitors (SSRIs) are typically the first choice in medication treatment.
    - Serotonin and Norepinephrine Reuptake Inhibitors (SNRIs) and Benzodiazepines might also be used.

- Lifestyle Modifications and Coping Strategies: Stress management techniques, regular physical exercise, avoiding caffeine, alcohol, and smoking can help reduce symptoms.
- Education: Understanding panic disorder can empower patients to manage their symptoms better.

9.27. Substance Use Disorder

> ➤ *Substance Use Disorder (SUD) is a condition characterized by an uncontrollable use of substances despite harmful consequences, leading to significant impairment in health, social, and occupational functioning.*
>
> ➤ *It encompasses a range of substances, including alcohol, nicotine, and illicit drugs.*
>
> ➤ *Treatment involves a combination of detoxification, behavioral therapies, medication, and support groups.*

Symptoms:

- Increased Tolerance: Needing more of the substance to achieve the same effect.
- Withdrawal Symptoms: Experiencing physical or psychological symptoms when not using the substance.
- Loss of Control: Using more of the substance or for longer than intended.
- Desire to Cut Down: Persistent desire or unsuccessful efforts to reduce or control substance use.
- Time Spent: A lot of time is spent obtaining, using, or recovering from the substance.
- Social Impairment: Continued use despite having persistent or recurrent social or interpersonal problems caused or exacerbated by the effects of the substance.
- Neglected Major Roles: Failure to fulfill major role obligations at work, school, or home due to substance use.
- Activities Given Up: Important social, occupational, or recreational activities are given up or reduced because of substance use.
- Hazardous Use: Use in situations in which it is physically hazardous.
- Continued Use Despite Problems: Continued substance use despite knowing it has caused or exacerbated physical or psychological problems.

- Craving: A strong desire or urge to use the substance.

Risk Factors:
- Genetic Predisposition: Family history of addiction.
- Environmental Influences: Peer pressure, lack of family involvement, and availability of drugs.
- Early Use: Starting drug use at an early age can increase the risk of developing SUD.
- Mental Health Disorders: Co-occurring disorders such as depression and anxiety can increase risk.
- Method of Use: Smoking or injecting drugs can increase addiction potential due to rapid onset of effects.

Epidemiology:
- Substance use disorders affect millions worldwide, with prevalence rates varying by substance, age, gender, and geography.
- Alcohol, nicotine, and illicit drugs are the most common substances involved.
- SUDs can start at any age but most commonly develop in adolescence and young adulthood.

Diagnosis:
- <u>Clinical Assessment:</u> Based on criteria outlined in the Diagnostic and Statistical Manual of Mental Disorders, Fifth Edition (DSM-5), which includes the symptoms listed above.
- <u>Screening Tools:</u> Instruments like the Alcohol Use Disorders Identification Test (AUDIT) or Drug Abuse Screening Test (DAST) can help identify individuals at risk.
- <u>Comprehensive Evaluation:</u> Includes a physical exam and often toxicology testing, along with an assessment of the individual's medical history, to rule out other conditions.

Treatment:
- <u>Detoxification:</u> The first step, usually under medical supervision, to safely withdraw from the substance.
- <u>Behavioral Therapies:</u> Cognitive-behavioral therapy, contingency management, motivational interviewing, and group therapy are effective in treating SUDs.
- <u>Medications:</u> Used to manage withdrawal symptoms, prevent relapse, or treat co-occurring disorders.

- **Support Groups:** Peer support from groups like Alcoholics Anonymous (AA) or Narcotics Anonymous (NA) can provide ongoing encouragement and guidance.
- **Comprehensive Care:** Treatment plans should address other possible mental health conditions and provide holistic support for recovery, including vocational and social rehabilitation.
- **Symptoms:** Dependence on substances (alcohol, prescription drugs, illicit drugs), impacting social, occupational, and health aspects of life.
- **Management:** Detoxification, counseling, support groups, and sometimes medication to reduce cravings.

9.28. Attention Deficit Hyperactivity Disorder

> ➤ *Attention Deficit Hyperactivity Disorder (ADHD) is a neurodevelopmental disorder characterized by patterns of inattention, hyperactivity, and impulsivity that impair functioning or development.*
> ➤ *It affects both children and adults, with symptoms often appearing in early childhood.*
> ➤ *Treatment typically involves medication, behavioral therapies, and educational support.*

Symptoms:

- Two types: (1) Inattention and (2) Hyperactivity-impulsivity
- **Inattention:**
    - Difficulty sustaining attention in tasks or play
    - Often does not seem to listen when spoken to directly
    - Struggles to follow through on instructions and fails to finish schoolwork or chores
    - Has difficulty organizing tasks and activities
    - Avoids or dislikes tasks that require sustained mental effort
    - Often loses things necessary for tasks and activities
    - Easily distracted by extraneous stimuli
    - Forgetful in daily activities
- **Hyperactivity-Impulsivity:**
    - Often fidgets with or taps hands or feet, or squirms in seat
    - Leaves seat in situations when remaining seated is expected

- Runs about or climbs in situations where it is inappropriate
- Unable to play or engage in leisure activities quietly
- Is often "on the go" or acts as if "driven by a motor"
- Talks excessively
- Blurts out answers before questions have been completed
- Has difficulty waiting their turn
- Interrupts or intrudes on others (e.g., butts into conversations or games)

Risk Factors:
- Genetics: Family history of ADHD or other mental health disorders.
- Environmental: Exposure to environmental toxins (e.g., lead) during pregnancy or at a young age.
- Developmental: Low birth weight, premature birth.
- Brain Structure and Function: Differences in certain areas of the brain that control attention, decision-making, and impulse control.

Epidemiology:
- ADHD is one of the most common neurodevelopmental disorders of childhood, with symptoms often first appearing between the ages of 3 and 6.
- It affects approximately 5% of children and 2.5% of adults worldwide.
- The condition is more frequently diagnosed in males than in females in childhood, though the gender gap may narrow in adulthood.

Diagnosis:
- Clinical Evaluation: Based on the American Psychiatric Association's Diagnostic and Statistical Manual of Mental Disorders, 5th edition (DSM-5) criteria.
  - *Inattention*: six (or more) of the following symptoms must have persisted for at least 6 months:
    - Often fails to give close attention to details or makes careless mistakes in schoolwork, work, or other activities.
    - Often has difficulty sustaining attention in tasks or play activities.
    - Often does not seem to listen when spoken to directly.
    - Often does not follow through on instructions and fails to finish schoolwork, chores, or duties in the workplace.

- Often has difficulty organizing tasks and activities.
            - Often avoids, dislikes, or is reluctant to engage in tasks that require sustained mental effort.
            - Often loses things necessary for tasks and activities.
            - Is often easily distracted by extraneous stimuli.
            - Is often forgetful in daily activities.
        - *Hyperactivity and Impulsivity*: six (or more) of the following symptoms must have persisted for at least 6 months:
            - Often fidgets with or taps hands or feet or squirms in seat.
            - Often leaves the seat in situations when remaining seated is expected.
            - Often runs about or climbs in situations where it is inappropriate.
            - Often unable to play or engage in leisure activities quietly.
            - Is often "on the go," acting as if "driven by a motor."
            - Often talks excessively.
            - Often blurts out an answer before a question has been completed.
            - Often has difficulty waiting his or her turn.
            - Often interrupts or intrudes on others.
- <u>Parent and Teacher Reports</u>: Often used to gather information on the child's behavior across different settings.
- <u>Physical Examination:</u> To rule out other possible causes of symptoms.

Treatment:
- <u>Medication</u>:
    - Stimulant medications (e.g., methylphenidate, amphetamines) are commonly used to improve symptoms of inattention and hyperactivity.
    - Non-stimulant medications may also be used.
- <u>Behavioral Therapy</u>: Especially for younger children, focusing on behavior management strategies for parents and teachers.
- <u>Psychoeducation</u>: Teaching individuals with ADHD and their families about the condition and how to manage symptoms.

- Cognitive Behavioral Therapy (CBT): For adults with ADHD to improve time management, organization, and planning skills.

9.29. Bipolar Disorder

> ➢ *Bipolar disorder is a mental health condition characterized by extreme mood swings, including emotional highs (mania or hypomania) and lows (depression).*
> ➢ *It affects a person's energy, activity levels, judgment, and ability to think clearly.*
> ➢ *Treatment typically involves a combination of medication, psychotherapy, and lifestyle changes to manage symptoms and prevent relapse.*

Symptoms:
- Manic episodes include:
    - Elevated or irritable mood
    - Over-activity, increased energy
    - Reduced need for sleep
    - Grandiosity or inflated self-esteem
    - Increased talkativeness
    - Racing thoughts
    - Poor judgment leading to risky behavior
    - Possible psychotic symptoms (delusions or hallucinations)
- Depressive episodes include:
    - Persistent sad, anxious, or "empty" mood
    - Feelings of hopelessness or pessimism
    - Irritability
    - Loss of interest in activities once enjoyed
    - Fatigue or loss of energy
    - Changes in sleep patterns
    - Changes in weight or appetite
    - Thoughts of death or suicide

Risk Factors:
- Genetics: A family history of bipolar disorder is the most significant risk factor.

- Brain Structure and Function: Changes in the brain's structure and neurotransmitter imbalances.
- Environmental: Stressful life events, trauma, and substance abuse.

Epidemiology:
- Bipolar disorder affects about 1% to 2.5% of the global population, with nearly equal prevalence among men and women.
- The condition typically begins in late adolescence or early adulthood.

Diagnosis:
- Clinical Evaluation: Diagnosis is based on the person's history of symptoms, including the severity, length, and frequency of manic and depressive episodes.
- Physical Examination: To rule out other medical conditions that might be causing similar symptoms of bipolar.
- DSM-5 Criteria: Divided primarily into Bipolar I Disorder, Bipolar II Disorder.
- Bipolar I Disorder:
    - Criteria have been met for at least one manic episode.
    - The manic episode may have been preceded by and may be followed by hypomanic or major depressive episodes.
- Manic Episode:
    - A distinct period of abnormally and persistently elevated, expansive, or irritable mood and abnormally and persistently increased goal-directed activity or energy, lasting at least one week (or any duration if hospitalization is necessary).
    - During the period of mood disturbance and increased energy or activity, three (or more) of the following symptoms (four if the mood is only irritable) are present to a significant degree and represent a noticeable change from usual behavior:
        - Inflated self-esteem or grandiosity.
        - Decreased need for sleep.
        - More talkative than usual or pressure to keep talking.
        - Flight of ideas or subjective experience that thoughts are racing.
        - Distractibility.
        - Increase in goal-directed activity or psychomotor agitation.

- - - Excessive involvement in activities that have a high potential for painful consequences.
  - The mood disturbance is sufficiently severe to cause marked impairment in social or occupational functioning or to necessitate hospitalization to prevent harm to self or others, or there are psychotic features.
- Bipolar II Disorder:
  - Criteria have been met for at least one hypomanic episode and at least one major depressive episode.
  - There has never been a manic episode.
- Hypomanic Episode:
  - A distinct period of abnormally and persistently elevated, expansive, or irritable mood and abnormally and persistently increased activity or energy, lasting at least four consecutive days and present most of the day, nearly every day.
  - The episode is not severe enough to cause marked impairment in social or occupational functioning or to necessitate hospitalization, and there are no psychotic features.
  - The episode represents a clear change in the person's usual behavior.
- Major Depressive Episode:
  - Five (or more) of the following symptoms have been present during the same 2-week period and represent a change from previous functioning; at least one of the symptoms is either (1) depressed mood or (2) loss of interest or pleasure.
    - Depressed mood most of the day, nearly every day.
    - Markedly diminished interest or pleasure in all, or almost all, activities most of the day, nearly every day.
    - Significant weight loss when not dieting, weight gain, or decrease or increase in appetite.
    - Insomnia or hypersomnia nearly every day.
    - Psychomotor agitation or retardation nearly every day.
    - Fatigue or loss of energy nearly every day.
    - Feelings of worthlessness or excessive or inappropriate guilt.
    - Diminished ability to think or concentrate, or indecisiveness.

> Recurrent thoughts of death, recurrent suicidal ideation without a specific plan, or a suicide attempt.

Treatment:

- Medication: Mood stabilizers (e.g., lithium, valproate), antipsychotics, and antidepressants can be used to control symptoms.
- Psychotherapy: Cognitive behavioral therapy (CBT), psychoeducation, and family therapy can help manage the disorder and prevent relapse.
- Lifestyle Modifications: Regular sleep patterns, avoiding substance abuse, and stress management are crucial.
- Electroconvulsive Therapy (ECT): For severe cases where medication and therapy have not been effective.

9.30. Post-Traumatic Stress Disorder

> *Post-Traumatic Stress Disorder (PTSD) is a psychiatric condition triggered by witnessing or experiencing a traumatic event, leading to symptoms like flashbacks, avoidance of trauma reminders, negative changes in thoughts and mood, and increased reactivity.*
>
> *It affects individuals of all ages and is diagnosed based on specific criteria including symptom duration and impact on functioning.*
>
> *Treatment typically involves psychotherapy, medication, and supportive care.*

Symptoms:

- Grouped into four categories:
    - *Intrusion:* Recurrent, involuntary, and intrusive distressing memories of the traumatic event, nightmares, flashbacks, and severe emotional distress or physical reactions to reminders of the traumatic event.
    - *Avoidance:* Persistent efforts to avoid thoughts, feelings, or conversations about the traumatic event, and avoidance of places, people, and activities that remind the person of the trauma.
    - *Negative alterations in cognition and mood:* Inability to remember important aspects of the traumatic event, negative beliefs about oneself or the world, distorted thoughts leading to blame of self or others, persistent negative emotional state,

- diminished interest in activities, feelings of detachment or estrangement, and inability to experience positive emotions.
    - *Arousal and reactivity:* Marked alterations in arousal and reactivity associated with the traumatic event, including irritable behavior and angry outbursts, reckless or self-destructive behavior, hypervigilance, exaggerated startle response, concentration problems, and sleep disturbance.

Risk Factors:
- Direct exposure to trauma as a victim or a witness.
- Personal history of mental illness or substance abuse.
- Lack of support after the trauma.
- Occupations that increase the risk of being exposed to traumatic events (military personnel, first responders).
- Gender, with women being more likely to develop PTSD than men.

Epidemiology:
- PTSD can affect individuals of any age, including children.
- The prevalence of PTSD varies widely, depending on the population studied and the methods used to assess PTSD.
- Studies suggest that about 6-9% of the general population will experience PTSD at some point in their lives, with higher rates in populations exposed to severe trauma.

Diagnosis:
- PTSD is diagnosed based on the Diagnostic and Statistical Manual of Mental Disorders, Fifth Edition (DSM-5), which requires that symptoms last for more than one month and cause significant distress or impairment in social, occupational, or other important areas of functioning.

Treatment:
- <u>Psychotherapy:</u> Especially effective treatments include cognitive-behavioral therapy (CBT), which encompasses various approaches like prolonged exposure therapy, cognitive processing therapy, and Eye Movement Desensitization and Reprocessing (EMDR).
- <u>Medications:</u> Antidepressants, particularly selective serotonin reuptake inhibitors (SSRIs) and serotonin-norepinephrine reuptake inhibitors (SNRIs), are commonly used to help alleviate symptoms of PTSD.
- <u>Supportive Care:</u> Peer support groups and education about the disorder can also be beneficial.

9.31. Obsessive-Compulsive Disorder

> ➤ *Obsessive-Compulsive Disorder (OCD) is characterized by persistent, unwanted thoughts (obsessions) and repetitive, ritualistic behaviors (compulsions) performed to alleviate the stress caused by these obsessions.*
>
> ➤ *It can significantly impair daily functioning and quality of life.*
>
> ➤ *Treatment typically involves a combination of cognitive-behavioral therapy, specifically exposure and response prevention, and medication, such as SSRIs.*

Symptoms:
- Obsessions are repetitive, unwanted, intrusive thoughts, images, or urges that cause distress or anxiety.
- Compulsions are repetitive behaviors or mental acts that a person feels driven to perform in response to an obsession or according to rules that must be applied rigidly, aimed at reducing distress or preventing some dreaded event or situation.

Risk Factors:
- Genetics: Family history of OCD increases risk.
- Brain Structure and Function: Changes in the body's natural chemistry or brain functions.
- Environmental Factors: Traumatic or stressful life events may trigger OCD in people with a predisposition toward the disorder.
- Behavioral Factors: Certain behaviors that increase or reinforce the anxiety or distress associated with obsessions can exacerbate the condition.

Epidemiology:
- OCD affects both adults and children.
- It is estimated that approximately 1-2% of the population will be diagnosed with OCD at some point in their lives, with roughly equal prevalence among men and women.
- Symptoms typically begin in adolescence or early adulthood, though they can start in childhood.

Diagnosis:
- <u>Clinical Diagnosis:</u> The DSM-5 criteria require that these obsessions and compulsions are time-consuming (e.g., take more than 1 hour

per day) or cause clinically significant distress or impairment in social, occupational, or other important areas of functioning.
- Differential Diagnosis: It's important to differentiate OCD from other mental health disorders, including anxiety disorders, depression, and tic disorders, among others.

Treatment:
- Cognitive Behavioral Therapy (CBT): Specifically, Exposure and Response Prevention (ERP) is considered the most effective form of psychotherapy for OCD.
- Medication: Selective Serotonin Reuptake Inhibitors (SSRIs) are commonly used to help manage OCD symptoms.
- Deep Brain Stimulation (DBS) and Transcranial Magnetic Stimulation (TMS): For severe cases not responding to conventional treatments.
- Support Groups and Education: Understanding OCD and connecting with others facing similar challenges can be beneficial.

9.32. Eating Disorders

> ➢ *Eating disorders are serious mental health conditions characterized by abnormal or disturbed eating habits, including Anorexia Nervosa, Bulimia Nervosa, and Binge-Eating Disorder.*
> ➢ *They stem from a complex mix of psychological, social, and biological factors, leading to severe consequences for health and well-being.*
> ➢ *Treatment often involves a multidisciplinary approach, including psychotherapy, nutritional counseling, and sometimes medication.*

Symptoms:
- Anorexia Nervosa: Restriction of food intake leading to a significantly low body weight, intense fear of gaining weight, and a distorted perception of body weight or shape.
- Bulimia Nervosa:
  - Recurrent episodes of binge eating followed by compensatory behaviors like vomiting, excessive exercise, or misuse of laxatives.
  - Individuals often feel a lack of control over their eating.
- Binge-Eating Disorder:

- Recurrent episodes of eating large quantities of food in a short period, a sense of lack of control during the episodes, and guilt or distress afterward.
- Unlike bulimia, there are no regular compensatory behaviors.

Risk Factors:
- Genetic Predisposition: Family history of eating disorders or other mental health disorders.
- Psychological Factors: Low self-esteem, perfectionism, impulsive behavior, and troubled relationships.
- Sociocultural Influences: Societal pressure to be thin, which can be intensified through media and cultural practices.
- Other Risk Factors: Early childhood trauma, bullying related to size or weight, and chronic dieting.

Epidemiology:
- Eating disorders affect people of all ages, racial/ethnic backgrounds, body weights, and genders.
- They commonly emerge during adolescence or young adulthood, but can also develop during childhood or later in life.
- Anorexia and Bulimia Nervosa are more prevalent among females, while Binge-Eating Disorder is more evenly distributed between genders.
- The lifetime prevalence of eating disorders varies, with estimates suggesting around 1-2% for Anorexia Nervosa, 1-3% for Bulimia Nervosa, and 1-5% for Binge-Eating Disorder in the general population.

Diagnosis:
- <u>Clinical Assessment</u>: Involves a detailed medical history, physical exam, and psychiatric evaluation based on DSM-5 criteria matched above symptoms.
- <u>Laboratory Tests</u>: May be used to rule out other medical conditions that mimic eating disorder symptoms or to identify complications.

Treatment:
- <u>Psychotherapy</u>: Cognitive-behavioral therapy (CBT) is the most effective treatment for Bulimia Nervosa and Binge-Eating Disorder. Anorexia Nervosa may require more intensive treatment, including hospitalization.
- <u>Nutritional Counseling and Support:</u> Essential for restoring healthy eating patterns and addressing misconceptions about food and diet.

- **Medication:** Can be used to treat co-occurring conditions like anxiety or depression but is not a primary treatment for Anorexia Nervosa.
- **Family-Based Treatment (FBT):** Particularly effective for adolescents with eating disorders, involving the family in treatment.

9.33. Insomnia

> ➢ *Insomnia is a common sleep disorder characterized by difficulty falling asleep, staying asleep, or obtaining restorative sleep, leading to daytime impairments such as fatigue and decreased performance.*
> ➢ *Risk factors include stress, mental health disorders, certain medical conditions, and lifestyle choices.*
> ➢ *Treatment often involves cognitive behavioral therapy for insomnia (CBT-I), medication for short-term relief, and lifestyle modifications to improve sleep hygiene.*

Symptoms:
- Difficulty falling asleep
- Difficulty staying asleep (including waking up frequently during the night or waking up early and being unable to return to sleep)
- Poor quality of sleep (non-restorative sleep)
- These difficulties occur despite adequate opportunity and circumstances for sleep, leading to daytime impairment or distress, such as fatigue, mood disturbances, decreased performance at work or school, and impaired social functioning.

Risk Factors:
- Age: Older adults are more likely to experience insomnia.
- Gender: Women are more likely to report insomnia symptoms.
- Psychological Stress: High levels of stress or traumatic events.
- Mental Health Disorders: Such as depression, anxiety, bipolar disorder, and others.
- Physical Conditions: Chronic pain, respiratory conditions, neurological diseases, hormonal changes (e.g., menopause), and other medical conditions.
- Substance Use: Consumption of caffeine, alcohol, nicotine, and certain medications.
- Lifestyle: Irregular sleep schedules, sedentary lifestyle, and poor sleep environment.

Epidemiology:
- Insomnia is the most common sleep disorder, affecting a significant portion of the adult population worldwide.
- Epidemiological studies suggest that about 10-30% of adults suffer from chronic insomnia, with higher rates observed in women and older adults.

Diagnosis:
- Clinical Interview: To gather comprehensive information about sleep habits, sleep environment, and daytime symptoms.
- Sleep Diary: Recording sleep and wake times to identify patterns or behaviors contributing to insomnia.
- Questionnaires: Such as the Insomnia Severity Index (ISI), to assess the severity of insomnia.
- Polysomnography (PSG) and Actigraphy: Rarely needed for diagnosis, but may be used to rule out other sleep disorders.

Treatment:
- Cognitive Behavioral Therapy for Insomnia (CBT-I): The first-line treatment, focusing on changing sleep habits and patterns of thought related to sleep.
- Medication: Used cautiously for short-term relief; includes non-benzodiazepine hypnotics, benzodiazepines, and certain antidepressants.
- Sleep Hygiene Education: Involves modifying lifestyle and environmental factors to promote better sleep (e.g., regular sleep schedule, comfortable sleep environment).
- Relaxation Techniques: Such as meditation, deep breathing exercises, and progressive muscle relaxation, to reduce bedtime anxiety and facilitate sleep onset.

9.34. Personality Disorders

> ➢ *Personality disorders are characterized by enduring, inflexible patterns of thinking, feeling, and behaving that deviate significantly from cultural expectations and cause distress or impairment.*
>
> ➢ *These disorders are categorized into three clusters based on similar characteristics and symptoms.*
>
> ➢ *Treatment typically involves psychotherapy, with medication used to manage specific symptoms or co-occurring conditions.*

Symptoms:
- Vary widely among the different types of personality disorders, which are grouped into three clusters:
    - Cluster A (Odd or Eccentric Disorders):
        - Including Paranoid, Schizoid, and Schizotypal Personality Disorders.
        - Symptoms include social awkwardness, social withdrawal, and distorted thinking.
    - Cluster B (Dramatic, Emotional, or Erratic Disorders):
        - Including Antisocial, Borderline, Histrionic, and Narcissistic Personality Disorders.
        - Symptoms involve impulsive and erratic behaviors, emotional instability, and exaggerated self-perception.
    - Cluster C (Anxious or Fearful Disorders):
        - Including Avoidant, Dependent, and Obsessive-Compulsive Personality Disorders.
        - Symptoms feature anxiety, fearfulness, and a pattern of dependent and perfectionist behaviors.

Risk Factors:
- Genetic: Family history of personality disorders or other mental health disorders.
- Environmental: Experiences of trauma, abuse, or neglect during childhood; unstable family life; loss; and cultural factors.
- Neurobiological: Changes in brain structure and function affecting emotion regulation, impulse control, and cognition.

Epidemiology:
- Personality disorders affect about 9-15% of the adult population.
- Prevalence varies by disorder and can be influenced by demographic factors such as age and gender.
- Cluster B disorders, for example, are more frequently diagnosed in younger individuals.

Diagnosis:
- <u>Clinical Assessment</u>: Diagnosis is based on a detailed interview, including a thorough history of symptoms and their impact on life functioning.

- **Diagnostic Criteria:** The DSM-5 provides specific criteria for each personality disorder, focusing on pervasive patterns of experience and behavior.
- **Psychological Evaluation:** May include questionnaires, self-assessments, and, in some cases, interviews with friends or family members.

Treatment

- **Psychotherapy:** The primary treatment method, especially Dialectical Behavior Therapy (DBT) for Borderline Personality Disorder, and other modalities like Cognitive Behavioral Therapy (CBT) and psychoanalytic therapy for other types.
- **Medication:** While there are no medications specifically approved to treat personality disorders, certain medications may help with symptoms or co-occurring conditions, such as depression or anxiety.
- **Support Groups:** Can provide additional support and coping strategies.
- **Lifestyle Modifications:** Encouraging healthy relationships, regular exercise, and adequate sleep can help improve symptoms.

References

- Dodick, D. W. (2018). A phase-by-phase review of migraine pathophysiology. Headache: The Journal of Head and Face Pain, 58(S1), 4-16.
- Jensen, R. (2019). Tension-type headache—The normal and most prevalent headache. Headache: The Journal of Head and Face Pain, 59(1), 114-115.
- Goadsby, P. J. (2018). Pathophysiology of cluster headache: A trigeminal autonomic cephalgia. The Lancet Neurology, 17(10), 858-868.
- Rizzoli, P. (2018). Acute and preventive treatment of migraine. Continuum: Lifelong Learning in Neurology, 24(4), 1032-1051.
- Easton, J. D., Saver, J. L., & et al. (2009). Definition and evaluation of transient ischemic attack: A scientific statement for healthcare professionals from the American Heart Association/American Stroke Association Stroke Council; Council on Cardiovascular Surgery and Anesthesia; Council on Cardiovascular Radiology and Intervention; Council on Cardiovascular Nursing; and the Interdisciplinary Council on Peripheral Vascular Disease. Stroke, 40(6), 2276-2293.
- Scheffer, I. E., Berkovic, S., & et al. (2017). ILAE classification of the epilepsies: Position paper of the ILAE Commission for Classification and Terminology. Epilepsia, 58(4), 512-521.

- England, J. D., & Gronseth, G. S. (2008). Practice parameter: Evaluation of distal symmetric polyneuropathy: Role of autonomic testing, nerve biopsy, and skin biopsy (an evidence-based review). Neurology, 69(9), 873-880.
- Thompson, A. J., Banwell, B. L., & et al. (2018). Diagnosis of multiple sclerosis: 2017 revisions of the McDonald criteria. The Lancet Neurology, 17(2), 162-173.
- Kalia, L. V., & Lang, A. E. (2015). Parkinson's disease. The Lancet, 386(9996), 896-912.
- Cummings, J., Lee, G., & et al. (2019). Alzheimer's disease drug development pipeline: 2019. Alzheimer's & Dementia: Translational Research & Clinical Interventions, 5, 272-293.
- Bhattacharyya, N., Gubbels, S. P., & et al. (2017). Clinical practice guideline: Benign paroxysmal positional vertigo (update). Otolaryngology–Head and Neck Surgery, 156(3_suppl), S1-S47.
- Nevoux, J., Barbara, M., & et al. (2018). International consensus (ICON) on treatment of Ménière's disease. European Annals of Otorhinolaryngology, Head and Neck Diseases, 135(1S), S29-S32.
- Brown, R. H., & Al-Chalabi, A. (2017). Amyotrophic lateral sclerosis. New England Journal of Medicine, 377(2), 162-172.
- Willison, H. J., & Jacobs, B. C. (2016). Guillain-Barré syndrome. The Lancet, 388(10045), 717-727.
- Gilhus, N. E. (2019). Myasthenia gravis. New England Journal of Medicine, 381(18), 1713-1723.
- Finsterer, J., & Grisold, W. (2016). Disorders of the peripheral nerves. Journal of Neurology, 263(1), 1-21.
- Benoliel, R., & Sharav, Y. (2012). Trigeminal neuralgia, neurovascular cross-compression, and habitual chewing. Muscle & Nerve, 46(6), 832-835.
- Padua, L., Coraci, D., & et al. (2016). Carpal tunnel syndrome: Clinical features, diagnosis, and management. The Lancet Neurology, 15(12), 1273-1284.
- Allen, R. P., Picchietti, D. L., & et al. (2014). Restless legs syndrome/Willis-Ekbom disease diagnostic criteria: Updated International Restless Legs Syndrome Study Group (IRLSSG) consensus criteria—history, rationale, description, and significance. Sleep Medicine, 15(8), 860-873.
- Bhatia, K. P., Bain, P., & et al. (2018). Consensus statement on the classification of tremors. from the task force on tremor of the International Parkinson and Movement Disorder Society. Movement Disorders, 33(1), 75-87.

Chapter 10: Rheumatologic and Musculoskeletal Disorders

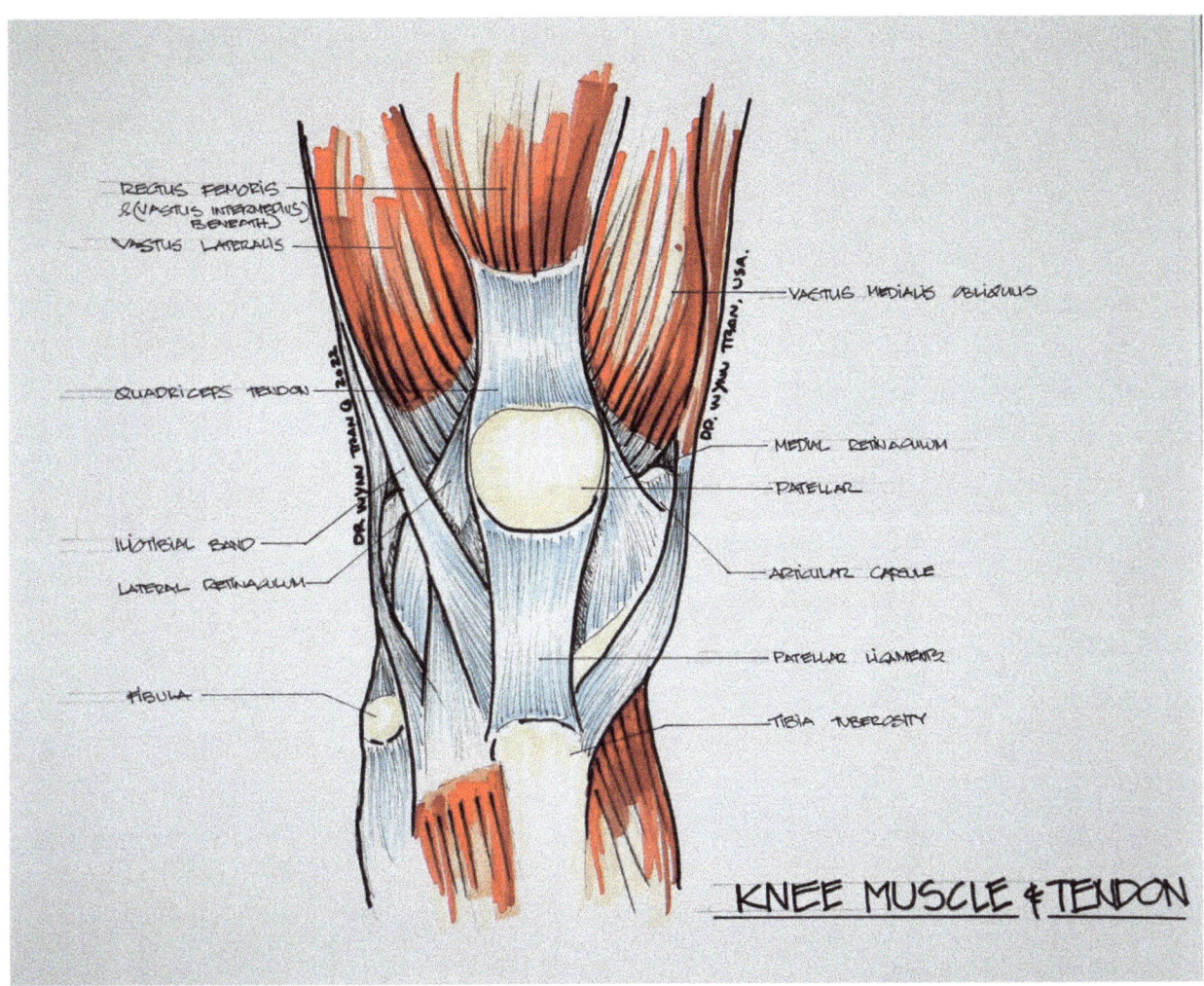

The APP should be familiar with the presentation, diagnosis, and management of these common musculoskeletal and rheumatologic disorders to provide appropriate care and referral to the rheumatologist when necessary.

10.1. Osteoarthritis

> ➢ *Osteoarthritis is a degenerative joint disease characterized by the breakdown of cartilage in the joints, leading to pain, stiffness, and reduced mobility.*
>
> ➢ *It commonly affects weight-bearing joints such as the knees, hips, and spine. Risk factors include aging, obesity, joint injuries, and genetics.*
>
> ➢ *Management involves a combination of lifestyle modifications, pain management, physical therapy, and in severe cases, surgical joint replacements.*

Symptoms

- Joint Pain: Osteoarthritis typically causes joint pain, which worsens with activity and improves with rest.
- Stiffness: Joints affected by osteoarthritis may feel stiff, especially in the morning or after periods of inactivity.
- Decreased Range of Motion: Osteoarthritis can lead to reduced flexibility and range of motion in the affected joints.
- Swelling: Inflammation and swelling may occur around the affected joints.
- Joint Deformity: Over time, osteoarthritis can cause changes in joint shape and structure, leading to deformities such as bony spurs or nodules.
- Grating Sensation: Some patients may experience a grating or crepitus when moving the affected joint.

Risk Factors

- Age: Osteoarthritis is more common in older adults, with the risk increasing with age.
- Gender: Women are more likely to develop osteoarthritis, particularly after menopause.
- Obesity: Excess body weight puts additional stress on weight-bearing joints such as the knees and hips, increasing the risk of osteoarthritis.
- Joint Injury: Previous joint injuries or trauma, such as fractures or ligament tears, can increase the risk of osteoarthritis in the affected joint.
- Genetics: Family history of osteoarthritis may predispose patients to develop the condition.

- Occupational Factors: Jobs or activities that involve repetitive stress on the joints, such as heavy lifting or kneeling, may increase the risk of osteoarthritis.
- Joint Alignment: Poor joint alignment or structural abnormalities can contribute to the development of osteoarthritis.
- Other Medical Conditions: Certain medical conditions, such as rheumatoid arthritis, gout, or metabolic disorders, may increase the risk of osteoarthritis.

Epidemiology
- Osteoarthritis is the most common form of arthritis and a leading cause of disability worldwide.
- It primarily affects weight-bearing joints such as the knees, hips, and spine, as well as the hands and fingers.
- Prevalence increases with age, with a significant proportion of older adults affected by osteoarthritis.
- It is estimated that more than 30 million adults in the United States have osteoarthritis.

Osteoarthritis Score
- Osteoarthritis severity can be assessed through various scoring systems, such as:
    - **Kellgren-Lawrence Radiology Grading Scale:** Classifies osteoarthritis severity based on X-ray findings, ranging from 0 (normal) to 4 (severe joint space narrowing, osteophyte formation, and sclerosis).
    - **WOMAC** (Western Ontario and McMaster Universities Arthritis Index): A patient-reported outcome measure assessing pain, stiffness, and physical function in osteoarthritis. The score typically ranges from 0 to 96, with higher scores indicating greater severity of osteoarthritis symptoms.
        - Pain: Score range typically from 0 to 20.
        - Stiffness: Score range typically from 0 to 8.
        - Physical Function: Score range typically from 0 to 68
    - **Lequesne Index:** Evaluates pain, maximum walking distance, and activities of daily living in patients with knee osteoarthritis. The scoring typically ranges from 0 to 24, with higher scores indicating more severe symptoms and functional limitations associated with knee osteoarthritis.

- ➢ Pain: Score range typically from 0 to 10, with higher scores indicating more severe pain.
- ➢ Maximum Walking Distance: Score range typically from 0 to 6, with higher scores indicating shorter walking distances.
- ➢ Activities of Daily Living: Scores range typically from 0 to 8, with higher scores indicating greater difficulty in performing daily activities.
  - ○ **OARSI** (Osteoarthritis Research Society International) Score: Incorporates imaging findings, pain, and function to assess osteoarthritis severity and progression.
  - ○ **ICOAP** (Intermittent and Constant Osteoarthritis Pain) Score: Assesses the frequency and severity of intermittent and constant pain in knee and hip osteoarthritis. The scoring for each subscale typically ranges from 0 to 100, with higher scores indicating greater pain severity and frequency.

Diagnosis

- Medical History and Physical Examination: The APP will assess symptoms, medical history, and perform a physical examination to evaluate joint function and mobility.
- Imaging Studies: X-rays, MRI, or CT scans may be ordered to visualize joint damage, cartilage loss, and other changes characteristic of osteoarthritis.
- Joint Fluid Analysis: In some cases, joint fluid analysis (arthrocentesis) may be performed to rule out other causes of joint pain or inflammation, such as infection or gout.

Treatment:

- Lifestyle Modifications: Weight management, regular exercise (including low-impact activities such as swimming or biking), and joint protection strategies can help reduce symptoms and improve joint function.
- Medications: Over-the-counter pain relievers such as acetaminophen or nonsteroidal anti-inflammatory drugs (NSAIDs) may provide relief from pain and inflammation. Topical treatments such as creams or patches containing NSAIDs or capsaicin may also be used.
- Physical Therapy: Physical therapy can help improve joint flexibility, strength, and function through targeted exercises and techniques.

- **Assistive Devices**: Braces, splints, or orthotic devices may be recommended to support and stabilize affected joints and reduce pain.
- **Injections**: Corticosteroid injections or hyaluronic acid injections (viscosupplementation) may be used to reduce inflammation and improve joint lubrication in certain cases.
- **Surgery**: In severe cases of osteoarthritis that do not respond to conservative treatments, surgical options such as joint replacement (arthroplasty) may be considered to alleviate pain and restore joint function.

10.1.1. Knee Osteoarthritis

Symptoms

- Persistent knee pain, worsening with activity, particularly with weight-bearing one or after prolonged periods of inactivity.
- Stiffness: Reduced range of motion and stiffness, especially after rest or in the morning.
- Swelling: Joint swelling or effusion, often due to inflammation or fluid accumulation.
- Crepitus: A grating or grinding sensation with movement, caused by friction between damaged knee joint surfaces.
- Instability: Feeling of knee instability or buckling, particularly during weight-bearing activities.
- Decreased Function: Difficulty walking, climbing stairs, or performing daily activities due to pain and joint dysfunction.

Risk Factors:

- Age: Older age is a significant risk factor, as knee OA becomes more prevalent with advancing age.
- Obesity: Excess body weight places increased stress on the knee joints, contributing to cartilage degeneration and OA progression.
- Joint Injury or Trauma: Previous knee injuries, such as ligament tears or fractures, elevate the risk of developing OA later in life.
- Joint Overuse: Repetitive stress on the knees from activities such as running, kneeling, or heavy lifting may accelerate joint degeneration.
- Genetics: Family history of OA or genetic predisposition may increase susceptibility to developing knee OA.
- Occupational Factors: Certain occupations involving repetitive kneeling, squatting, or heavy lifting may raise the risk of knee OA.

- Gender: Knee OA is more common in women, although the precise reasons for this gender disparity are not fully understood.

Diagnosis:

- Medical History and Physical Examination: Assessment of symptoms, functional limitations, knee joint tenderness, swelling, and range of motion.
- Imaging Studies: X-rays may reveal joint space narrowing, osteophyte formation, subchondral sclerosis, and other characteristic features of knee OA.
- Laboratory Tests: Blood tests are typically not necessary for diagnosing knee OA but may be performed to rule out other conditions or assess disease severity (e.g., inflammatory markers).

Treatment:

- Lifestyle Modifications: Weight loss, regular exercise (e.g., low-impact activities such as walking, swimming, cycling), and joint protection strategies.
- Physical Therapy: Strengthening exercises, stretching, and range-of-motion exercises to improve joint function and alleviate pain.
- Medications: Analgesics (e.g., acetaminophen), nonsteroidal anti-inflammatory drugs (NSAIDs), and intra-articular corticosteroid injections for pain management.
- Orthotic Devices: Shoe inserts, knee braces, or assistive devices to reduce joint stress and improve stability.
- Surgical Interventions: In cases of severe pain or functional impairment, surgical options such as arthroscopy, osteotomy, partial or total knee arthroplasty may be considered.

Disease Management:

- Knee OA is a chronic condition that requires long-term management aimed at reducing pain, preserving joint function, and improving quality of life.
- Regular follow-up visits with The APP to monitor disease progression, adjust treatment strategies, and address any complications or comorbidities.

10.1.2. Shoulder OA

Symptoms

- Pain: Persistent shoulder pain, particularly with movement or weight-bearing activities.

- Stiffness: Reduced range of motion, especially in external rotation and abduction.
- Crepitus: A grating or grinding sensation with shoulder movement.
- Weakness: Weakness or difficulty with activities requiring shoulder strength, such as lifting or reaching.
- Instability: Feeling of shoulder instability or subluxation, particularly in advanced stages of OA.
- Decreased Function: Difficulty performing daily activities, such as dressing, grooming, or lifting objects overhead.

Risk Factors

- Age: Increasing age is a significant risk factor for shoulder OA, as cartilage degeneration occurs over time.
- Gender: Shoulder OA is more common in women, although the reasons for this gender disparity are not fully understood.
- Joint Overuse: Repetitive stress on the shoulder joint from activities such as overhead lifting, throwing, or sports participation may accelerate joint degeneration.
- Trauma or Injury: Previous shoulder injuries, fractures, dislocations, or repetitive microtrauma increase the risk of developing OA.
- Genetics: Family history of OA or genetic predisposition may influence susceptibility to shoulder OA.
- Occupational Factors: Certain occupations involving repetitive overhead movements or heavy lifting may elevate the risk of shoulder OA.
- Obesity: Excess body weight can contribute to shoulder OA by placing increased stress on the joint and accelerating cartilage wear.

Diagnosis:

- Medical History and Physical Examination: Evaluation of symptoms, functional limitations, joint tenderness, range of motion, and shoulder strength.
- Imaging Studies: X-rays may reveal joint space narrowing, osteophyte formation, subchondral sclerosis, and other characteristic features of shoulder OA.
- Magnetic Resonance Imaging (MRI): MRI may be used to assess soft tissue structures, cartilage integrity, and identify other shoulder pathologies.

Treatment:

- Conservative Management: Initial treatment typically includes rest, activity modification, physical therapy, and analgesic medications (e.g., acetaminophen, NSAIDs).
- Corticosteroid Injection: Intra-articular corticosteroid injections may provide short-term pain relief and reduce inflammation.

- **Viscosupplementation**: Hyaluronic acid injections may be considered to improve joint lubrication and reduce pain.
- **Surgical Options**: In cases of severe pain or functional impairment refractory to conservative measures, surgical interventions such as arthroscopy, joint debridement, or shoulder arthroplasty (total or partial) may be recommended.

Disease Management

- Long-term management of shoulder OA focuses on pain relief, preserving joint function, and optimizing quality of life.
- Regular follow-up visits with The APP are important for monitoring disease progression, adjusting treatment strategies, and addressing any complications or comorbidities

10.1.3. Hand and Wrist OA

Symptoms

- Pain: Persistent pain in the affected joints, often worsening with activity and improving with rest.
- Stiffness: Joint stiffness, especially after periods of inactivity or upon waking in the morning.
- Swelling: Swelling around the affected joints, which may be accompanied by warmth and tenderness.
- Reduced range of motion: Difficulty bending, straightening, or fully moving the fingers, hands, or wrists.
- Crepitus: A sensation of grinding, clicking, or cracking in the affected joints during movement.

Diagnosis

- Medical history: Discussing symptoms, onset, and any relevant risk factors with a healthcare provider.
- Physical examination: Assessing joint tenderness, swelling, range of motion, and other signs of OA.
- Imaging studies: X-rays are commonly used to visualize joint structures, including joint space narrowing, osteophyte formation (bone spurs), and cartilage loss, which are indicative of OA.

Treatments

- Medications: Nonsteroidal anti-inflammatory drugs (NSAIDs), acetaminophen, or topical analgesics to relieve pain and inflammation.
- Splinting: Using splints or braces to support and stabilize the affected joints, reducing pain and improving function.

- **Physical therapy:** Specific exercises and stretches to improve joint flexibility, strength, and range of motion, and reduce pain and stiffness.
- **Lifestyle modifications:** Maintaining a healthy weight, avoiding repetitive stress on the joints, and using ergonomic tools or adaptive devices to reduce strain on the hands and wrists.
- **Assistive devices:** Using assistive devices such as ergonomic tools, jar openers, or specialized utensils to minimize joint stress during daily activities.
- **Injections:** Corticosteroid injections may be considered to reduce inflammation and pain in the affected joints, especially if conservative measures are ineffective.
- **Surgery:** In severe cases of hand and wrist OA that do not respond to conservative treatments, surgical options such as joint fusion, joint replacement, or arthroscopic debridement may be considered to relieve pain and improve joint function.

10.2. Rheumatoid Arthritis

> *Rheumatoid arthritis (RA) is a chronic autoimmune disorder causing inflammation primarily in the joints, leading to pain, swelling, and stiffness.*
>
> *It can affect any joint but often targets the hands, wrists, and knees symmetrically.*
>
> *Treatment involves medications, physical therapy, and lifestyle modifications to manage symptoms and prevent joint damage.*

Symptoms

- Joint pain, swelling, and stiffness: often worse in the morning or after periods of inactivity.
- Symmetrical joint involvement: such as both wrists, both knees, or multiple joints on both sides of the body.
- Fatigue: can be chronic which can be debilitating and affect daily activities.
- Joint deformity: Over time, RA can cause joint damage, deformities, and loss of function, particularly in the hands, wrists, and feet.
- Systemic symptoms: RA can affect other organs and systems in the body, leading to symptoms such as fever, weight loss, and general malaise.

Risk Factors:

- Genetics: family history of RA increases the risk of developing the condition, suggesting a genetic predisposition.
- Gender: RA is more common in women than in men.
- Age: While RA can occur at any age, it most commonly begins between the ages of 30 and 60.
- Smoking: Smoking increases the risk of developing RA, particularly in patients with a genetic predisposition.
- Environmental Factors: Exposure to certain environmental factors, such as infections or pollutants, may trigger the immune system to attack the joints in susceptible patients.

Epidemiology

- RA is a chronic autoimmune disease that affects approximately 1% of the population worldwide.
- It is more common in women, with a female-to-male ratio of about 3:1.
- RA can develop at any age, but it most commonly occurs between the ages of 30 and 60.
- The prevalence of RA varies geographically, with higher rates reported in certain regions.

Workup and Diagnosis

- <u>Clinical Evaluation</u>: Diagnosis of RA is based on a combination of clinical symptoms, physical examination findings, and laboratory tests.
- <u>Diagnostic Criteria</u>: The 2010 American College of Rheumatology (ACR)/European League Against Rheumatism (EULAR) classification criteria for rheumatoid arthritis (RA) involve a scoring system where each component is assigned a score.
  - The maximum score is 10, with points allocated as follows:
    - Joint involvement: 0 to 5 points
      - *0 points: No joint involvement*
      - *1 point: 1 large joint*
      - *2 points: 2–10 large joints*
      - *3 points: 1–3 small joints (with or without involvement of large joints)*
      - *4 points: 4–10 small joints (with or without involvement of large joints)*
      - *5 points: >10 joints (at least 1 small joint)*

- ➤ Serology (rheumatoid factor or anti-citrullinated protein antibodies): 0 to 3 points
- ➤ Acute phase reactants (CRP or ESR): 0 to 1 point
- ➤ Duration of symptoms: 0 to 1 point (less than 66 wks
    - The total score is calculated based on the presence and severity of these components. A score of 6 or higher indicates a classification of RA, while scores below 6 are less suggestive of RA.
    - It's important to note that these criteria are used for classification rather than diagnosis, and they are primarily intended for research purposes to identify patients likely to have RA for inclusion in studies and clinical trials.
- Imaging Studies: X-rays, ultrasound, or MRI may be used to assess joint damage, inflammation, and erosion in patients with suspected RA.

Treatment:
- Disease-Modifying Antirheumatic Drugs (DMARDs): DMARDs such as methotrexate, hydroxychloroquine, sulfasalazine, and biologic agents (such as tumor necrosis factor inhibitors, interleukin-6 inhibitors, and T-cell co-stimulation modulators) are the mainstay of treatment for RA.
- Nonsteroidal Anti-Inflammatory Drugs (NSAIDs): NSAIDs may be used to provide symptomatic relief from pain and inflammation in RA.
- Corticosteroids: Short-term use of corticosteroids may be prescribed to rapidly reduce inflammation and alleviate symptoms during disease flares.
- Physical Therapy: Physical therapy can help improve joint function, range of motion, and muscle strength, and may include exercises, stretching, and joint protection techniques.
- Occupational Therapy: Occupational therapy focuses on strategies and adaptations to help patients with RA perform daily activities and tasks more easily.
- Surgery: In cases of severe joint damage or deformity, surgical interventions such as joint replacement surgery (arthroplasty) may be considered to restore function and alleviate pain.

10.3. Reactive Arthritis

> ➤ *Reactive arthritis, also known as Reiter's syndrome, is an inflammatory condition that develops in response to an infection, typically in the genital, urinary, or gastrointestinal tract.*
>
> ➤ *It presents with joint pain, swelling, and stiffness, along with other symptoms such as urethritis and conjunctivitis.*
>
> ➤ *Treatment focuses on managing symptoms, addressing the underlying infection, and reducing inflammation with medications.*

Symptoms

- Joint inflammation: Typically affects the lower extremities, especially the knees, ankles, and feet. Joints may be swollen, warm, and tender.
- Urethritis: Inflammation of the urethra, leading to pain or burning during urination.
- Conjunctivitis: Redness, itching, and discharge from the eyes.
- Skin rash: Characteristic lesions may develop on the palms, soles, or trunk, called *Keratoderma blennorrhagicum*.
- Mouth ulcers: Painful sores may appear in the mouth, resembling aphthous ulcers.
- Enthesitis: Inflammation of the tendons, ligaments, or joint capsules, often at their insertion points into bone.
- Back pain: Some patients may experience low back pain due to inflammation of the sacroiliac joints or spine.

Risk Factors

- Genetic predisposition: Certain genetic factors may increase susceptibility to reactive arthritis, particularly the presence of the HLA-B27 gene.
- Infections: Previous or concurrent infections with certain bacteria, such as Chlamydia trachomatis, Salmonella, Shigella, Yersinia, or Campylobacter, are common triggers.
- Age and sex: Reactive arthritis most commonly affects young to middle-aged adults and is more prevalent in males.

Epidemiology

- Reactive arthritis is relatively uncommon but may occur following certain infections, particularly sexually transmitted infections or gastrointestinal infections.

- The exact prevalence varies depending on geographical location, ethnicity, and other factors.
- It typically affects patients between the ages of 20 and 40, with a male predominance.

Diagnosis
- Clinical evaluation: Based on a thorough medical history and physical examination, including assessment of joint involvement, urogenital symptoms, skin lesions, and eye inflammation.
- Laboratory tests: Blood tests may show evidence of inflammation (elevated ESR and CRP) and HLA-B27 positivity in some cases. Tests for specific infectious agents may be performed based on clinical suspicion.
- Imaging studies: X-rays, CT, or MRI may be used to assess joint inflammation and rule out other causes of arthritis.
- Urethral or joint fluid analysis: Examination of urethral or joint fluid may reveal signs of inflammation or the presence of infectious agents.

Treatment
- Nonsteroidal anti-inflammatory drugs (NSAIDs): First-line treatment to relieve pain and reduce inflammation.
- Antibiotics: If an underlying infection is identified, appropriate antibiotic therapy may be prescribed.
- Corticosteroids: In severe cases or when NSAIDs are ineffective, corticosteroid injections or oral corticosteroids may be considered to suppress inflammation.
- Disease-modifying antirheumatic drugs (DMARDs): Methotrexate or sulfasalazine may be used in refractory cases to help control symptoms and prevent disease progression.
- Physical therapy: Exercises to maintain joint mobility, strengthen muscles, and improve posture may be beneficial.
- Supportive measures: Rest, joint protection, and orthotics may help alleviate symptoms and improve functional status.

10.4. Gout Arthritis

> ➤ *Gout is a form of arthritis caused by the buildup of uric acid crystals in the joints, leading to sudden and severe attacks of pain, swelling, and redness, often in the big toe.*
>
> ➤ *It is associated with high levels of uric acid in the blood, which can be influenced by diet, genetics, kidney functions, and other factors.*
>
> ➤ *Treatment involves medications to manage symptoms, dietary changes, and lifestyle modifications to prevent future attacks.*

Symptoms

- Sudden onset of intense joint pain: Typically affects the big toe, although other joints such as the ankles, knees, elbows, wrists, and fingers may also be affected.
- Swelling and warmth: Affected joints may become swollen, tender, and warm to the touch during a gout attack.
- Redness: The skin over the affected joint may appear red or purplish.
- Limited mobility: Pain and swelling may limit the range of motion in the affected joint.
- Recurrent attacks: Gout attacks may recur periodically, with symptom-free intervals between episodes.

Risk Factors

- Hyperuricemia: Elevated levels of uric acid in the blood are a primary risk factor for gout. Uric acid crystallizes and deposits in the joints, leading to inflammation and pain.
- Diet: Consumption of purine-rich foods (e.g., red meat, shellfish, organ meats) and sugary beverages increases the risk of gout.
- Alcohol consumption: Excessive alcohol intake, particularly beer and spirits, is associated with an increased risk of gout.
- Obesity: Being overweight or obese increases the risk of developing gout.
- Genetics: Family history of gout increases the likelihood of developing the condition.

Epidemiology

- Gout is common, affecting approximately 4% of adults in the United States.
- The prevalence of gout has been increasing worldwide, likely due to changes in diet and lifestyle factors.

Diagnosis
- Clinical evaluations: Diagnosis is based on clinical presentation, medical history, physical examination, and laboratory tests.
- Laboratory tests: Blood tests to measure serum uric acid levels during an acute attack may reveal hyperuricemia. Joint fluid analysis may show the presence of urate crystals.
- Imaging studies: X-rays and ultrasound may be used to assess joint damage and monitor disease progression.

Treatment
- Acute gout treatment: Nonsteroidal anti-inflammatory drugs (NSAIDs), colchicine, and corticosteroids are commonly used to relieve pain and inflammation during acute gout attacks.
- Long-term management: Medications such as allopurinol, febuxostat, and probenecid may be prescribed to lower uric acid levels and prevent recurrent gout attacks.
- Lifestyle modifications: Dietary changes, weight loss, limiting alcohol consumption, and staying hydrated can help reduce the frequency and severity of gout attacks.
- Avoidance of trigger foods: Limiting intake of purine-rich foods and sugary beverages can help prevent gout flare-ups.

10.5. Fibromyalgia

> *Fibromyalgia is a chronic disorder characterized by widespread musculoskeletal pain, fatigue, and tenderness in specific areas of the body.*
>
> *Its exact cause is unknown, but factors like genetics, infections, and physical or emotional trauma may contribute.*
>
> *Treatment typically involves a multidisciplinary approach including medications, therapy, and lifestyle changes to alleviate symptoms and improve quality of life.*

Symptoms
- Widespread musculoskeletal pain: Pain typically affects both sides of the body, above and below the waist, and along the spine.
- Fatigue and sleep disturbances: Patients often experience non-restorative sleep, waking up feeling tired or unrefreshed.
- Cognitive difficulties: Often referred to as "fibro fog," patients may experience problems with memory, concentration, and attention.

- Other symptoms: Headaches, irritable bowel syndrome (IBS), temporomandibular joint (TMJ) disorders, anxiety, and depression are commonly associated with fibromyalgia.

Risk Factors

- Gender: Fibromyalgia is more common in women than in men.
- Family history: A family history of fibromyalgia increases the risk of developing the condition.
- Other disorders: Rheumatic diseases, such as rheumatoid arthritis and systemic lupus erythematosus, and psychological conditions, such as post-traumatic stress disorder (PTSD), are associated with an increased risk of fibromyalgia.

Epidemiology

- Fibromyalgia affects an estimated 2% to 8% of the population worldwide.
- It commonly affects adults of working age, with a higher prevalence in women.

Diagnosis

- Diagnosis is primarily based on clinical criteria, including widespread pain lasting for at least three months and the presence of tender points on physical examination.
- The American College of Rheumatology (ACR) criteria include widespread pain in combination with tenderness in at least 11 of 18 specified tender points.
- Blood tests and imaging studies may be performed to rule out other conditions with similar symptoms.

Treatment

- Multidisciplinary approach: Treatment typically involves a combination of medications, lifestyle modifications, and therapies tailored to patient symptoms.
- Medications: Pain relievers, antidepressants, and anticonvulsants may be prescribed to manage pain, improve sleep, and alleviate other symptoms.
- Lifestyle modifications: Regular exercise, stress management techniques, and maintaining a healthy sleep routine can help improve symptoms.
- Therapies: Physical therapy, cognitive-behavioral therapy (CBT), and complementary therapies such as acupuncture and massage therapy may provide symptom relief.

10.6. Systemic Lupus Erythematosus

> ➤ *Systemic lupus erythematosus (SLE) is a chronic autoimmune disease where the body's immune system attacks its own tissues, leading to inflammation and damage in various organs and tissues.*
>
> ➤ *Symptoms can range from mild to severe, affecting joints, skin, kidneys, heart, and other organs.*
>
> ➤ *Treatment involves medications to control inflammation, manage symptoms, and prevent flares, along with lifestyle adjustments and regular medical monitoring.*

Symptoms

- Fatigue
- Fever
- Joint pain and swelling
- Butterfly-shaped rash across the cheeks and bridge of the nose
- Skin lesions that worsen with sun exposure
- Raynaud's phenomenon
- Chest pain or shortness of breath
- Headaches, confusion, or memory loss
- Mouth sores
- Hair loss
- Photosensitivity
- Kidney problems
- Neuropsychiatric symptoms such as anxiety, depression, or seizures

Risk Factors

- Gender: SLE is more common in women, particularly during childbearing years.
- Genetics: Family history of autoimmune diseases, including SLE, increases the risk.
- Ethnicity: SLE is more prevalent in patients of African, Asian, and Hispanic descent.
- Environmental factors: Sunlight exposure, infections, certain medications, and hormonal factors may trigger or exacerbate SLE.

Epidemiology

- SLE affects approximately 0.1% to 0.2% of the population worldwide.
- It can occur at any age but most commonly develops in patients aged 15 to 44.
- Women are affected more than men, with a female-to-male ratio ranging from 7:1 to 15:1.

Diagnosis and Criteria
- Diagnosis is based on a combination of clinical symptoms, laboratory tests, and imaging studies.
- Diagnostic criteria The ACR classification criteria for SLE include 11 criteria. A patient is classified as having SLE if they satisfy 4 or more of the following criteria, not necessarily simultaneously:
  - *Malar rash*: Fixed erythema, flat or raised, over the malar eminences, tending to spare the nasolabial folds.
  - *Discoid rash*: Erythematous raised patches with adherent keratotic scaling and follicular plugging, scarring may occur.
  - *Photosensitivity*: Skin rash as a result of unusual reaction to sunlight, by patient history or physician observation.
  - *Oral ulcers*: Oral or nasopharyngeal ulceration, usually painless, observed by a physician.
  - *Arthritis*: Nonerosive arthritis involving two or more peripheral joints, characterized by tenderness, swelling, or effusion.
  - *Serositis*: Pleuritis or pericarditis, documented by clinical evaluation or imaging studies.
  - *Renal disorder*: Persistent proteinuria >0.5 g/day or >3+ if quantitation not performed, or cellular casts (red cell, hemoglobin, granular, tubular, or mixed).
  - *Neurologic disorder*: Seizures or psychosis, in the absence of offending drugs or known metabolic derangements; cranial neuropathy (e.g., optic neuritis, cranial nerve palsies) or peripheral neuropathy (e.g., sensory or motor seizures, cranial or peripheral neuropathy).
  - *Hematologic disorder*: Hemolytic anemia with reticulocytosis, or leukopenia (<4000/mm^3 total on two or more occasions), or lymphopenia (<1500/mm^3 on two or more occasions), or thrombocytopenia (<100,000/mm^3) in the absence of offending drugs.
  - *Immunologic disorder*: Positive antinuclear antibody (ANA) on immunofluorescence microscopy of HEp-2 cells or equivalent assay at a titer ≥1:80 OR an equivalent positive test at any point in time OR Anti-dsDNA antibody, antibody to Sm nuclear antigen, or antiphospholipid antibodies (including anticardiolipin IgG or IgM, or lupus anticoagulant).
  - *Antinuclear antibody (ANA) level:* Abnormal titer of antinuclear antibody by immunofluorescence or an equivalent assay at any

point in time and in the absence of drugs known to be associated with drug-induced lupus syndrome.
- Laboratory tests: SLE panel including Antinuclear antibody (ANA), anti-double-stranded DNA (anti-dsDNA) antibody, anti-Smith (anti-Sm) antibody, and complement levels.
- Imaging studies: Such as chest X-ray, echocardiogram, or kidney biopsy may be performed to assess organ involvement.

Treatment
- Treatment aims to control symptoms, prevent flares, and minimize organ damage.
- Medications: May include nonsteroidal anti-inflammatory drugs (NSAIDs), antimalarial drugs (e.g., hydroxychloroquine), corticosteroids, immunosuppressants (e.g., methotrexate, azathioprine), and biologic agents (e.g., belimumab).
- Lifestyle modifications: Such as sun protection, regular exercise, and smoking cessation are recommended.
- Close monitoring by a rheumatologist and other healthcare providers is essential to adjust treatment as needed and manage potential complications.

10.7. Ankylosing Spondylitis

> - *Ankylosing spondylitis is a chronic inflammatory arthritis primarily affecting the spine and sacroiliac joints, causing stiffness, pain, and eventual fusion of the spine.*
> - *It often begins in young adulthood, with symptoms worsening over time and potentially leading to spinal deformity and reduced mobility.*
> - *Treatment focuses on pain management, physical therapy, and medications to reduce inflammation and slow disease progression.*

Symptoms
- Lower back pain and stiffness: Gradual onset of dull, aching pain and stiffness in the lower back, which may worsen with rest and improve with movement.
- Morning stiffness decreased mobility, particularly in the morning or after periods of inactivity.
- Pain and stiffness in other joints: AS can also affect other joints such as the hips, shoulders, knees, and ankles.

- Fatigue: Persistent fatigue and malaise are common symptoms, particularly during disease flares.
- Loss of flexibility: As the disease progresses, the spine may become less flexible, leading to a stooped posture.
- Eye inflammation: Some patients with AS may develop inflammation of the eyes (uveitis), causing eye pain, redness, and sensitivity to light.

Risk Factors

- Genetic predisposition: AS is strongly associated with the human leukocyte antigen (HLA)-B27 gene. Patients who carry the HLA-B27 gene have an increased risk of developing AS.
- Family history: Having a first-degree relative with AS increases the risk of developing the condition.
- Gender: AS is more common in men than in women.
- Age: Symptoms typically begin in late adolescence or early adulthood, but AS can develop at any age.

Epidemiology

- AS is estimated to affect approximately 0.1% to 0.5% of the population worldwide.
- It most commonly affects patients aged 15 to 40 years.
- Men are affected more frequently than women, with a male-to-female ratio ranging from 2:1 to 3:1.

Diagnosis

- Diagnosis is based on a combination of clinical symptoms, medical history, physical examination, and imaging studies.
- Criteria such as the modified New York criteria are commonly used to diagnose AS, which include radiographic evidence of sacroiliitis and specific clinical features.
- Imaging studies such as X-rays, MRI, and CT scans may be used to assess sacroiliac joint involvement and spinal changes.

Treatment

- <u>Medications:</u>
  - Nonsteroidal anti-inflammatory drugs (NSAIDs) are commonly used to reduce pain and inflammation.
  - Disease-modifying antirheumatic drugs (DMARDs) and biologic agents may be prescribed to slow disease progression in patients with active inflammation and structural damage.

- **Physical therapy**: Exercises and stretching techniques can help improve flexibility, posture, and overall function.
- **Lifestyle modifications**: Maintaining a healthy weight, practicing good posture, and avoiding smoking can help manage symptoms and prevent complications.
- **Surgery**: In severe cases of AS with spinal fusion or joint damage, surgical interventions such as joint replacement or spinal fusion surgery may be considered to improve mobility and quality of life.

10.8. Enteropathic Arthritis

> ➢ *Enteropathic arthritis is a form of chronic, inflammatory arthritis associated with inflammatory bowel disease (IBD), such as Crohn's disease and ulcerative colitis, affecting joints and potentially the spine.*
>
> ➢ *It occurs in about 10-20% of individuals with IBD, with symptoms including joint pain, swelling, and gastrointestinal issues related to the underlying bowel condition.*
>
> ➢ *Treatment strategies focus on managing IBD symptoms, reducing joint inflammation, and maintaining joint function through medications and physical therapy.*

Symptoms
- Joint pain and swelling, particularly affecting the peripheral joints and the spine.
- Gastrointestinal symptoms related to the underlying inflammatory bowel disease (IBD), such as abdominal pain, diarrhea, and weight loss.
- Other possible symptoms include skin problems, eye inflammation, and fatigue.

Risk Factors
- Having an underlying inflammatory bowel disease (IBD), such as Crohn's disease or ulcerative colitis.
- Genetic predisposition: Family history of IBD or arthritis increases risk.
- Age: Most commonly diagnosed in young adults, but it can occur at any age.

Epidemiology
- Enteropathic arthritis occurs in about 10% to 20% of people with inflammatory bowel disease.

- Both men and women with IBD are equally at risk of developing enteropathic arthritis.
- The condition can develop before, after, or simultaneously with the diagnosis of IBD.

Diagnosis
- Diagnosis involves a combination of clinical evaluation, medical history (including IBD diagnosis), and imaging tests (X-rays, MRI) to assess joint and spinal inflammation.
- Blood tests may be done to rule out other types of arthritis (e.g., rheumatoid arthritis, ankylosing spondylitis) and to check for markers of inflammation.
- There's no single test for enteropathic arthritis; diagnosis is based on the presence of IBD and arthritis symptoms.

Treatment
- Medications:
    - Nonsteroidal anti-inflammatory drugs (NSAIDs)- used cautiously due to potential gastrointestinal side effects.
    - Disease-modifying antirheumatic drugs (DMARDs) like sulfasalazine and methotrexate
    - TNF inhibitors and other biologics for both joint and GI symptoms.
- Physical Therapy: Helps maintain joint flexibility and strength.
- Management of IBD: Treatment of the underlying IBD often helps alleviate the joint symptoms. This may involve a combination of medications, diet changes, and sometimes surgery.
- Lifestyle Modifications: Regular exercise, smoking cessation, and maintaining a healthy diet can help manage symptoms and improve overall health.

10.9. Psoriatic arthritis

> ➢ *Psoriatic arthritis is a chronic inflammatory arthritis that affects individuals with psoriasis, causing joint pain, stiffness, and swelling.*
> ➢ *It can also lead to nail changes, fatigue, and inflammation in other organs.*
> ➢ *Treatment includes medications to manage symptoms, control inflammation, and slow joint damage, along with lifestyle modifications and physical therapy.*

Symptoms
- Joint pain and stiffness: PsA typically causes joint pain, swelling, and stiffness, often affecting the fingers, toes, wrists, knees, and ankles.
- Psoriasis: Many patients with PsA also have skin symptoms of psoriasis, including red, scaly patches of skin, particularly on the scalp, elbows, knees, and lower back.
- Enthesitis: Inflammation at the sites where tendons and ligaments attach to bone, leading to pain and swelling, commonly seen in the heels, bottoms of the feet, and elbows.
- Dactylitis: Swelling of an entire finger or toe, giving it a sausage-like appearance.
- Nail changes: Psoriatic nail changes such as pitting, ridges, or separation of the nail from the nail bed may occur.
- Fatigue: Persistent fatigue and malaise are common symptoms, particularly during disease flares.

Risk Factors
- Psoriasis: patients with psoriasis have an increased risk of developing PsA.
- Family history: Having a first-degree relative with PsA or psoriasis increases the risk of developing the condition.
- Genetics: Certain genetic factors, including the presence of the HLA-B27 gene, may predispose patients to PsA.
- Environmental factors: Infections, injuries, and stress may trigger or exacerbate PsA symptoms in genetically susceptible patients.

Epidemiology
- PsA affects approximately 20% to 30% of patients with psoriasis.

- It typically develops in adults aged 30 to 50 years but can occur at any age.
- Both men and women are affected, with PsA having a slightly higher prevalence in men.

Diagnosis

- Diagnosis is based on a combination of clinical symptoms, medical history, physical examination, and laboratory tests.
- The Classification Criteria for Psoriatic Arthritis (CASPAR) criteria are commonly used to diagnose PsA, which include evidence of current psoriasis, a history of psoriasis, or a family history of psoriasis in combination with specific clinical features.
- Imaging studies such as X-rays, MRI, and ultrasound may be used to assess joint and entheseal involvement.

Treatment

- <u>Medications</u>: Nonsteroidal anti-inflammatory drugs (NSAIDs), disease-modifying antirheumatic drugs (DMARDs), biologic agents, and corticosteroids are commonly used to reduce inflammation and control symptoms.
- <u>Physical therapy</u>: Exercises, stretching techniques, and posture training can help improve flexibility, strength, and overall function.
- <u>Lifestyle modifications</u>: Maintaining a healthy weight, practicing good posture, and avoiding smoking can help manage symptoms and improve outcomes.
- <u>Patient education</u>: Providing education about the disease, its management, and the importance of adherence to treatment is essential for empowering patients to actively participate in their care.

10.10. Osteoporosis

> ➢ *Osteoporosis is a condition characterized by weakened bones, increasing the risk of fractures, especially in the spine, hip, and wrist.*
>
> ➢ *It typically develops silently without symptoms until a fracture occurs and is more common in older adults, particularly postmenopausal women.*
>
> ➢ *Treatment involves medications to prevent bone loss, dietary changes to promote bone health, weight-bearing exercise, and fall prevention strategies.*

Symptoms
- Osteoporosis is often referred to as a "silent disease" because it typically progresses without symptoms until a fracture occurs.
- Fractures: The most common symptom, especially in the hip, spine, and wrist. These fractures may occur with minimal trauma or even spontaneously.
- Back pain: Compression fractures of the spine may cause back pain, height loss, and kyphosis.
- Loss of height: Osteoporosis-related fractures in the spine can lead to a gradual loss of height over time.

Risk Factors
- Age: Risk of osteoporosis increases with age, particularly after menopause in women.
- Gender: Women are at a higher risk of developing osteoporosis than men.
- Family history: Having a family history of osteoporosis or fractures increases the risk.
- Menopause: Estrogen levels decrease after menopause, leading to accelerated bone loss in women.
- Low body weight: Being underweight or having a BMI less than 20 increases the risk of osteoporosis.
- Sedentary lifestyle: Lack of physical activity or prolonged immobilization increases the risk.
- Smoking and excessive alcohol consumption: Both smoking and heavy alcohol intake can weaken bones and increase fracture risk.
- Certain medications: Long-term use of corticosteroids, anticonvulsants, and some cancer treatments can contribute to bone loss.

Epidemiology
- Osteoporosis is a common condition, particularly in older adults.
- Women are more commonly affected than men, especially postmenopausal women.
- The prevalence of osteoporosis increases with age, with estimates suggesting that over 50% of women over 50 years old will experience an osteoporotic fracture.

Diagnosis

- DEXA measures bone mineral density (BMD) at various sites, usually the spine, hip, or wrist, and provides a T-score comparing an individual's BMD to that of a young, healthy adult.
    - A T-score of -2.5 or lower indicates osteoporosis, while scores between -1.0 and -2.5 indicate osteopenia, a precursor to osteoporosis.
- Fracture risk assessment: FRAX (Fracture Risk Assessment Tool) calculates the 10-year probability of a major osteoporotic fracture based on clinical risk factors and BMD.
- Laboratory tests: Blood tests may be performed to evaluate calcium, vitamin D, and other markers of bone health.

Treatment

- Lifestyle modifications: Regular weight-bearing exercise, adequate calcium and vitamin D intake, smoking cessation, and limiting alcohol consumption are essential for maintaining bone health.
- Pharmacological therapy: Medications such as bisphosphonates, selective estrogen receptor modulators (SERMs), denosumab, and teriparatide may be prescribed to prevent further bone loss and reduce fracture risk.
- Fall prevention strategies: Measures to reduce the risk of falls, such as home modifications, balance exercises, and vision correction, can help prevent fractures in patients with osteoporosis.

10.11. Juvenile idiopathic arthritis

> *Juvenile idiopathic arthritis (JIA) is the most common chronic rheumatic disease in children, causing joint inflammation, pain, and stiffness.*
>
> *It encompasses several subtypes with varying symptoms and disease courses*
>
> *Treatment often requires a multidisciplinary approach involving medications, physical therapy, and regular monitoring to manage symptoms and prevent joint damage.*

Symptoms

- Joint pain: Persistent pain, swelling, and stiffness in one or more joints, often accompanied by warmth and redness.

- Joint stiffness: Morning stiffness that improves with movement or as the day progresses.
- Joint swelling: Swelling of affected joints, which may limit range of motion.
- Fever: Some children with JIA may experience intermittent fever, especially during disease flares.
- Fatigue: Chronic fatigue and malaise are common symptoms, particularly during active disease.

Risk Factors

- Genetics: There is evidence of a genetic predisposition to JIA, with certain genetic factors increasing the risk of developing the condition.
- Environmental factors: Infections, particularly viral infections, have been implicated as potential triggers for JIA in genetically susceptible patients.
- Autoimmune factors: Dysregulation of the immune system leading to inflammation and joint damage is believed to play a central role in the development of JIA.

Epidemiology

- JIA affects approximately 1 in 1,000 children, making it the most common rheumatic disease in childhood.
- The condition can occur at any age, but onset is most commonly between the ages of 1 and 3 years old or during early adolescence.
- JIA affects both boys and girls, with some subtypes more common in one gender than the other.

Diagnosis

- Diagnosis of JIA is based on a combination of clinical symptoms, physical examination findings, laboratory tests, and imaging studies.
- Classification criteria such as *the International League of Associations for Rheumatology (ILAR)* criteria are used to categorize different subtypes of JIA based on clinical features and disease course.
- Laboratory tests may include complete blood count (CBC), erythrocyte sedimentation rate (ESR), C-reactive protein (CRP), rheumatoid factor (RF), and antinuclear antibody (ANA) testing.

Treatment

- Treatment of JIA aims to control symptoms, prevent joint damage, and improve quality of life.
- Nonsteroidal anti-inflammatory drugs (NSAIDs) are often used to relieve pain and inflammation.

- Disease-modifying antirheumatic drugs (DMARDs), such as methotrexate, may be prescribed to suppress the underlying immune response and reduce disease activity.
- Biologic agents, including tumor necrosis factor (TNF) inhibitors, interleukin-6 (IL-6) inhibitors, and other targeted therapies, are used in more severe or refractory cases.
- Physical therapy and occupational therapy are important components of JIA management, helping to improve joint function, mobility, and muscle strength.

10.12. Sjögren's syndrome

> ➤ *Sjögren's syndrome is an autoimmune disorder characterized by dry eyes and mouth due to damage to the glands that produce tears and saliva.*
>
> ➤ *It can also affect other organs, leading to fatigue, joint pain, and systemic complications.*
>
> ➤ *Treatment focuses on relieving symptoms with eye drops, saliva substitutes, medications to reduce inflammation, and managing associated conditions.*

Symptoms

- Dry eyes: Persistent dryness, grittiness, or a burning sensation in the eyes.
- Dry mouth: Difficulty swallowing, altered taste, and increased dental decay due to reduced saliva production.
- Other symptoms: Fatigue, joint pain, dry skin, and vaginal dryness are common. Some patients may experience systemic manifestations such as fever, rash, or lung and kidney involvement.

Risk Factors

- Gender: Sjögren's syndrome is more common in women than men, with a female to male ratio of around 9:1.
- Age: Although Sjögren's syndrome can occur at any age, it most commonly affects patients between 40 and 60 years old.
- Autoimmune diseases: patients with other autoimmune diseases such as rheumatoid arthritis, systemic lupus erythematosus (SLE), or scleroderma have an increased risk of developing Sjögren's syndrome.

Epidemiology
- Sjögren's syndrome is estimated to affect 0.5% to 1% of the general population.
- It is one of the most common autoimmune rheumatic diseases.
- The prevalence varies among different populations and ethnic groups.

Diagnosis
- Diagnosis of Sjögren's syndrome involves a combination of clinical evaluation, laboratory tests, and imaging studies.
- <u>Diagnostic criteria</u>: The American College of Rheumatology (ACR) and the European League Against Rheumatism (EULAR) have established classification criteria for the diagnosis of Sjögren's syndrome, which include symptoms, serological markers, and salivary gland biopsy findings.
- <u>Laboratory tests</u>: Blood tests may reveal autoantibodies such as anti-SSA (Ro) and anti-SSB (La) antibodies, rheumatoid factor (RF), and antinuclear antibodies (ANA).
- <u>Imaging studies</u>: Salivary gland ultrasound or sialography may be performed to assess glandular involvement.

Treatment
- <u>Symptomatic management</u>:
  - Treatment focuses on relieving symptoms of dry eyes and dry mouth.
  - Artificial tears, lubricating eye drops, and saliva substitutes can help alleviate dryness.
- <u>Immunomodulatory therapy</u>: For patients with systemic manifestations or significant organ involvement, medications such as corticosteroids, hydroxychloroquine, and immunosuppressants may be prescribed to suppress the immune response and reduce inflammation.
- <u>Supportive care</u>: Regular dental visits, good oral hygiene practices, and use of fluoride products can help prevent dental complications associated with dry mouth.
- <u>Patient education</u>: Patients should be educated about the chronic nature of the disease, the importance of symptom management, and strategies for coping with dryness-related issues.

10.13. Polymyalgia Rheumatica

> ➤ *Polymyalgia rheumatica (PMR) is an inflammatory disorder causing pain and stiffness, typically in the shoulders, neck, and hips, especially in older adults.*
>
> ➤ *It often presents with morning stiffness and can be associated with symptoms like fatigue, weight loss, and fever.*
>
> ➤ *Treatment involves corticosteroids to manage inflammation, with gradual tapering of doses over time, along with lifestyle modifications and regular monitoring for potential complications.*

Symptoms

- Muscle pain and stiffness: Symmetrical pain and stiffness, usually affecting the shoulders, neck, upper arms, hips, and thighs. The stiffness is typically worse in the morning or after periods of inactivity.
- Fatigue: Many patients with PMR experience profound fatigue and weakness.
- Other symptoms: Some patients may also experience mild fever, loss of appetite, weight loss, and depression.

Risk Factors

- Age: Polymyalgia rheumatica primarily affects patients over the age of 50, with the highest incidence in those over 70.
- Genetic factors: There may be a genetic predisposition to PMR, as it tends to cluster in families.
- Environmental triggers: Infections or other environmental factors may trigger the immune system to attack the body's own tissues, leading to PMR.

Epidemiology

- Polymyalgia rheumatica is relatively common, especially in older adults.
- It is estimated to affect 50 to 100 patients per 100,000 population over the age of 50.
- PMR is more common in women than in men.

Diagnosis

- Diagnosis of PMR is based on a combination of clinical symptoms, physical examination findings, laboratory tests, and imaging studies.

- Typical clinical features include bilateral shoulder pain and stiffness lasting for at least one month, morning stiffness lasting more than 45 minutes, and age over 50.
- Laboratory tests may show elevated markers of inflammation, such as erythrocyte sedimentation rate (ESR) and C-reactive protein (CRP).
- Imaging studies such as ultrasound or magnetic resonance imaging (MRI) may be used to evaluate for signs of inflammation in the affected muscles and joints.

Treatment
- Corticosteroids: The mainstay of treatment for PMR is oral corticosteroids, such as prednisone or prednisolone. These medications are usually started at a relatively high dose and gradually tapered down as symptoms improve.
- Other medications: In some cases, other immunosuppressive medications may be used in combination with corticosteroids to help reduce the dose and duration of steroid therapy.
- Physical therapy: Gentle exercises and stretching can help improve flexibility and strength and reduce stiffness.
- Lifestyle modifications: Adequate rest, proper nutrition, and regular exercise can help manage symptoms and improve overall well-being.

10.14. Systemic Sclerosis

> *Systemic sclerosis (scleroderma) is a rare autoimmune disease characterized by excessive collagen production, leading to thickening and hardening of the skin and internal organs.*
>
> *It can affect various body systems, causing symptoms such as skin tightness, Raynaud's phenomenon, digestive issues, and organ dysfunction.*
>
> *Treatment aims to manage symptoms, prevent complications, and improve quality of life through medications, physical therapy, and lifestyle modifications.*

Symptoms
- Skin changes: The hallmark symptom is thickening and hardening of the skin, typically starting in the fingers and hands and spreading to other areas of the body. This can lead to tight, shiny skin, skin ulcers, and loss of flexibility.

- Raynaud's phenomenon: Almost all patients with systemic sclerosis experience Raynaud's phenomenon, characterized by episodes of cold-induced color changes in the fingers and toes, often accompanied by pain or numbness.
- Internal organ involvement: Systemic sclerosis can affect various internal organs, leading to symptoms such as esophageal dysmotility, heartburn, shortness of breath, cough, joint pain, muscle weakness, and kidney problems.
- Other symptoms: Fatigue, weight loss, and symptoms related to specific organ involvement may also occur.

Risk Factors

- Gender: Systemic sclerosis is more common in women than men, with a female to male ratio of about 3:1.
- Age: Although systemic sclerosis can occur at any age, it most commonly affects patients between 30 and 50 years old.
- Genetic factors: There may be a genetic predisposition to systemic sclerosis, as it tends to cluster in families.
- Environmental factors: Exposure to certain environmental factors, such as silica dust or certain chemicals, may increase the risk of developing systemic sclerosis.

Epidemiology

- Systemic sclerosis is relatively rare, with an estimated prevalence of 50 to 300 cases per million adults.
- It affects patients of all ethnic backgrounds but is more common in certain populations, such as African Americans and Native Americans.
- The incidence and prevalence of systemic sclerosis vary geographically, with higher rates reported in certain regions of the world.

Diagnosis

- Diagnosis of systemic sclerosis is based on clinical features, laboratory tests, and imaging studies.
- Specific criteria, such as those developed by the American College of Rheumatology (ACR) or the European League Against Rheumatism (EULAR), are used to classify the disease.
- Laboratory tests may reveal autoantibodies such as anti-centromere antibody (ACA), anti-topoisomerase antibody (anti-Scl-70), and anti-RNA polymerase III antibody.

- Imaging studies, such as chest X-ray, echocardiogram, or high-resolution computed tomography (HRCT) scan, may be performed to evaluate for internal organ involvement.

Treatment
- Treatment of systemic sclerosis focuses on managing symptoms, slowing disease progression, and preventing complications.
- <u>Medications</u>: Immunosuppressive medications, such as corticosteroids, methotrexate, mycophenolate mofetil, or cyclophosphamide
- <u>Symptomatic treatment</u>: Medications may be prescribed to manage symptoms such as Raynaud's phenomenon (e.g., calcium channel blockers), heartburn (e.g., proton pump inhibitors), and joint pain (e.g., nonsteroidal anti-inflammatory drugs).
- <u>Physical therapy</u>: Physical and occupational therapy can help improve joint mobility, muscle strength, and overall function.
- <u>Lifestyle modifications</u>: Avoiding tobacco smoke, maintaining a healthy diet, staying physically active, and protecting the skin from injury and excessive sun exposure are important for managing systemic sclerosis.

10.15. Temporal Arteritis

> - *Temporal arteritis, also known as giant cell arteritis (GCA), is a type of vasculitis affecting medium and large arteries, particularly the temporal arteries.*
> - *It commonly presents with headaches, jaw pain, scalp tenderness, and vision changes, and if left untreated, can lead to serious complications such as blindness or stroke.*
> - *Diagnosis is made through clinical evaluation, blood tests, imaging, and often confirmed with a temporal artery biopsy.*

Symptoms
- Severe headache, often localized to the temple area
- Scalp tenderness, especially over the temporal arteries
- Jaw pain or claudication
- Vision changes, including sudden vision loss, double vision, or blurry vision
- Fever

- Fatigue
- Muscle aches and stiffness, especially in the neck, shoulders, and hips
- Unintended weight loss
- Loss of appetite
- Generalized malaise

Risk Factors
- Age: GCA primarily affects patients over the age of 50, with the highest incidence in those over 70.
- Sex: Women are more commonly affected than men.
- Caucasian ethnicity: GCA is more prevalent in patients of Northern European descent.
- Genetic factors: Certain genetic variants may predispose patients to develop GCA.
- Smoking: Cigarette smoking has been identified as a risk factor for GCA.

Epidemiology
- GCA is relatively rare, with an estimated annual incidence of 10 to 20 cases per 100,000 patients over the age of 50.
- The prevalence increases with age, peaking in the seventh and eighth decades of life.
- The condition is more common in populations of Northern European ancestry.

Diagnosis
- <u>Clinical evaluation</u>: Based on characteristic symptoms and physical examination findings, such as scalp tenderness and decreased temporal artery pulse.
- <u>Laboratory tests</u>: Including erythrocyte sedimentation rate (ESR) and C-reactive protein (CRP) levels, which are typically elevated in GCA.
- <u>Imaging studies</u>: Doppler ultrasound or magnetic resonance angiography (MRA) may show characteristic changes in the temporal arteries, such as wall thickening or skip lesions.
- <u>Temporal artery biopsy</u>: Considered the gold standard for diagnosis, demonstrating inflammatory infiltrates and giant cells in the arterial wall.

Treatment
- High-dose corticosteroids: The mainstay of treatment to reduce inflammation and prevent complications. Prednisone is typically initiated at a dose of 40-60 mg/day.
- Long-term corticosteroid taper: Once symptoms are controlled, the dose of prednisone is gradually tapered over several months to lower maintenance levels.
- Adjunctive therapy: Methotrexate or other immunosuppressive agents may be added in patients requiring prolonged corticosteroid therapy or who experience relapses.
- Monitoring: Regular follow-up with The APP is essential to monitor for disease activity, treatment response, and potential complications of corticosteroid therapy, such as osteoporosis and infection.

10.16. Polymyositis and Dermatomyositi

> - *Polymyositis and dermatomyositis are autoimmune diseases characterized by muscle inflammation leading to weakness and fatigue, with dermatomyositis additionally involving skin rash.*
> - *Both conditions can affect mobility and daily activities.*
> - *Treatment typically involves corticosteroids and immunosuppressive medications to manage inflammation and symptoms, along with physical therapy to improve muscle strength and function.*

Symptoms
- Muscle weakness, typically symmetric and affecting proximal muscles (shoulders, hips, thighs, upper arms).
- Difficulty rising from a seated position, climbing stairs, lifting objects, or reaching overhead.
- Fatigue and general malaise.
- Skin involvement in dermatomyositis, including characteristic rash:
    - Gottron's papules: Raised, scaly patches over the knuckles.
    - Heliotrope rash: Purple or reddish discoloration of the eyelids.
    - Shawl sign: Rash over the shoulders and upper back.
    - Gottron's sign: Reddish patches over bony prominences, such as elbows and knees.

Risk Factors
- Autoimmune diseases: patients with other autoimmune disorders, such as lupus or rheumatoid arthritis, may have an increased risk.
- Environmental factors: Certain infections or exposures may trigger the immune response.
- Genetic predisposition: Some genetic factors may contribute to the development of these conditions.

Epidemiology
- Polymyositis and dermatomyositis are relatively rare disorders, with an estimated annual incidence of 2-10 cases per million patients.
- Dermatomyositis is more common in females and typically presents in childhood or adulthood, whereas polymyositis affects adults and has a slight male predominance.
- The prevalence varies among different populations and ethnic groups.

Diagnosis
- Clinical evaluation: Based on characteristic symptoms, physical examination findings (muscle weakness, skin rash), and medical history.
- Laboratory tests: Elevated levels of muscle enzymes (creatine kinase, aldolase) and markers of inflammation (ESR, CRP).
- Electromyography (EMG): Measures electrical activity in muscles to assess muscle function.
- Muscle biopsy: Often necessary to confirm the diagnosis and assess the extent of muscle inflammation and damage.
- Imaging studies: MRI or CT scans may show muscle inflammation and help differentiate polymyositis/dermatomyositis from other conditions.

Treatment
- Corticosteroids: High-dose prednisone is typically the first-line treatment to suppress inflammation and improve muscle strength.
- Immunosuppressive agents: Methotrexate, azathioprine, mycophenolate, or rituximab may be added in cases of refractory disease or to allow for steroid tapering.
- Physical therapy: Helps maintain muscle strength and function, improve mobility, and prevent muscle atrophy.
- Sun protection: Important for patients with dermatomyositis to minimize skin rash exacerbations.

- Supportive measures: Adequate rest, balanced nutrition, and psychosocial support may also be beneficial.

10.17. Paget's Disease of Bone

> ➤ *Paget's disease of bone is a chronic condition characterized by abnormal bone remodeling, leading to weakened, enlarged, and deformed bones.*
> ➤ *It often presents with bone pain, fractures, and skeletal deformities, and can involve multiple bones.*
> ➤ *Treatment aims to alleviate symptoms and prevent complications through medications to regulate bone turnover and, in some cases, surgical interventions.*

Symptoms
- Bone pain: Paget's disease may cause bone pain, especially in the affected bones, such as the pelvis, spine, skull, or long bones of the legs.
- Bone deformities: Overgrowth and remodeling of bones can lead to deformities, such as bowing of the legs, skull enlargement, or spinal curvature.
- Fractures: Weakened bones are more prone to fractures, which may occur spontaneously or with minor trauma.
- Joint stiffness: Paget's disease can affect adjacent joints, leading to stiffness and reduced range of motion.
- Neurological symptoms: Compression of nerves due to enlarged bones, especially in the spine, may cause neurological symptoms like numbness, tingling, or weakness.

Risk Factors
- Age: Paget's disease is more common in older adults, with onset typically occurring after the age of 50.
- Genetic factors: There may be a genetic predisposition to Paget's disease, as it tends to run in families.
- Ethnicity: The condition is more common in patients of European descent, particularly those from the UK.
- Viral infection: Some studies suggest that certain viral infections, such as paramyxovirus infections, may be associated with the development of Paget's disease.

Epidemiology

- Paget's disease is relatively common in Western countries, particularly in the UK, where it affects around 2-3% of patients over the age of 55.
- Its prevalence varies depending on geographical location and ethnicity, with lower rates reported in Asian and African populations.
- The exact cause of Paget's disease is unknown, but both genetic and environmental factors likely play a role.

Diagnosis

- Imaging studies: X-rays, CT scans, or MRI may reveal characteristic changes in affected bones, such as bone enlargement, sclerosis, or lytic lesions.
- Blood tests: Elevated levels of alkaline phosphatase (ALP) are often observed due to increased bone turnover.
- Bone biopsy: Rarely needed but may be performed to confirm the diagnosis and rule out other bone disorders.

Treatment

- Bisphosphonates: These medications are the mainstay of treatment for Paget's disease, as they help to reduce bone turnover and prevent further bone enlargement and deformity.
- Pain management: Analgesics may be prescribed to relieve bone pain associated with Paget's disease.
- Physical therapy: Exercises to improve joint mobility and strengthen muscles may be beneficial, especially for patients with joint stiffness or deformities.
- Surgery: In severe cases or when complications like fractures or neurological compression occur, surgical intervention may be necessary to stabilize bones or decompress nerves.

10.18. Behçet's Disease

> ➢ Behçet's disease is a rare autoimmune disorder causing recurrent oral and genital ulcers, along with inflammation in the eyes, skin, and other organs.
> ➢ It is characterized by a triad of symptoms: oral ulcers, genital ulcers, and uveitis, though it can also involve joints, blood vessels, and central nervous system.
> ➢ Treatment focuses on managing symptoms with medications to suppress inflammation and immune response.

Symptoms
- Oral ulcers: Recurrent mouth ulcers are one of the hallmark symptoms of Behçet's disease, often painful and recurring.
- Genital ulcers: Ulcers may also develop on the genitals, typically in the form of painful sores.
- Skin lesions: Behçet's disease can cause various skin manifestations, including erythema nodosum, papulopustular lesions, and acneiform nodules.
- Eye inflammation: Uveitis, inflammation of the middle layer of the eye, is a common complication of Behçet's disease and can lead to vision loss if untreated.
- Joint pain and swelling: Arthritis may occur, resulting in joint pain, stiffness, and swelling.
- Gastrointestinal symptoms: Some patients may experience abdominal pain, diarrhea, and other gastrointestinal symptoms due to inflammation of the intestines.
- Neurological symptoms: In severe cases, Behçet's disease can affect the central nervous system, leading to headaches, meningitis, and stroke-like symptoms.

Risk Factors
- Genetic predisposition: Behçet's disease has a strong genetic component, with certain genetic factors increasing susceptibility to the condition.
- Environmental triggers: Infections, particularly viral or bacterial, may trigger the onset or exacerbation of Behçet's disease in genetically susceptible patients.

Epidemiology

- Behçet's disease is relatively rare, with higher prevalence rates reported in certain regions, including the Middle East, Mediterranean countries, and East Asia.
- The condition typically affects patients in their 20s to 40s, although it can occur at any age.
- Behçet's disease affects both men and women, but some studies suggest a slightly higher prevalence in males.

Diagnosis

- There is no specific diagnostic test for Behçet's disease, and diagnosis is based on clinical criteria and exclusion of other conditions.
- Diagnostic criteria include the presence of recurrent oral ulcers plus two of the following: genital ulcers, eye inflammation, skin lesions, or a positive pathergy test.
- Additional tests may be performed to evaluate organ involvement and rule out other conditions, including blood tests, eye exams, and imaging studies.

Treatment

- Treatment aims to reduce inflammation, alleviate symptoms, and prevent complications.
- Corticosteroids: Oral or topical corticosteroids may be used to control inflammation during acute flare-ups.
- Immunosuppressive medications: Drugs like colchicine, azathioprine, methotrexate, or biologic agents may be prescribed to suppress the immune system and reduce disease activity.
- Symptomatic treatment: Medications may be prescribed to manage specific symptoms, such as pain relievers for joint pain or topical treatments for skin lesions.
- Ocular treatment: Eye inflammation requires prompt treatment with corticosteroid eye drops and may also involve immunosuppressive therapy to prevent vision loss.

10.19. Raynaud's Phenomenon

> ➢ *Raynaud's phenomenon is a condition characterized by episodes of reduced blood flow to extremities, typically triggered by cold or stress, leading to color changes in fingers or toes, followed by numbness or pain.*
>
> ➢ *It's caused by spasms in small blood vessels and can occur on its own or as a secondary condition to other underlying disorders.*
>
> ➢ *Treatment and management includes avoiding triggers, keeping warm, and sometimes medications to improve blood flow.*

Symptoms

- Color changes in the skin: During episodes of reduced blood flow, the affected fingers or toes may turn white due to lack of oxygenated blood, followed by blue due to decreased oxygen levels, and then red as blood flow returns.
- Cold sensation: Patients may experience cold or numbness in the affected extremities during episodes.
- Pain or tingling: Some patients may feel pain, throbbing, or tingling sensations in the fingers or toes during or after episodes.
- Episodes triggered by cold or stress: Raynaud's phenomenon is often triggered by exposure to cold temperatures or emotional stress.

Risk Factors

- Gender: Raynaud's phenomenon is more common in women than in men, especially during childbearing years.
- Age: Symptoms typically first appear between the ages of 15 and 30, although Raynaud's can occur at any age.
- Family history: There may be a genetic predisposition to developing Raynaud's phenomenon, as it often occurs in families.
- Underlying conditions: Raynaud's phenomenon may occur secondary to other medical conditions, such as autoimmune diseases (e.g., lupus, scleroderma), connective tissue disorders, or vascular diseases.

Epidemiology

- Raynaud's phenomenon is relatively common, affecting an estimated 5-10% of the general population.
- Primary Raynaud's phenomenon, where symptoms occur without an underlying medical condition, is more common than secondary Raynaud's, which is associated with other diseases.

- The condition can occur in patients of all ages and ethnicities, although it is more prevalent in colder climates.

Diagnosis

- Diagnosis is based on clinical symptoms and medical history, including the presence of characteristic color changes in response to cold or stress.
- Tests may be performed to rule out underlying conditions associated with secondary Raynaud's phenomenon, such as blood tests for autoimmune markers or imaging studies to evaluate blood flow.
- A cold stimulation test, where the hands are immersed in cold water to induce an episode, may be performed to confirm the diagnosis.

Treatment

- Avoiding triggers: Patients are advised to avoid cold temperatures and take measures to keep warm, such as wearing gloves and socks.
- Lifestyle modifications: Smoking cessation, stress reduction techniques, and regular exercise may help improve symptoms.
- Medications: In severe cases or secondary Raynaud's phenomenon, medications such as calcium channel blockers (e.g., nifedipine), vasodilators, or topical nitroglycerin may be prescribed to improve blood flow and reduce the frequency and severity of episodes.
- Biofeedback therapy: Some patients may benefit from biofeedback techniques to learn to control body temperature and reduce the frequency of attacks.

10.20. Ehlers-Danlos Syndrome

> *Ehlers-Danlos syndrome (EDS) is a group of rare genetic connective tissue disorders characterized by joint hypermobility, skin hyperextensibility, and tissue fragility.*
>
> *Symptoms vary widely but may include chronic pain, easy bruising, and joint dislocations.*
>
> *Treatment and management involves symptom-specific interventions, physical therapy, and lifestyle adjustments to minimize complications and improve quality of life.*

Symptoms

- Joint hypermobility: Affected patients may have joints that extend beyond the normal range of motion, leading to joint instability, dislocations, or frequent sprains.

- Skin hyperextensibility: The skin may be stretchy and fragile, with increased elasticity that allows it to be pulled further than normal.
- Tissue fragility: Connective tissues such as blood vessels, ligaments, and internal organs may be fragile and prone to injury or rupture.
- Easy bruising: Due to the fragility of blood vessels, patients with EDS may bruise easily and experience prolonged bleeding after minor injuries.
- Chronic pain: Joint pain, muscle pain, and headaches are common symptoms associated with EDS.
- Gastrointestinal issues: Some patients may experience gastrointestinal problems such as constipation, diarrhea, or gastroesophageal reflux disease (GERD).
- Cardiovascular complications: In some cases, EDS can affect the structure and function of blood vessels, leading to conditions such as aortic aneurysms or dissections.

Risk Factors
- Genetic mutations: EDS is caused by mutations in genes responsible for producing collagen or other proteins involved in connective tissue structure and function.
- Family history: EDS can be inherited in an autosomal dominant or autosomal recessive pattern, meaning that patients with a family history of the condition may be at increased risk.
- Environmental factors: While genetic factors play a primary role, certain environmental factors or lifestyle choices may influence the severity of symptoms or complications associated with EDS.

Epidemiology
- EDS is considered a rare disorder, with an estimated prevalence of 1 in 5,000 to 20,000 patients worldwide.
- The prevalence of EDS may be underestimated due to variability in symptoms and challenges in diagnosis.

Diagnosis
- Clinical evaluation: A healthcare provider will perform a physical examination and review the patient's medical history to assess symptoms such as joint hypermobility, skin elasticity, and tissue fragility.
- Genetic testing: Molecular genetic testing can confirm the diagnosis of EDS by identifying specific genetic mutations associated with the condition.

- Diagnostic criteria: EDS is classified into different subtypes based on clinical features and genetic findings, with the most common types including classical, hypermobile, vascular, and kyphoscoliotic EDS.

Treatment
- Management of symptoms: Focuses on addressing patient symptoms and complications, such as pain management, physical therapy, and bracing to support unstable joints.
- Multidisciplinary care: A team-based approach involving healthcare specialists such as geneticists, rheumatologists, orthopedic surgeons, and physical therapists, may be necessary to manage the diverse manifestations of EDS.
- Lifestyle modifications: Lifestyle modifications such as avoiding high-impact activities, maintaining a healthy weight, and practicing joint protection techniques to minimize the risk of injury.

10.21 Lumbar Radiculopathy

> ➤ Lumbar radiculopathy, also known as sciatica, is a condition characterized by pain, numbness, or weakness that radiates from the lower back down the leg, following the path of the affected nerve root.
>
> ➤ It's often caused by compression or irritation of the lumbar spinal nerve roots due to conditions like herniated discs or spinal stenosis.
>
> ➤ Treatment includes pain management, physical therapy, and addressing the underlying cause, which may involve medications or surgical intervention.

Symptoms
- Sharp, shooting pain: Patients with lumbar radiculopathy often experience a sharp, shooting pain that radiates from the lower back down one leg.
- Numbness or tingling: Sensations of numbness, tingling, or "pins and needles" may be felt along the affected leg, often extending into the foot or toes.
- Weakness: Weakness or difficulty moving the leg or foot may occur, especially when attempting to stand from a seated position or lift the leg.
- Worsening with certain activities: Symptoms may worsen with activities that involve prolonged sitting, standing, bending, or twisting of the spine.

Risk Factors
- Age: Lumbar radiculopathy is more common in older adults, as degenerative changes in the spine, such as disc herniation or spinal stenosis, become more prevalent with age.
- Occupation and lifestyle: Jobs or activities that involve heavy lifting, prolonged sitting, or repetitive twisting motions may increase the risk of developing lumbar radiculopathy.
- Obesity: Excess body weight can place added strain on the spine, increasing the risk of disc herniation and nerve compression.
- Trauma or injury: Traumatic events such as falls, accidents, or sports injuries may damage the structures of the spine, leading to nerve compression and radicular symptoms.

Epidemiology
- Lumbar radiculopathy is a common condition, with estimates suggesting that up to 40% of adults will experience sciatica at some point in their lifetime.
- The prevalence of lumbar radiculopathy tends to increase with age, peaking in patients aged 45 to 64 years.

Diagnosis
- Clinical evaluation: A healthcare provider will perform a physical examination to assess the patient's symptoms, range of motion, reflexes, and muscle strength.
- Imaging studies: Diagnostic imaging tests such as X-rays, MRI, or CT scans may be ordered to visualize the structures of the spine and identify any abnormalities, such as disc herniation or spinal stenosis.
- Electromyography (EMG) and nerve conduction studies: These tests may be used to assess nerve function and identify the location and severity of nerve compression or damage.

Treatment
- Conservative measures: Initial treatment typically involves conservative measures such as rest, activity modification, and over-the-counter pain relievers (e.g., NSAIDs) to alleviate pain and inflammation.
- Physical therapy: Physical therapy exercises and stretching techniques can help improve flexibility, strengthen the muscles supporting the spine, and alleviate pressure on the affected nerve.
- Epidural steroid injections: In cases of severe or persistent pain, epidural steroid injections may be recommended to deliver anti-

inflammatory medication directly to the affected area, providing temporary relief of symptoms.

- Surgery:
    - Surgery may be considered for patients who do not experience significant improvement with conservative treatment or who develop progressive neurological deficits.
    - Surgical options may include discectomy or decompression surgery to alleviate nerve compression.

10.22. Cervical Radiculopathy

> *Cervical radiculopathy is a condition characterized by pain, numbness, or weakness that radiates from the neck down the arm, following the path of the affected nerve root in the cervical spine.*
>
> *It's typically caused by compression or irritation of the nerve roots due to conditions such as herniated discs, degenerative changes, or spinal stenosis.*
>
> *Treatment includes pain management, physical therapy, and addressing the underlying cause through medications or, in some cases, surgical intervention.*

Symptoms

- Neck pain: Patients may experience pain in the neck, which may radiate into the shoulders, arms, or hands.
- Radicular pain: Sharp, shooting pain may travel down the arm, often following a specific dermatomal pattern corresponding to the affected nerve root.
- Numbness or tingling: Sensations of numbness, tingling, or "pins and needles" may be felt in the arms, hands, or fingers.
- Muscle weakness: Weakness or difficulty moving the arms, hands, or fingers may occur, affecting grip strength or fine motor skills.
- Sensory changes: Patients may notice changes in sensation, such as hypersensitivity or loss of sensation, in the affected areas.
- Reflex changes: Reflexes may be diminished or absent in the affected limbs.

Risk Factors

- Age-related changes: Degenerative changes in the cervical spine, such as disc herniation, osteophytes, or cervical spondylosis, are common risk factors for cervical radiculopathy.

- Occupation and lifestyle: Jobs or activities that involve repetitive neck movements, heavy lifting, or prolonged sitting may increase the risk of developing cervical radiculopathy.
- Trauma or injury: Traumatic events such as whiplash injuries, falls, or sports-related injuries may damage the structures of the cervical spine, leading to nerve compression and radicular symptoms.
- Smoking: Tobacco use has been associated with an increased risk of cervical spine degeneration and disc herniation, predisposing patients to radicular symptoms.

Epidemiology
- Cervical radiculopathy is a relatively common condition, with estimates suggesting that it affects approximately 83 per 100,000 patients per year.
- The prevalence of cervical radiculopathy tends to increase with age, peaking in patients aged 50 to 54 years.

Diagnosis
- Clinical evaluation: A healthcare provider will perform a physical examination to assess the patient's symptoms, neck mobility, reflexes, and muscle strength.
- Imaging studies: Diagnostic imaging tests such as X-rays, MRI, or CT scans may be ordered to visualize the structures of the cervical spine and identify any abnormalities, such as disc herniation or spinal stenosis.
- Electromyography (EMG) and nerve conduction studies: These tests may be used to assess nerve function and identify the location and severity of nerve compression or damage.

Treatment
- Conservative measures: Initial treatment typically involves conservative measures such as rest, activity modification, and over-the-counter pain relievers (e.g., NSAIDs) to alleviate pain and inflammation.
- Physical therapy: Physical therapy exercises and stretching techniques can help improve neck flexibility, strengthen the muscles supporting the cervical spine, and alleviate pressure on the affected nerve roots.
- Epidural steroid injections: In cases of severe or persistent pain, epidural steroid injections may be recommended to deliver anti-inflammatory medication directly to the affected area, providing temporary relief of symptoms.

- Surgery:
  - Surgery may be considered for patients who do not experience significant improvement with conservative treatment or who develop progressive neurological deficits.
  - Options may include discectomy or decompression surgery to alleviate nerve compression.

10.23. Baker's Cyst

> ➤ Baker's cyst, also known as a popliteal cyst, is a fluid-filled swelling behind the knee, often caused by excess synovial fluid production within the knee joint due to conditions like arthritis or meniscus tears.
> ➤ It can cause discomfort, stiffness, and a feeling of tightness behind the knee, especially when bending or straightening the leg.
> ➤ Treatment may involve managing the underlying condition, pain relief, physical therapy, or, in severe cases, drainage or surgical removal.

Symptoms
- Swelling behind the knee: Baker's cyst typically presents as a noticeable bulge or lump at the back of the knee joint.
- Knee pain: Patients may experience discomfort or pain behind the knee, particularly when bending or straightening the leg.
- Stiffness: Some patients may notice stiffness or limitation of movement in the affected knee joint.
- Occasionally, the cyst may rupture, causing sudden onset of sharp pain, swelling, and redness in the calf area.

Risk Factors
- Knee injuries: Previous knee injuries, such as meniscal tears, ligamentous injuries, or osteoarthritis, are common risk factors for the development of Baker's cyst.
- Knee arthritis: patients with underlying knee arthritis, particularly osteoarthritis or rheumatoid arthritis, have an increased risk of developing Baker's cyst.
- Age: Baker's cysts are more common in adults, especially those over the age of 40.
- Occupation and activity: Jobs or activities that involve repetitive knee movements or prolonged standing may predispose patients to Baker's cyst formation.

Epidemiology
- Baker's cysts are relatively common, with a prevalence estimated to be around 5% in the general population.
- While Baker's cysts can occur at any age, they are more commonly seen in older adults, particularly those with degenerative knee conditions.

Diagnosis
- Physical examination: A healthcare provider may perform a physical examination to assess the size, location, and consistency of the swelling behind the knee.
- Imaging studies: Diagnostic imaging tests such as ultrasound, MRI, or occasionally X-rays may be ordered to confirm the diagnosis and evaluate the extent of the cyst and any underlying knee pathology.

Treatment
- Conservative management: In many cases, Baker's cysts resolve on their own without specific treatment. Conservative measures such as rest, ice, elevation, and over-the-counter pain relievers (e.g., NSAIDs) may help alleviate symptoms and reduce inflammation.
- Physical therapy: Physical therapy exercises focused on strengthening the muscles surrounding the knee joint and improving flexibility may be beneficial for some patients.
- Injection therapy: Injections of corticosteroids or hyaluronic acid into the cyst may help reduce inflammation and relieve symptoms in some cases.
- Aspiration: Draining the fluid from the cyst using a needle (aspiration) may be performed to alleviate symptoms and reduce the size of the cyst.
- Surgery: cystectomy or repair underlying knee joint pathology may be considered for patients with large, symptomatic cysts or persistent symptoms despite conservative treatment.

10.24. Ganglion Cyst

> ➤ *Ganglion cyst is a lump filled with thick, jelly-like fluid, often found near joints or tendons, typically in the wrist or hand.*
>
> ➤ *The exact cause is unknown, but they may form due to joint or tendon irritation or trauma.*
>
> ➤ *Treatment options include observation, aspiration to drain fluid, or surgical removal if the cyst causes pain or limits movement.*

Symptoms

- Visible lump: Ganglion cysts usually present as a noticeable lump or bump beneath the skin. The size of the lump can vary from small to large.
- Pain or discomfort: Some patients may experience pain or discomfort, particularly if the cyst presses on nearby nerves or tendons.
- Changes in sensation: In some cases, ganglion cysts may cause tingling, numbness, or weakness in the affected area.
- Increased size: The size of the cyst may fluctuate over time, becoming larger or smaller spontaneously.

Risk Factors

- Age and gender: Ganglion cysts are most commonly seen in young to middle-aged adults, particularly women.
- Joint or tendon trauma: Previous joint or tendon injuries or repetitive stress on the affected area may increase the risk of developing ganglion cysts.
- Joint or tendon degeneration: Conditions such as osteoarthritis or rheumatoid arthritis, which affect the joints and tendons, may predispose patients to ganglion cyst formation.
- Genetic predisposition: There may be a genetic component involved in the development of ganglion cysts, as they often occur in families.

Epidemiology

- Ganglion cysts are among the most common soft tissue masses found in the hand and wrist.
- They are more prevalent in certain populations, such as manual laborers or patients involved in activities that place repetitive stress on the joints.

Diagnosis
- Clinical examination: A healthcare provider may perform a physical examination to assess the size, location, and characteristics of the cyst.
- Imaging studies: While ganglion cysts are often diagnosed based on clinical examination alone, imaging tests such as ultrasound or MRI may be ordered to confirm the diagnosis and evaluate the extent of the cyst and any associated soft tissue or joint pathology.

Treatment
- Watchful waiting: Small, asymptomatic ganglion cysts may not require treatment, and a healthcare provider may recommend monitoring the cyst over time for changes.
- Aspiration: may be performed to alleviate symptoms and reduce the size of the cyst. However, recurrence of the cyst is common with this approach.
- Immobilization: Immobilizing the affected joint with a splint or brace may help alleviate symptoms and prevent further irritation of the cyst.
- Surgery: cyst excision may be recommended for patients with large, symptomatic cysts or persistent symptoms despite conservative treatment.

10.25. Frozen Shoulder

> ➤ *Frozen shoulder, or adhesive capsulitis, is a condition characterized by stiffness, pain, and limited range of motion in the shoulder joint.*
>
> ➤ *It typically develops gradually and may follow a period of immobilization or injury.*
>
> ➤ *Treatment involves physical therapy, pain management, and in some cases, corticosteroid injections or surgical intervention to release the tight capsule.*

Symptoms
- Pain: Gradual onset of shoulder pain, often worsened by movement or pressure.
- Stiffness: Progressive loss of shoulder mobility, typically affecting both active and passive range of motion.
- Difficulty with Activities: Difficulty reaching overhead, behind the back, or across the body.

- Sleep Disturbance: Pain and discomfort may interfere with sleep, particularly when lying on the affected side.

Risk Factors
- Age: Frozen shoulder most commonly affects patients between the ages of 40 and 60, with peak incidence in the 50s.
- Gender: Women are more likely than men to develop frozen shoulders.
- Diabetes: Patients with diabetes are at increased risk of developing frozen shoulders, with prevalence rates up to 20% among diabetic patients.
- Shoulder Trauma or Surgery: Previous shoulder injury or surgery may predispose patients to adhesive capsulitis.
- Other Health Conditions: Certain medical conditions such as thyroid disorders, cardiovascular disease, and autoimmune diseases may increase the risk.

Epidemiology
- Frozen shoulder affects approximately 2-5% of the general population.
- It is more common in patients with certain risk factors, such as diabetes, thyroid disorders, or previous shoulder injury.

Diagnosis
- <u>Medical History and Physical Examination</u>: The healthcare provider will inquire about symptoms and perform a physical examination to assess shoulder range of motion and identify areas of tenderness.
- <u>Imaging Studies</u>: X-rays may be obtained to rule out other shoulder conditions such as arthritis or fractures. MRI may be used to visualize soft tissues and assess for inflammation or structural changes.
- <u>Diagnostic Tests</u>: In some cases, diagnostic tests such as blood tests or joint aspiration may be performed to rule out underlying medical conditions or infections.

Treatment
- <u>Conservative Management</u>: Initial treatment typically involves conservative measures such as physical therapy, stretching exercises, and anti-inflammatory medications (e.g., NSAIDs) to reduce pain and improve mobility.
- <u>Corticosteroid Injections</u>: Injections of corticosteroids into the shoulder joint may provide temporary relief of pain and inflammation.

- **Joint Distension**: Hydrodilatation involves injecting sterile fluid into the shoulder joint to stretch the capsule and improve range of motion.
- **Manipulation Under Anesthesia (MUA)**: MUA is a procedure performed under anesthesia to forcibly manipulate the shoulder joint to break up adhesions and improve mobility.
- **Surgery**: In severe cases where conservative treatments fail to provide relief, surgical intervention such as arthroscopic capsular release may be considered to release tight or thickened tissues within the shoulder joint.

10.26. Hip Avascular Necrosis

> ➤ *Hip avascular necrosis is a condition where blood supply to the femoral head is disrupted, leading to bone tissue death and eventual collapse of the hip joint.*
>
> ➤ *It can result from factors like trauma, corticosteroid use, or underlying health conditions.*
>
> ➤ *Treatment may involve medications, physical therapy, or surgical interventions such as core decompression or hip replacement.*

Symptoms
- **Hip Pain**: The most common symptom is hip pain, which may be mild initially but can worsen over time and become severe.
- **Restricted Range of Motion**: Patients may experience stiffness and decreased range of motion in the affected hip joint.
- **Pain with Weight-Bearing**: Pain may worsen with weight-bearing activities such as walking or standing.
- **Groin Pain**: Pain may radiate to the groin area or buttocks.
- **Limping**: Some patients may develop a limp due to pain and difficulty walking.

Risk Factors
- **Corticosteroid Use**: Long-term or high-dose corticosteroid therapy is a significant risk factor for AVN.
- **Trauma**: Traumatic injury to the hip joint, such as a fracture or dislocation, can disrupt blood flow and increase the risk of AVN.
- **Alcohol Abuse**: Excessive alcohol consumption is associated with AVN, possibly due to its toxic effects on bone cells and blood vessels.

- Smoking: Smoking is a known risk factor for AVN, as it can impair blood flow to the bones.
- Medical Conditions: Certain medical conditions such as sickle cell disease, lupus, HIV/AIDS, and coagulation disorders increase the risk of AVN.
- Radiation Therapy: Radiation therapy for cancer treatment can damage blood vessels and increase the risk of AVN in nearby bones.

Epidemiology
- Avascular necrosis of the hip is relatively rare but can occur at any age.
- It is more common in males than females and tends to affect patients in their 30s to 50s.

Diagnosis
- Physical Examination: The healthcare provider will perform a physical examination to assess hip joint function and range of motion and evaluate for signs of tenderness or swelling.
- Imaging Studies: X-rays, magnetic resonance imaging (MRI), or computed tomography (CT) scans may be used to visualize changes in the bone structure and assess the extent of bone damage.
- Blood Tests: Blood tests may be performed to evaluate for underlying medical conditions such as coagulation disorders or autoimmune diseases.
- Bone Biopsy: In some cases, a bone biopsy may be performed to confirm the diagnosis and assess the extent of bone necrosis.

Treatment
- Conservative Management: In the early stages of AVN, conservative measures such as rest, activity modification, and pain management may be recommended to relieve symptoms and slow disease progression.
- Medications: Nonsteroidal anti-inflammatory drugs (NSAIDs), pain relievers, and bisphosphonates may be prescribed to alleviate pain and reduce inflammation.
- Physical Therapy: Physical therapy exercises and stretches may help improve joint mobility, strengthen surrounding muscles, and alleviate pain.
- Surgical Interventions: In advanced cases of AVN or when conservative treatments fail, surgical interventions such as core decompression, bone grafting, osteotomy, or total hip replacement

may be necessary to alleviate pain, restore function, and prevent further joint damage.

10.27. Tennis Elbow

> ➢ Tennis elbow, or lateral epicondylitis, is a painful condition caused by overuse of the forearm muscles and tendons, resulting in inflammation at the outer elbow.
> ➢ It commonly occurs due to repetitive motions, not just in tennis, but also in activities like typing or gardening.
> ➢ Treatment includes rest, icing, physical therapy, bracing, and sometimes corticosteroid injections for pain relief.

Symptoms
- Pain and tenderness on the outer aspect of the elbow.
- Pain worsens with activities such as gripping, lifting, or twisting movements of the wrist or forearm.
- Weakness in gripping objects or performing certain movements.
- Stiffness or difficulty extending the forearm fully.

Risk Factors
- Repetitive Strain: Activities involving repetitive wrist extension or gripping motions, such as tennis, painting, plumbing, or carpentry.
- Age: Most common in patients aged 30 to 50 years, but can occur at any age.
- Occupation: Certain occupations that involve repetitive arm movements or use of vibrating tools may increase the risk.
- Sports: Participation in racquet sports, particularly tennis, increases the risk.
- Poor Technique: Improper technique during sports or activities can contribute to the development of tennis elbow.

Epidemiology
- Tennis elbow is a common condition, affecting both men and women.
- It is estimated to occur in 1-3% of the general population annually.
- Prevalence is higher among patients who engage in activities or occupations that involve repetitive arm movements.

Diagnosis
- Clinical Examination: Diagnosis is typically based on a thorough history and physical examination. Pain localized to the lateral epicondyle during resisted wrist extension or gripping maneuvers is characteristic.
- Imaging: X-rays may be ordered to rule out other causes of elbow pain, such as fractures or arthritis. MRI or ultrasound may be used if there is uncertainty about the diagnosis or to assess the extent of soft tissue involvement.

Treatment
- Rest: Avoid activities that exacerbate symptoms to allow for healing.
- Ice: Apply ice packs to the affected area for 15-20 minutes several times a day to reduce inflammation and pain.
- Bracing: Wearing a counterforce brace or strap around the forearm just below the elbow can help reduce strain on the tendon.
- Physical Therapy: Stretching and strengthening exercises for the forearm muscles can help improve flexibility and reduce pain. Techniques such as massage, ultrasound, or dry needling may also be beneficial.
- Medications: Over-the-counter pain relievers such as ibuprofen or naproxen may help reduce pain and inflammation.
- Corticosteroid Injections: Injections of corticosteroids into the affected area may provide temporary relief of symptoms.
- Platelet-Rich Plasma (PRP) Therapy: Injection of concentrated platelets from the patient's own blood may promote healing of the tendon.
- Surgery: In severe cases that do not respond to conservative treatment, surgical options such as tendon repair or debridement may be considered.

Prevention:
- Proper Technique: Use proper form and technique during sports or activities to avoid excessive strain on the elbow.
- Warm-up: Perform a proper warm-up routine before engaging in physical activities to prepare the muscles and tendons.
- Equipment: Use properly fitted equipment and tools to minimize strain on the elbow.

10.28. Falls in the Elderly

> ➢ *Falls in the elderly are common and can result from various factors including muscle weakness, balance issues, vision problems, medication side effects, and environmental hazards.*
> ➢ *They often lead to serious injuries such as fractures, head trauma, and loss of independence.*
> ➢ *Prevention strategies include exercise, home modifications, regular vision and medication assessments, and minimizing fall risks.*

Symptoms
- Actual or near-fall incidents, where the patient loses balance but catches themselves before falling.
- Slips, trips, or stumbling while walking or moving around.
- Injuries resulting from falls, such as bruises, fractures (e.g., hip fractures), head trauma, or lacerations.
- Fear of falling, leading to decreased mobility, social isolation, and functional decline.
- Changes in gait or balance, including shuffling gait, unsteady walking, or difficulty with posture and stability.

Risk Factors
- Advanced age: The risk of falls increases with age, particularly in patients over 65 years old.
- Muscle weakness and balance impairment: Weakness in the lower extremities, impaired balance, and gait instability contribute to the risk of falls.
- Chronic medical conditions: Conditions such as arthritis, osteoporosis, Parkinson's disease, stroke, dementia, and sensory impairments (e.g., vision or hearing loss) increase fall risk.
- Medication side effects: Certain medications, such as sedatives, hypnotics, antihypertensives, and psychotropic drugs, can cause dizziness, orthostatic hypotension, or impaired cognition, increasing the risk of falls.
- Environmental hazards: Poor lighting, slippery floors, uneven surfaces, clutter, and inadequate footwear increase the risk of falls.
- History of falls: patients with a history of previous falls are at increased risk of future falls.

- Functional impairment: Activities of daily living (ADL) impairment, mobility limitations, and decreased physical activity contribute to fall risk.
- Cognitive impairment: Cognitive decline, confusion, and dementia increase the risk of falls due to impaired judgment and decision-making.
- Fear of falling: Fear or anxiety about falling can lead to decreased physical activity, muscle weakness, and increased fall risk.
- Vitamin D deficiency: Inadequate vitamin D levels are associated with muscle weakness and increased fall risk.

Epidemiology

Falls are a leading cause of injury-related morbidity and mortality among older adults.

Approximately one in four adults aged 65 and older experience a fall each year, and the risk increases with age.

Falls are the leading cause of fatal and non-fatal injuries among older adults, with hip fractures being the most common fall-related injury.

Falls often result in hospitalizations, nursing home admissions, functional decline, and increased healthcare costs.

Diagnosis

- Comprehensive assessment: Evaluation of medical history, medication use, functional status, mobility, balance, gait, cognition, and sensory function.
- Physical examination: Assessment of muscle strength, joint range of motion, proprioception, and neurological function.
- Assessment of fall risk factors: Identification of modifiable and non-modifiable risk factors contributing to fall risk.
- Gait and balance testing: Evaluation of gait patterns, balance control, and postural stability using standardized assessments such as the Timed Up and Go test, Berg Balance Scale, or Tinetti Balance Assessment Tool.
- Medication review: Assessment of medications for potential side effects, drug interactions, and appropriateness in older adults.
- Environmental assessment: Identification of environmental hazards in the home or community that may increase fall risk.

Treatment
- Multifactorial interventions: Comprehensive fall prevention programs targeting multiple risk factors, including exercise, balance training, medication management, home modifications, and education.
- Physical therapy: individualized exercise programs focusing on strength, flexibility, balance, and gait training to improve mobility and reduce fall risk.
- Occupational therapy: Assessment and modification of the home environment, adaptive equipment provision, and strategies to improve functional independence and safety.
- Medication management: Review and adjustment of medications to minimize side effects, drug interactions, and sedative use.
- Vision assessment and correction: Regular eye examinations and appropriate corrective lenses to optimize vision and reduce fall risk.
- Environmental modifications: Removal of hazards, installation of grab bars, handrails, and improved lighting to enhance safety in the home environment.
- Assistive devices: Use of mobility aids such as canes, walkers, or orthotics to improve stability and reduce fall risk.
- Education and counseling: Provision of fall prevention education, safety tips, and strategies to minimize fall risk in daily activities.
- Community resources: Referral to community-based programs, support groups, or senior centers offering fall prevention initiatives and social activities.

10.29. Low Back Pain

> ➤ *Low back pain is a common ailment characterized by discomfort or pain in the lumbar region of the spine, often extending to the buttocks and legs.*
>
> ➤ *It can result from various factors such as muscle strain, poor posture, injury, or underlying medical conditions.*
>
> ➤ *Treatment typically involves a combination of pain management, physical therapy, and lifestyle modifications tailored to individual needs.*

Symptoms
- Pain and discomfort: Usually localized in the lower back area, but can radiate to buttocks, thighs, or even further down the leg.

- Stiffness: Difficulty moving, especially after waking up or sitting for prolonged periods.
- Muscle spasms: Sudden, involuntary muscle contractions that can be painful.
- Decreased range of motion and flexibility in the back.

Risk Factors
- Age: Incidence increases with age, particularly after 30 or 40.
- Fitness level: Poor physical fitness can contribute to low back pain due to weak back and abdominal muscles.
- Weight gain: Being overweight or obese puts additional stress on the back.
- Genetics: Some causes of low back pain, such as certain types of arthritis, may have a genetic component.
- Occupational hazards: Jobs that require heavy lifting, bending, or twisting can increase the risk, as can sitting at a desk all day without proper back support.
- Smoking: It can reduce blood flow to the lower spine and contribute to disk degeneration.

Epidemiology
- Low back pain is a leading cause of disability worldwide. It affects people of all ages, from adolescents to the elderly, making it a significant public health challenge. The prevalence varies by region, but it is estimated that up to 80% of the population will experience low back pain at some point in their lives.

Diagnostic Approach
- Differential diagnosis for low back pain (LBP) involves considering various potential causes of the pain, as the symptom can result from a wide range of conditions.
- *Musculoskeletal Causes*
  - Muscle strain: Often due to overuse, poor posture, or improper lifting techniques.
  - Lumbar disc herniation: The soft material inside a disc can bulge or rupture, pressing on a nerve.
  - Degenerative disc disease: The discs between the vertebrae lose hydration and elasticity with age.
  - Facet joint osteoarthritis: Wear-and-tear arthritis affecting the joints of the vertebrae.

- ○ Spondylolisthesis: One vertebra slips forward over the one below it, often due to a fracture or degeneration.
  - ○ Spinal stenosis: Narrowing of the spinal canal, often due to aging, putting pressure on spinal nerves and the spinal cord.
- *Inflammatory* Causes
  - ○ Ankylosing spondylitis: A type of arthritis affecting the spine, causing inflammation of the spinal joints.
  - ○ Other spondyloarthropathies: Such as psoriatic arthritis or reactive arthritis, which can also affect the spine.
- *Infectious* Causes
  - ○ Osteomyelitis: Infection of the vertebrae.
  - ○ Discitis: Infection in the intervertebral disc space.
  - ○ Epidural abscess: An infection that develops in the space around the dura mater.
- *Neoplastic* Causes
  - ○ Primary spinal tumors: Originating in the spine.
  - ○ Metastatic tumors: Cancer that has spread to the spine from another part of the body.
- *Vascular* Causes
  - ○ Abdominal aortic aneurysm: An enlarged area in the lower part of the major vessel that supplies blood to the body (aortic) can sometimes cause back pain.
- *Other* Causes
  - ○ Kidney stones or kidney infections: These can cause pain that radiates to the lower back.
  - ○ Endometriosis: A condition in which tissue similar to the lining inside the uterus is found outside the uterus, causing pain.
  - ○ Pelvic inflammatory disease: Infection of the female reproductive organs can sometimes manifest as back pain.
  - ○ Pregnancy: The added weight and pressure on the back can cause discomfort.
- ★ Determining the exact cause of low back pain typically involves a combination of patient history (including symptom duration, intensity, and any exacerbating or alleviating factors), physical examination (focusing on the back, neurological examination, and sometimes examination of other areas like the abdomen), and

diagnostic testing (such as X-rays, MRI, CT scans, and blood tests) when necessary.

Treatment
- Self-care: Rest, ice/heat therapy, and over-the-counter pain relievers can help manage symptoms.
- Physical therapy: Exercises to strengthen back muscles and improve flexibility can be effective.
- Medications: Nonsteroidal anti-inflammatory drugs (NSAIDs) or, in some cases, muscle relaxants.
- Injections: Corticosteroid injections may be considered for pain relief in specific cases.
- Surgery: Typically reserved for cases where there is a specific cause that can be addressed surgically, such as a herniated disk, and conservative treatments have failed.
- Alternative therapies: Acupuncture, chiropractic adjustments, and massage therapy may offer relief for some people.

10.30. Vasculitis

> *Vasculitis is a group of diseases characterized by inflammation of blood vessels.*
>
> *Symptoms vary depending on the type and affected organs but may include fever, fatigue, and organ dysfunction.*
>
> *Treatment typically involves immunosuppressive drugs to reduce inflammation and manage symptoms.*

Symptoms
- Fever, fatigue, and weight loss
- Muscle and joint pain
- Loss of appetite
- Skin manifestations, such as rashes or purpura (small, raised purple spots)
- Nerve problems, such as numbness or weakness
- Abdominal pain or kidney issues
- Shortness of breath or cough

Risk Factors
- Genetic predisposition: Some vasculitis types have a genetic component.
- Age: Certain types are more common in specific age groups.
- Sex: Some vasculitis are more prevalent in either males or females.
- Environmental factors: Infections, exposure to chemicals, and drugs can trigger vasculitis in susceptible individuals.
- Autoimmune conditions like rheumatoid arthritis and systemic lupus erythematosus may increase the risk.

Epidemiology
- The prevalence and incidence of vasculitis vary widely among different types and populations. Some forms are relatively rare, while others may be more common. For example, giant cell arteritis predominantly affects older adults, especially those over 50 years of age, and is more common in people of Northern European descent.
- Vasculitis subtypes categorized from large to small vessels:
    - Giant cell arteritis (Temporal arteritis)
    - Takayasu arteritis
    - Polyarteritis nodosa
    - Kawasaki disease
    - Behçet's disease
    - Medium-sized vessel vasculitis
        - Granulomatosis with polyangiitis (Wegener's granulomatosis)
        - Eosinophilic granulomatosis with polyangiitis (Churg-Strauss syndrome)
    - Microscopic polyangiitis
    - Henoch-Schönlein purpura
    - Cryoglobulinemic vasculitis

Diagnosis
- Diagnosing vasculitis involves a combination of clinical evaluation, laboratory tests, imaging studies, and sometimes a biopsy of affected tissue.
- Blood tests: Looking for markers of inflammation (e.g., ESR, CRP) and antibodies associated with specific types of vasculitis.

- **Imaging tests**: MRI, CT scans, and ultrasound can identify abnormal blood vessels and affected organs.
- **Biopsy**: Examining a small sample of tissue from an affected organ can confirm the presence of vasculitis.

Treatment

- Treatment for vasculitis aims to reduce inflammation, manage symptoms, and prevent further organ damage. It can vary significantly depending on the type and severity of the disease, as well as the organs involved.
- **Corticosteroids**: To quickly reduce inflammation.
- **Immunosuppressive drugs**: Such as cyclophosphamide, methotrexate, and azathioprine, to control the immune system's activity.
- **Biologic therapies**: Targeted drugs like rituximab that are used for certain types of vasculitis.
- **Management of underlying conditions**: Addressing any diseases or factors contributing to vasculitis.

References

- Bijlsma, J. W., Berenbaum, F., & et al. (2011). Osteoarthritis: An update with relevance for clinical practice. The Lancet, 377(9783), 2115-2126.
- Smolen, J. S., Aletaha, D., & et al. (2016). Rheumatoid arthritis. The Lancet, 388(10055), 2023-2038.
- Clauw, D. J., Häuser, W., & et al. (2014). Fibromyalgia. Nature Reviews Disease Primers, 1(1), 15022.
- Richette, P., Doherty, M., & et al. (2017). 2016 updated EULAR evidence-based recommendations for the management of gout. Annals of the Rheumatic Diseases, 76(1), 29-42.
- Tsokos, G. C. (2011). Systemic lupus erythematosus. New England Journal of Medicine, 365(22), 2110-2121.
- Braun, J., Sieper, J., & et al. (2007). Ankylosing spondylitis. The Lancet, 369(9570), 1379-1390.
- Rudwaleit, M., & van der Heijde, D. (2011). Spondyloarthritis including psoriatic arthritis. Rheumatic Disease Clinics, 37(3), 521-537.
- Ritchlin, C. T., Colbert, R. A., & et al. (2017). Psoriatic arthritis. New England Journal of Medicine, 376(10), 957-970.
- Cosman, F., de Beur, S. J., & et al. (2014). Clinician's guide to prevention and treatment of osteoporosis. Osteoporosis International, 25(10), 2359-2381.

- Petty, R. E., & Southwood, T. R. (2016). Classification of childhood arthritis: Entering a new era. Annals of the Rheumatic Diseases, 75(6), 991-994.
- Ramos-Casals, M., & Tzioufas, A. G. (2014). Systemic Sjögren's syndrome: Diagnosis and treatment. Rheumatic Disease Clinics, 40(2), 155-177.
- Dejaco, C., Singh, Y. P., & et al. (2015). 2015 recommendations for the management of polymyalgia rheumatica: A European League Against Rheumatism/American College of Rheumatology collaborative initiative. Arthritis & Rheumatology, 67(10), 2569-2580.
- Denton, C. P., Khanna, D., & et al. (2017). EULAR recommendations for the treatment of systemic sclerosis: A report from the EULAR Scleroderma Trials and Research group (EUSTAR). Annals of the Rheumatic Diseases, 76(8), 1327-1339.
- Salvarani, C., & Cantini, F. (2012). Treatment and prognosis in elderly-onset (≥ 65 years) polymyalgia rheumatica and temporal arteritis. Rheumatic Disease Clinics, 38(4), 795-804.
- Rider, L. G., & Miller, F. W. (2019). Classification and epidemiology of juvenile idiopathic inflammatory myopathies. Rheumatic Disease Clinics, 45(4), 529-542.
- Zochling, J., & Smith, E. U. (2010). Seronegative spondyloarthritis. Best Practice & Research Clinical Rheumatology, 24(6), 747-756.
- Ralston, S. H., Langston, A. L., & et al. (2017). Paget's disease of bone: Diagnosis and management. BMJ, 356, j418.
- Hatemi, G., Christensen, R., & et al. (2018). 2018 update of the EULAR recommendations for the management of Behçet's syndrome. Annals of the Rheumatic Diseases, 77(6), 808-818.
- Herrick, A. L., & Wigley, F. M. (2012). Raynaud's phenomenon. Best Practice & Research Clinical Rheumatology, 26(6), 715-728.
- Malfait, F., Francomano, C., & et al. (2017). The 2017 international classification of the Ehlers–Danlos syndromes. American Journal of Medical Genetics Part C: Seminars in Medical Genetics, 175(1), 8-26.
- Kreiner, D. S., Hwang, S. W., & et al. (2014). An evidence-based clinical guideline for the diagnosis and treatment of lumbar disc herniation with radiculopathy. Spine Journal, 14(1), 180-191.
- Chou, R., Loeser, J. D., & et al. (2015). Interventional therapies, surgery, and interdisciplinary rehabilitation for low back pain: An evidence-based clinical practice guideline from the American Pain Society. Spine, 40(10), 1060-1077.
- Maffulli, N., Papalia, R., & et al. (2012). Baker's cyst. Best Practice & Research Clinical Rheumatology, 26(5), 673-682.

- Spicer, D. D., & Pedowitz, D. I. (2014). Ganglion cysts of the wrist. Clinical Orthopaedics and Related Research®, 472(6), 1856-1865.
- Hand, G. C., Athanasou, N. A., & et al. (2008). The pathology of frozen shoulder. Journal of Bone and Joint Surgery, 90(3), 336-342.
- Mont, M. A., Jones, L. C., & et al. (2006). Nontraumatic osteonecrosis of the femoral head: Ten years later. Journal of Bone and Joint Surgery, 88(5), 1117-1132.
- Krogh, T. P., Bartels, E. M., & et al. (2013). Comparative effectiveness of injection therapies in lateral epicondylitis: A systematic review and network meta-analysis of randomized controlled trials. American Journal of Sports Medicine, 41(6), 1435-1446.
- Tinetti, M. E., Speechley, M., & et al. (1988). Risk factors for falls among elderly persons living in the community. New England Journal of Medicine, 319(26), 1701-1707.

www.ingramcontent.com/pod-product-compliance
Lightning Source LLC
LaVergne TN
LVHW072117060526
838201LV00011B/257